The Malformed Infant *An Illustrated Guide*

Complim

Oxford   *einhardt*

                                             93

Teach thy tongue to say
"I do not know."

Moses ben Maimon (Maimonides)
(1135–1204)

THE MALFORMED INFANT AND CHILD

An Illustrated Guide

RICHARD M. GOODMAN, M.D.
Professor of Human Genetics
Sackler School of Medicine
Tel-Aviv University
The Chaim Sheba Medical Center
Tel-Hashomer, Israel

ROBERT J. GORLIN, D.D.S., M.S.
Regents' Professor and Chairman
Department of Oral Pathology and Genetics
School of Dentistry
University of Minnesota

Medical Illustrator

DEBORAH MEYER, B.A.
Ramat-Aviv, Israel

New York   Oxford
OXFORD UNIVERSITY PRESS
1983

Library of Congress Cataloging in Publication Data
Goodman, Richard Merle, 1932–
The malformed infant and child.
Bibliography: p.   , Includes index.
1. Children—Diseases—Diagnosis.
2. Infants—Diseases—Diagnosis.
3. Abnormalities, Human—Diagnosis.
I. Gorlin, Robert J. II. Title.
[DNLM: 1. Abnormalities. QS 675 G653m]
RJ50.G65 1983   618.92′0043   82-14085
ISBN 0-19-503254-3
ISBN 0-19-503255-1 (pbk.)

Printed in the United States of America

Printing (last digit): 9 8 7 6 5 4 3 2 1

Dedicated
To our patients who seek care
and
To those who must be aware

Preface

The number of new congenital malformation syndromes appearing in the literature seems to be endless, thus challenging to the maximum one's ability for recall. As a memory and coordinating aid, computers are now in vogue for use in the diagnosis of such disorders, but they have not proven to be the panacea. Through the years our students, house-physicians, and those who have contact with mentally retarded and congenitally malformed patients have urged us to synthesize our experience in a concise, well-illustrated text devoted to the more common disorders. We have accepted this challenge, realizing full well that it is impossible to obtain total agreement among our colleagues as to which conditions would be the most germane. For example, we have not included *thalidomide embryopathy* as this drug is no longer being given to pregnant women, but have elected to present the *battered child syndrome* since this environmental disorder unfortunately is being seen today.

Much thought has been given to the best way of presenting information on the 200 entities we have selected. Emphasis has been given to those conditions which appear at birth or in early childhood. The text for each disorder begins with a description of the clinical features followed by comments on specific and differential diagnosis. The current status of prenatal diagnosis is mentioned. In some instances we have even postulated that certain conditions may be recognized prenatally by chance when another disorder is being ruled out. Further remarks cover the basic defect, genetics, prognosis, and treatment. Schematic drawings have been used to achieve the clarity and simplicity we desire. These illustrations have been designed at times to explain, but mainly to show certain characteristic physical, radiographic and laboratory features, including the progression of the physical findings with age. It is our sincere hope that this text will serve as a guidebook in the diagnosis and care of affected patients and aid in counseling their families.

Knowing that improvement is always possible, we welcome all criticism and constructive suggestions.

Acknowledgments

We have been privileged to have as our medical illustrator Deborah Meyer. Her exceptional talent, meticulous effort, and unceasing dedication has been exemplary, and to Debby we express our deepest appreciation. Elizabeth Fall has been our research assistant from the beginning and her outstanding efforts and sincere devotion have indeed made lighter our task, and to Libby we are most grateful. Hannah Amir provided us with exceptional photographic assistance and to Hannah we are most appreciative. The typing of the manuscript was diligently done by Ruth Grossman, Virginia Hansen and Shani Hanft and to them we express our sincere thanks.

To our many colleagues at the Chaim Sheba Medical Center, the University of Minnesota and throughout the world who have so kindly shared their thoughts with us and willingly provided us with illustrative material—to them all we are much indebted. We extend to Dr. Murray Feingold a special thanks for permitting us to use his material on body measurements. Mr. Jeffrey W. House, editor at Oxford University Press, has not only been most understanding but has shared with us his experience and enthusiasm, and for these and more we are grateful to him and his excellent staff.

Financial support for this text has been most generously provided by the National Foundation for Jewish Genetic Diseases, the Lake Chemical Company, the Roucher Foundation and the Philip Hecht family and to these organizations and individuals we are most appreciative.

Our final thanks go to our wives, Audrey and Marilyn, for only they know the time spent, and without their devotion this endeavor would not have been possible.

Richard M. Goodman
Robert J. Gorlin

Contents

INTRODUCTION

Making a Diagnosis and Its Implications

Although the dysmorphologist is unable to make a precise diagnosis in the majority of children with congenital malformations, this has not impeded the continuing expansion of our diagnostic acumen in this area. New congenital malformation syndromes are being recognized and reported almost daily. This flood of diagnostic information has tended to make physicians (unfortunately even pediatricians) shy away from malformed children, and refer them instead to those specialists primarily interested in such disorders.

It could be rightly asked, how does one make a correct diagnosis (if such is possible) in a congenitally malformed child? We have been taught that all diagnoses in medicine rest on the three pillars of (1) history, (2) physical examination, and (3) various laboratory and investigative studies. Although this schema is sound and logical and must be employed, it does not always lead to the end point of a specific diagnosis when applied to the malformed child. Its failure is often not due to a lack of information or a sparsity of physical or radiographic findings, but rather resides in the interpretation of all the data. As alluded to earlier, the diagnostician commonly must resort to merely giving a description of the findings without a diagnosis. However, while the schema mentioned does work, there are special diagnostic pitfalls that arise when dealing with the subject of dysmorphology. For example, we are aware that not all students or physicians have been properly trained to recognize and interpret many malformation defects. The adage that we tend to diagnose what we know could be paraphrased to state that we see what we know. If we don't know what dystopia canthorum is, chances are we may not recognize it when present and therefore never understand its diagnostic significance.

Through the years we have developed a set of guidelines which we have found relevant in the diagnosis of the infant or child having multiple malformations. The diagnostic guidelines for the physical examination are as follows:

1. No child can be properly examined unless completely undressed.
2. Carefully observe the child before you begin to use your hands for the physical examination.
3. The longer you refrain from touching the child, the more you will observe.
4. Compare one side of the body with the other (even one nail with the other).
5. Consider each observation important until you know its proper significance.
6. Accurately and properly measure those physical features which lend themselves to being measured.
7. Compare your measurements with accepted and standardized tables, charts, and figures.
8. Try to use the proper terminology for each physical finding.
9. Accurately record all your observations and when possible document the more significant ones by means of photographs.
10. Never hesitate to reexamine a child if you are not certain about a finding.

Once a specific diagnosis is contemplated, what other considerations should come into play?

1. Even though you may be certain of the diagnosis, always let your mind be open to a differential diagnosis. What else could it be?
2. Only by insisting on a differential diagnosis can you expand your diagnostic abilities.

3. Diagnoses pertaining to malformation defects or syndromes can be grouped into three major categories:
   a. Known and established conditions.
   b. Recently described conditions or variants of known disorders (genetic heterogeneity).
   c. Entirely new malformations, syndromes, or variants which have not been previously reported.

Obviously the latter two categories (b and c) present a challenge to those not well versed in the literature. When faced with a possibility in these areas, not only is a search of the literature needed, but consultation with an authority is advisable, especially if an entirely new entity or variant is being considered.

After an accurate diagnosis has been made, the physician must be prepared to deal with a number of crucial problems. The two main areas of concern involve the child and the parents. What can and should be done to provide proper care for the child? This can be a complex and most difficult question, and often will require the opinions of a number of qualified individuals. Furthermore, the treatment process itself may extend over a number of years.

The parents must be properly informed as to the diagnosis and prognosis of their child's condition. If the disorder is of genetic etiology, family studies may be needed and genetic counseling should certainly be given. The key point to be emphasized is that proper management of the congenitally malformed child, regardless of the etiology of the disorder, usually requires the team efforts of various qualified individuals. Frequently, it will fall upon the one who made the diagnosis to be not only the initiator, but also the organizer of this team approach.

Concepts and Terminology
Relating to
Defects of Morphogenesis

Recently, Spranger and co-workers (1982) published their recommendations on concepts and terms pertaining to errors of morphogenesis. Since this publication may be helpful to the reader, we have elected to present a brief summary of its main concepts.

Spranger and colleagues emphasize definitions in their presentation, which is dictated by the intricate relationship between terminology and nosology: "naming is classifying" as, conversely, there is no useful classification without properly defined terms.

Individual Alterations of Form or Structure

Malformation: A malformation is a morphologic defect of an organ, part of an organ, or a larger region of the body resulting from an intrinsically abnormal developmental process.

"Intrinsic" means that the developmental potential of the organ—its anlage—is abnormal from the beginning, which can be diagrammed as follows:

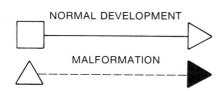

Most malformations are field defects. A morphogenetic field is a region or a part of an embryo which responds as a coordinated unit to embryonic interaction and results in complex or multiple anatomic structures. "Embryonic interaction" refers to the reciprocal (chemical or physical) influence of developing tissues on one another during embryogenesis.

Disruption: A disruption is a morphologic defect of an organ, part of an organ, or a larger region of the body resulting from the extrinsic breakdown of, or an interference with, an originally normal developmental process.

Some extrinsic factor such as an infection, teratogen, or trauma interferes with development, which thereafter proceeds abnormally. This can be depicted as follows:

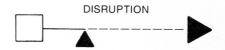

A disruption is not inherited, but inherited factors can predispose to and influence the development of a disruption.

Deformation: A deformation is an abnormal form, shape, or position of part of the body caused by mechanical forces.

The use of this term is restricted to aberrations of form considered a normal response of the affected tissue to unusual mechanical forces. This is diagrammed below:

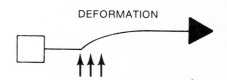

An example of a prenatal deformation is an equinovarus foot, resulting from extrinsic compression of the fetus due to oligohydramnios.

Introduction

Dysplasia: A dysplasia is an abnormal organization of cells into tissue(s) and the morphologic result(s). Thus, it involves the process of histogenesis.

Dysplastic lesions are usually not confined to single organs. In the heritable disorders of connective tissue, for example, the basic defect commonly involves many anatomic sites in which the affected tissue element is present. We represent dysplasia as:

DYSPLASIA

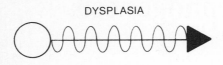

Patterns of Morphologic Defects

The terms we define here reflect our present-day knowledge regarding causation and genesis of pattern defects.

Polytopic field defect: A polytopic field defect is a pattern of anomalies derived from the disturbance of a single developmental field.

Unfortunately, little is known about developmental fields and their defects in man, but certain conditions strongly support the validity of this concept in human embryogenesis. For example, the multiple defects of holoprosencephaly may be traced to a disturbance of prechordal mesoderm, which normally migrates forward into the area anterior to the notochord and interacts with the development of the forebrain and midfacial structures. Defects in this field can produce a wide range of anomalies (see pages 60–61.).

Sequence: A sequence is a pattern of multiple anomalies derived from a single known or presumed prior anomaly or mechanical factor.

For example, a myelomeningocele may result in lower limb paralysis, muscle wasting, clubfeet, incontinence, urinary tract infection, renal damage, constipation, etc. Thus, the pattern may be termed myelomeningocele sequence.

Syndrome: A syndrome is a pattern of multiple anomalies thought to be pathogenetically related and not known to represent a single sequence or a polytopic field defect.

The term syndrome often implies a single cause, as in Down syndrome. Like "sequence," it is used only when the components of the given pattern of anomalies are known or thought to be pathogenetically related.

Association: An association is a nonrandom occurrence in two or more individuals of multiple anomalies not known to represent a polytopic field defect, sequence, or syndrome.

The term refers solely to statistically—not pathogenetically or causally—related anomalies.

These concepts should not be regarded as definitive, but merely represent a stage in our endeavor to better understand errors of morphogenesis. Undoubtedly, they will have to be revised as knowledge of the causes of altered prenatal development advances.

REFERENCE

Spranger, J., Benirschke, K., Hall, J.G., Lenz, W., Lowry, R.B., Opitz, J.M., Pinsky, L., Schwarzacher, H.G., and Smith, D.W. Errors of morphogenesis: concepts and terms. *J. Pediatr. 100:* 160–165,1982.

An Approach
to the Use of This Book

For those in search of diagnosis, it is suggested that this book be used in the following manner:

1. The customary information should be obtained from the medical and family histories which may serve as as guide to the etiology, be it environmental or genetic.

2. Observations from the physical examination should be considered according to (a) single or multiple system involvement, (b) symmetry of the anomalies (symmetrical anomalies tend to be of genetic etiology), and (c) presence or absence of mental retardation.

3. Based on information from the first two procedures, a tentative decision may be reached which would lead to one of the three categories:
   A. fetal environmental syndromes
   B. developmental defects, or
   C. genetic syndromes.
   (Not all disorders listed under genetic are known to be of definite genetic etiology; however, such conditions are in the minority.)

4. If the direction is toward a genetic syndrome, then further thought should be given to the various arbitrary clinical subdivisions:
   a. chromosomal,
   b. connective tissue,
   c. endocrine/metabolic,
   d. facial and/or skeletal,
   e. skeletal dysplasia, or
   f. skin and hair.

It is important to note that many of these genetic syndromes overlap in their clinical features, so there is an arbitrariness in classification. Furthermore, there is much discrepancy regarding the choice of terminology for each disorder, and although we have selected the term which we think is most appropriate, we know that unanimous agreement cannot be achieved.

5. Under each of the three main categories and under the six genetic subdivisions, the disorders are listed alphabetically. At the top of each illustrated page, M.R. stands for mental retardation; (+) means present and (−) means not present. If present, there is a further indication of prevalence: *all* (100%), *most* (50–100%), *some* (30–50%), or *few* (less than 30%). On the right are listed a few of the outstanding characteristics and early physical features of the disorder.

To provide the reader with a better means of understanding the terminology, and to delineate how to perform and interpret various body measurements, the following can be found in the appendix:

General principles for measuring body parts
Guidelines for head and facial measurements
Figures, tables, and charts on body measurements
Glossary of medical terms

In addition to the references found at the end of each disorder, a number of selected book references are grouped according to subject matter in the appendix.

THE DISORDERS

A. Fetal Environmental Syndromes

1. Amniotic Band Disruption Complex
2. Anti-Folic Acid Embryopathy
3. Battered Child Syndrome
4. Fetal Alcohol Syndrome
5. Fetal Cytomegalovirus Syndrome
6. Fetal Hydantoin Syndrome
7. Fetal Rubella Syndrome
8. Fetal Syphilis Syndrome
9. Fetal Toxoplasmosis Syndrome
10. Fetal Trimethadione, Paramethadione, and Primidone Syndromes
11. Perinatal Herpes Simplex Virus Infection
12. Warfarin Embryopathy

1. AMNIOTIC BAND DISRUPTION COMPLEX

Clinical Features The amniotic band disruption complex occurs in various forms. The most common involves the limbs only. The anomalies range from congenital ring constrictions of a digit or limb to complete amputation of one or more digits or limbs to major craniofacial and visceral defects. The absent parts are often multiple but rarely bilaterally symmetrical. Not uncommonly, there is associated terminal digital fusion (distal pseudosyndactyly), talipes (about 30%), and lymphedema below the ring constriction. Rarely, clubbing of the hands has been observed. Soft tissue depressions may be manifested on the neck, trunk, or abdomen. The most severe combination of anomalies in this disorder includes limb and craniofacial abnormalities acronymically termed the ADAM (*A*mniotic *D*eformity, *A*dhesions, *M*utilations) complex. Facial anomalies include cleft lip (usually bilateral), bizarre midfacial clefts, hydrocephalus, microcephalus, multiple anterior asymmetric encephaloceles, and occasionally meningoceles. Eye abnormalities include distorted or colobomatous palpebral fissures, microphthalmia, anophthalmia, and corneal opacity. The nasal malformations may be complex. Major visceral anomalies comprise omphalocele and gastroschisis.

Specific Diagnosis Diagnosis is clinical. Radiographs of the underlying bones generally are unremarkable except for the amputation.

Differential Diagnosis Intrauterine amputation must be differentiated from those cases that clearly are genetic. The genetic forms are usually bilaterally symmetrical and rudimentary digits are often present. Furthermore, genetic syndactyly is proximal, not distal.

Prenatal Diagnosis Severe cases of the ADAM complex may be associated with elevated alpha-fetoprotein and acetylcholinesterase in amniotic fluid and with sonographic findings.

Basic Defect and Other Considerations The most common hypothesis concerning the amniotic band syndrome is that the fetal deformities result from primary amnion rupture without chorionic sac damage at various stages of gestation. The placenta and membranes are often abnormal, that is, in separation of amnion from chorion. Fibrous strands attached to the amnion or chorion have been noted. Rarely, a band is attached to the infant. It is presumed that the duration and severity of compression by amniotic or chorionic strands determines whether there is simple ring constriction, a block to venous and lymphatic drainage, or interference with arterial blood supply with subsequent necrosis. In essence, the earlier the rupture, the more severe the anomalies. There is no evidence to indicate that a genetic factor is involved. Etiologic factors leading to amniotic disruption have not been well identified but a case has been reported following amniocentesis done with a large needle which may have caused disruption of the amnion, formation of bands, and attendant oligohydramnios. Estimates of its frequency range from 1 in 5,000 to 1 in 10,000 newborns. There must be at least 600 case reports. No sex predilection has been noted.

Prognosis and Treatment Prognosis depends upon the severity of anomalies; mental retardation may occur in those with more severe CNS involvement. The most severe examples are aborted or stillborn. Some infants have only a mild cosmetic deformity, while others exhibit severe amputations that require orthopedic prostheses. Many of those with the so-called ADAM complex die, while others may require the services of a team of specialists.

REFERENCES

Higginbottom, M.C., Jones, K.L., Hall, B.D. et al. The amniotic band disruption complex: timing of amniotic rupture and variable spectra of consequent defects. *J. Pediatr. 95:* 544–549, 1979.

Keller, H., Neuhauser, G., Durkin-Stamm, M.V., Kaveggia, E.G., Schaaff, A., and Sitzmann, F. "ADAM complex" (Amniotic Deformity, Adhesions, Mutilations)—a pattern of craniofacial and limb defects. *Am. J. Med. Genet. 2:* 81–98, 1978.

Moessinger, A.C., Blanc, W.A., Byrne, J. et al. Amniotic band syndrome associated with amniocentesis. *Am. J. Obstet. Gynecol. 141:* 588–591, 1981.

- **tissue bands**
- **unilateral limb anomalies**
- **facial clefting**
- **encephaloceles**

Amniotic Band Disruption Complex

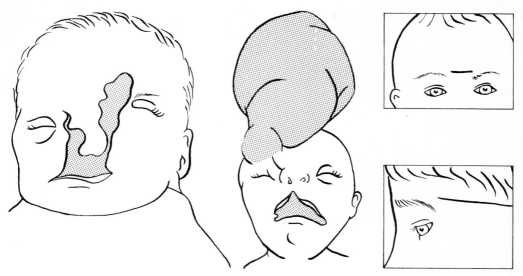

Altered facial morphogenesis, asymmetric encephalocele —
lines from frontal and temporal constriction bands

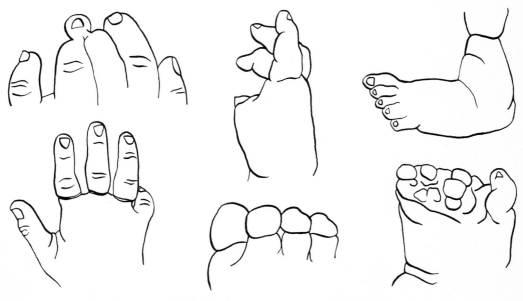

Limb anomalies due to aberrant bands

2. ANTI-FOLIC ACID EMBRYOPATHY

Clinical Features Aminopterin and its methyl derivative, methotrexate, have long been implicated as fetal teratogens, producing a classic clinical picture characterized by growth retardation and malformations of the skull, face, and limbs. It has been estimated that almost 25% of infants delivered at term after maternal ingestion of either of these folic acid antagonists taken between the eighth and ninth week of pregnancy had major abnormalities of bone growth and development. Other organ systems appear unaffected. There are approximately a dozen case reports of children who have survived the neonatal period. The mothers of several of these patients tried unsuccessfully to abort their pregnancies with one of the abovementioned drugs. Aminopterin was used as an abortifacient especially in Scandinavia in the 1960s.

Specific Diagnosis The clinical picture is remarkably characteristic and once seen can easily be identified during infancy. There are frontal and/or parietal bony defects which ultimately fill in, bitemporal flattening, and brachycephaly. Not uncommonly the hairline is bizarre. The supraorbital ridges are underdeveloped. There is marked pigmentation of the medial half of the eyebrows, the lateral half often being absent. Marked ocular hypertelorism, exophthalmos, blepharophimosis, an extremely prominent nose, micrognathia, and malformed posteriorly rotated pinnae characterize the facies. The palate is highly arched or, at times, cleft. The limbs are distally shortened, with the radial heads often subluxated. There is marked growth retardation, the stature being below the third percentile. Brachydactyly, syndactyly, and hypoplasia of digits are extremely variable. Intelligence is normal.

Differential Diagnosis The phenotype is so characteristic that differential diagnosis is virtually unnecessary. Problems in diagnosis arise largely when the mother denies using aminopterin or methotrexate to induce abortion.

Prenatal Diagnosis This is not currently available.

Basic Defect and Other Considerations The basic defect results from the ability of aminopterin and methotrexate to produce a folic acid deficiency in the embryo. If given in sufficient amounts during the first trimester, it causes suppression of fetal hematopoiesis, liver necrosis, and fetal death. If the fetus is approximately eight to nine weeks gestation, doses of 6 to 12 mg will produce the embryopathy.

Prognosis and Treatment Intelligence is normal. The bony defects of the skull eventually fill in. Prevention consists of avoidance of the drugs during the first trimester of pregnancy.

REFERENCES

Howard, N.J. and Rudd, N.L. The natural history of aminopterin-induced embryopathy. *Birth Defects 13(3C):* 85–93, 1977.

Reich, E.W., Cox, R.P., Becker, M.H., Genieser, N.B., et al. Recognition in adult patients of malformations induced by folic-acid antagonists. *Birth Defects 14(6B):* 139–160, 1978.

Warkany, J. Aminopterin and methotrexate: folic acid deficiency. *Teratology 17:* 353–357, 1978.

- **prominent nose**
- **absent lateral eyebrows**
- **hypertelorism**
- **bitemporal flattening**

Anti-Folic Acid Embryopathy

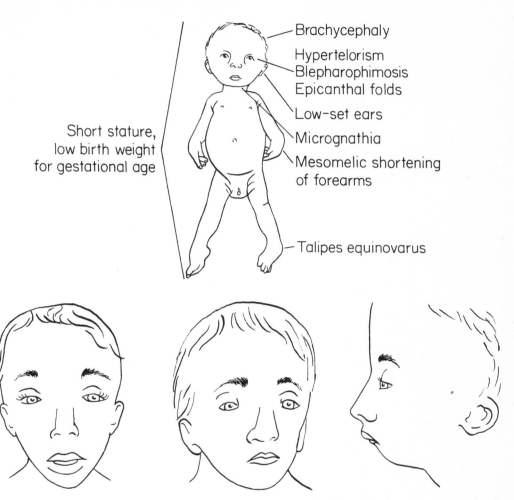

Brachycephaly

Hypertelorism
Blepharophimosis
Epicanthal folds

Low-set ears

Micrognathia

Mesomelic shortening
of forearms

Short stature,
low birth weight
for gestational age

Talipes equinovarus

Shallow supraorbital ridges, sparse eyebrows laterally,
blepharophimosis, prominent nose, low-set ears, micrognathia

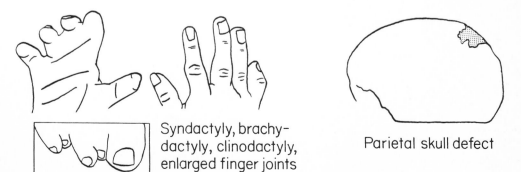

Syndactyly, brachy-
dactyly, clinodactyly,
enlarged finger joints

Parietal skull defect

15

3. BATTERED CHILD SYNDROME

Clinical Features The term has been expanded to encompass more than severe physical abuse; emotional and sexual abuse, nutritional deprivation, and medical care neglect are also included. Physical abuse may take several forms: bruises, head injuries, fractures, or burns and range in severity from a minor bruise to a fatal subdural hematoma. The agent producing the injury may be evident from characteristic marks such as human bites, bruises showing the attacker's finger and thumb marks, loop marks from doubled cord, lash marks from belts, choke marks or circumferential tie marks on ankles or wrists. Somewhat less commonly (10%) the child is burned with a cigarette or held against a hot radiator. Hot water burns result from dunking the child into scalding water. Ocular damage is especially severe, ranging from acute hyphema to the permanent damage produced by dislocated lens or detached retina. In the case of subdural hematoma, coma and convulsions often result. There may be multiple skull fractures which are secondary to violent shaking and may be associated with retinal hemorrhages. The most common cause of death is intra-abdominal injury; this is associated with recurrent vomiting, absent bowel sounds, localized tenderness, or abdominal distension. Most commonly one finds tears in the mesentery or small intestine. Many battered children fail to thrive. A characteristic pinched face due to loss of fat from the buccal pads, prominent ribs and wasted buttocks, redundant skin, and spindly extremities are common.

Specific Diagnosis Usually the individual presenting with the child gives an implausible explanation for the child's injuries or presents vague explanations. Frequently there is discrepancy between case histories presented by the two parents or history of a minor accident with finding of major injury. Often a considerable span of time exists between the injury and the child being brought to the doctor, sometimes several days. Radiological survey of long bones, skull, ribs, and pelvis should be obtained in cases of suspected physical abuse, although no fracture may be evident. While some children manifest multiple bone injuries at different stages of healing, others may show only thickened periosteum or chip or corner fracture at a metaphysis due to twisting or jerking.

Differential Diagnosis One must exclude *osteogenesis imperfecta, accidental trauma,* and *failure to thrive* due to numerous causes as well as *pseudobattering* (coin rubbing, cupping, etc.).

Basic Defect and Other Considerations Often individuals producing the physical abuse were themselves abused as children. Events leading to multiple ongoing crises or acute crises on the part of the parent or acute illness which leads to intractable crying on the part of the child will often precipitate the beating. Often the child was unwanted and frequently the father is absent. Physical abuse has been estimated at approximately 6 per 1000 live births with prevalence being estimated at about 500 cases per million population per year. Among children less than five years of age seen in hospital emergency rooms, approximately 10% of all injuries represent battered child syndrome. Usually about a third are less than six months of age, another third from six months to three years, and a third over three. A child with failure to thrive is usually less than two years. Both premature children and stepchildren are at increased risk. Women are more likely to be the abusers, but if the father is unemployed there tends to be no sex difference.

Prognosis and Treatment Mortality in the United States is approximately 3% or about 2000 deaths per year. If physical child abuse is suspected, the child should be hospitalized as "his injuries need to be watched." If hospitalization is refused, a court order can be obtained. The injuries or malnutrition should be treated after consultation with a team of specialists. State law requires that suspected cases of child abuse be reported. Cooperation with the parent is at best difficult, for the abuser already feels inadequate and unloved. The report must be made by phone within 24 hours to the children's protective service in the patient's county of residence and an official report written within 48 hours, thoroughly documenting history, and physical examination, and radiographic findings. A statement concerning why this does not represent nonaccidental trauma must be included. Hospital social service consultations should be obtained within 72 hours for evaluation of how safe the home is for the child. Medical and psychosocial follow-up are necessary. Among those returned to the parents without intervention, approximately 5% are killed and 35% seriously reinjured. Severe psychological damage is almost invariably done.

---

*Although this condition is not a fetal environmental syndrome, it is of an environmental nature and thus, is placed in this section.

REFERENCES

Caffey, J. On the theory and practice of shaking infants. *Am. J. Dis. Child. 124:* 161–169, 1972.
Jackson, G. Child abuse syndrome: the cases we miss. *Br. Med. J. 2:* 756–758, 1972.

Kempe, C.H. Paediatric implications of the battered baby syndrome. *Arch. Dis. Child. 46:* 28–37, 1971.

Battered Child Syndrome

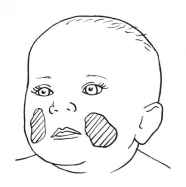
Bruising of face

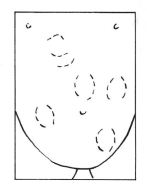
Bite marks

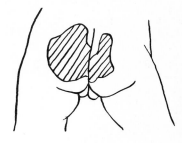
Hot pad burn

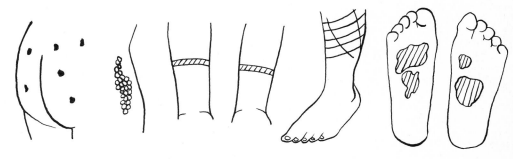
Burns about the body due to cigarette, rope, heater, and hot grid

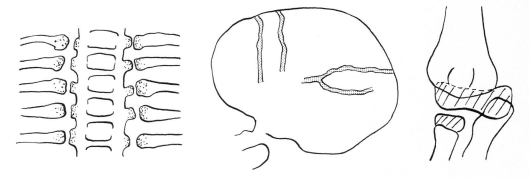
Fractures of costovertebral joints, skull and displacement of distal humeral epiphysis

4. FETAL ALCOHOL SYNDROME

Clinical Features The fetal alcohol syndrome is extremely variable and appears to be dose related. In over 80%, microcephaly, mild to moderate mental retardation, fine motor dysfunction, irritability in infancy, poor suck, growth retardation at birth with poor "catch-up" growth (birth length being severely retarded in comparison with birth weight and adult male height being 158–162 cm), short palpebral fissures, hypoplastic or shallow philtrum, and thinned vermilion of the upper lip are present. Noted in over 50% but less than 80% of infants are hypotonia, hyperactivity in childhood, sparse adipose tissue, sacral dimple, short upturned nose, and hypoplastic maxilla. Somewhat less common (26–50%) are strabismus, myopia, epicanthal folds, posterior rotation of the pinnae, hip dislocation, pectus excavatum, abnormally deep or accentuated palmar creases, clinodactyly of fifth finger and brachydactyly of index finger, hypoplasia of the labia, small raised cutaneous (strawberry) hemangiomas, and atrial or less often ventricular septal defect. Present in 1–25% of affected offspring are various eye problems (such as eyelid ptosis and microphthalmia), neural tube defect, cleft lip and/or cleft palate, limited joint movement of elbows and fingers, Klippel-Feil anomaly, scoliosis, hypoplasia of the fifth fingernail, hydronephrosis, small rotated kidneys, hypospadias, hernia and divarication of recti. There appears to be an increased association with neural crest tumors. Mild retinal aberrations are relatively common.

Specific Diagnosis Diagnosis is clinical. It should be borne in mind that not all severely chronic alcoholic mothers, even with excessive consumption of alcohol during their entire pregnancy, will necessarily give birth to affected infants. In severe cases, cerebellar hypoplasia and cerebral dysgenesis with heterotopic cell clusters are found. Palpebral fissure length is difficult to measure in the newborn (normal = 19.5 mm ± 1.5). Radiographic changes include "copperbeaten" skull, delayed bone age, carpal bone fusions, pseudoepiphyses of metacarpals, and, occasionally, radioulnar synostosis.

Differential Diagnosis In maternal malnutrition, birth length is not especially retarded in contrast to marked decrease in birth weight. Confusion is most likely to occur with *fetal hydantoin syndrome*. It is far less likely that various other disorders such as *Noonan syndrome, de Lange syndrome, Dubowitz syndrome, familial blepharophimosis, trisomy 18, 10q+,* or *Smith-Lemli-Opitz syndrome* need be excluded. Several children that we have seen have been diagnosed as having *cerebral palsy*. Conversely, the diagnosis has often been misapplied when no other one was forthcoming.

Prenatal Diagnosis We do not currently have a valid method of diagnosing the condition prenatally. Periodic serum acetaldehyde levels of the mother may be a possible monitor.

Basic Defect and Other Considerations Pathogenesis is not known, but is probably related to the toxic effect of a breakdown product of ethanol, most likely acetaldehyde. It is possible that genetic polymorphisms for acetaldehyde metabolism may alter fetal susceptibility. Some aspects (joint problems, abnormal palmar creases) may be secondary to lack of fetal movement. While the expression of the disease is related to the degree of alcohol consumption during the pregnancy, it has been estimated that approximately 30–50% of infants born to severely chronic alcoholic mothers exhibit signs of the disorder. If a daily consumption of 100 ml or more of alcohol is assumed to be teratogenic, then possibly 10% of females in the United States are at risk. Consumption of two shot-equivalents or less per day during the pregnancy appears to produce minimal stigmata and the data on "binge" drinking are conflicting. However, even as little as 35 to 45 ml/day may be associated with increased risk for prematurity and/or decreased birth weight. Estimates of the frequency of the disorder range from 1 in 600 to 1 in 1000 live births. There is no sex predilection. Perhaps the most susceptible period is the first trimester.

Prognosis and Treatment Prognosis is not good. Miscarriage is common, there is increased incidence of stillbirths, and perinatal mortality is enhanced tenfold. Catch-up growth does not progress satisfactorily and there is mild to moderate mental retardation. Surgery may be necessary for correction of the cardiac anomalies. Markedly reduced alcohol consumption should be encouraged, however the use of disulfiram (Antabuse) is contraindicated since it raises blood acetaldehyde levels.

REFERENCES

Clarren, S.K. and Smith, D.W. The fetal alcohol syndrome. *N. Engl. J. Med. 298:* 1063–1067, 1978.
Jones, K. L. and Smith, D.W. The fetal alcohol syndrome. *Teratology 12:* 1–10, 1975.
Little, R.E. and Streissguth, P. Effects of alcohol on the fetus: impact and prevention. *Can. Med. Assoc. J. 125:* 159–164, 1981.

- irritable infant
- growth (length) retardation
- shallow philtrum
- narrow palpebral fissures

Fetal Alcohol Syndrome

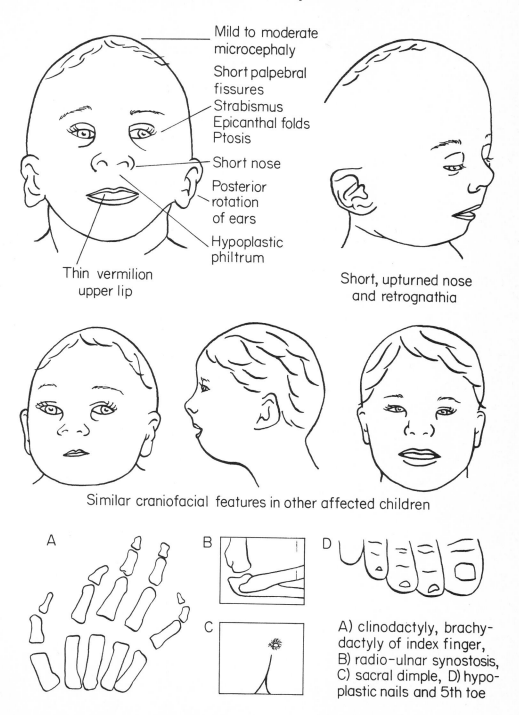

Mild to moderate microcephaly

Short palpebral fissures
Strabismus
Epicanthal folds
Ptosis

Short nose

Posterior rotation of ears

Hypoplastic philtrum

Thin vermilion upper lip

Short, upturned nose and retrognathia

Similar craniofacial features in other affected children

A

B

D

C

A) clinodactyly, brachy-dactyly of index finger, B) radio-ulnar synostosis, C) sacral dimple, D) hypo-plastic nails and 5th toe

5. FETAL CYTOMEGALOVIRUS SYNDROME

Clinical Features Fetal cytomegalovirus (CMV) syndrome is extremely variable in its expression. It may be congenital (occurring in 0.5–2.5% of newborns) or acquired, being found in almost 40% of infants during the first year of life. It can range from no clinical stigmata to a severe infection. Observed in about 60–75% of newborn symptomatic infants are hepatosplenomegaly, petechiae, jaundice, and anemia. Prematurity and intrauterine growth retardation are noted in approximately 30%. Occasionally there may be hydrocephaly. Microcephaly, while present at birth in about 50%, may not necessarily become apparent until the second year of life. Among symptomatic newborns, among those who survive, mental retardation (60%); hyperactivity, seizures, spasticity (35%), and hearing loss (30%) have been found. Pneumonia occurs in about 25%. While hepatosplenomegaly may persist for several years, chronic liver problems are not common. Inguinal hernia is noted in about 25%. Chorioretinitis or optic atrophy has been found in about 10% of these children. CMV infections have been associated with *Pneumocystis carinii, E. coli,* and *H. influenza* in immunocompetent infants.

Specific Diagnosis Thrombocytopenia (60%), hemolytic anemia (60%), increased cord serum IgM (85%), elevated SGOT (80%), and increased CSF protein (50%) are noted. Atypical lymphocytes have been observed during the first month in about 80%. Raised skin ("blueberry muffin") lesions are actually sites of extramedullary hemopoiesis. Radiographic studies have demonstrated cerebral calcifications and metaphysitis in approximately 25%. Biopsy of the liver has demonstrated varying degrees of hepatitis with giant cells, portal fibrosis, and cholangitis. Isolation of the cytomegalovirus is the most reliable method. Infants infected with CMV usually excrete the virus in the urine for several years. Characteristic inclusion cells are seen in only a third of the cases. Serologic tests: a simple fluorescent test has been developed to demonstrate macroglobulin specific antibodies.

Differential Diagnosis The clinical signs resemble those of *fetal rubella, toxoplasmosis, fetal syphilis,* or *herpes.* Almost any of the stigmata may be found as isolated findings of various etiology. Flat disseminated cerebral calcifications can also be noted in toxoplasmosis. Chorioretinitis occurs more frequently with toxoplasmosis. The cytomegalovirus can be cultured in vitro only on human fibroblasts.

Prenatal Diagnosis The cytomegalovirus is recoverable from the amniotic fluid during the first trimester, making possible the prenatal diagnosis of the condition. During the third trimester, a radiograph may show cerebral brain calcifications.

Basic Defect and Other Considerations Transmission of the human cytomegalovirus in utero to the conceptus usually occurs transplacentally in the third or fourth month, rarely by intrauterine transfusion. The virus causes cell necrosis. The acquired form usually results from maternal-infant interaction (cervical secretion, saliva, breast milk, urine, tears). Occasionally the infection may be acquired within the first 30 days of life by transfusion of whole fresh blood. The frequency for the syndrome is approximately 1 in 3500 live births.

Prognosis and Treatment There is no known effective drug therapy. If the infection is severe, death eventuates in the newborn period. In those in whom the disease is severe but who survive, seizures, mental retardation, or spasticity may occur. Most of those with a mild course recover completely.

REFERENCES

Pass, R.F., Stagno, S., Myers, G.J. et al. Outcome of symptomatic congenital CMV infection: results of long-term follow-up. *Pediatrics 66:* 758–762, 1980.

Stagno, S., Pass, R.F., Reynolds, D.W. et al. Comparative study of diagnostic procedures for congenital cytomegalovirus infection. *Pediatrics 65:* 251–257, 1980.

Weller, T.H. The cytomegaloviruses: ubiquitous agents with protean clinical manifestations. *N. Engl. J. Med. 285:* 203–214, 267–274, 1971.

- **hepatosplenomegaly**
- **petechiae**
- **jaundice**
- **anemia**

Fetal Cytomegalovirus Syndrome

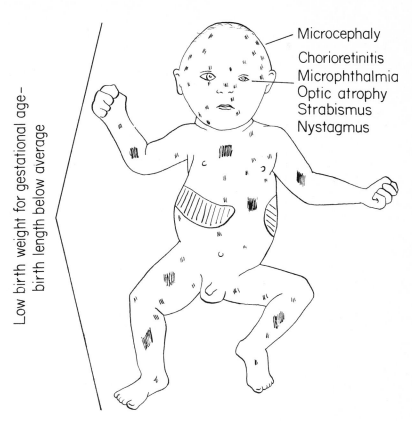

Low birth weight for gestational age-
birth length below average

— Microcephaly

Chorioretinitis
Microphthalmia
Optic atrophy
Strabismus
Nystagmus

Affected infant with petechiae, purpura,
jaundice and hepatosplenomegaly

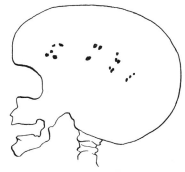

Cerebral calcification mainly
in the periventricular region

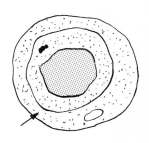

Intranuclear inclusion body
from urine sediment

6. FETAL HYDANTOIN SYNDROME

Clinical Features There appears to be basic agreement that epileptic mothers receiving hydantoin are two to three times more likely to have malformed infants than mothers who have never had a seizure; but there is considerable debate regarding whether the incidence of anomalies is greater in the offspring of treated and untreated epileptics. However, while the total of major anomalies appears to be about the same, difficulties arise because of lack of crucial untreated epileptic control groups. The anomalies most frequently cited include cleft lip, cleft palate, and congenital heart disease (septal defect, coarctation of aorta, tetralogy of Fallot). Pre- and postnatal growth deficiency have been reported. Mental deficiency and microcephaly have also been noted to be increased. However, there has been a general lack of assessment of parental intelligence and head circumference and differences between children of treated epileptics and those of nonepileptic controls are small (0.5 cm in head circumference, 92 versus 97 IQ). Environmental factors may play a significant role when mothers have a serious chronic illness. There is no general agreement concerning increased fetal wastage or neonatal mortality. A characteristic facies has been suggested: metopic suture ridging, depressed nasal bridge, short nose, ocular hypertelorism, epicanthal folds, ptosis of eyelid, strabismus, wide mouth, and short neck. Limb anomalies include hypoplasia of nails and distal phalanges, fingerlike thumbs, and increased numbers of fingerprint arches.

Specific Diagnosis It has been stated that at least 10% of exposed infants exhibit a full pattern of the anomalies noted above with perhaps 30% exhibiting some of the stigmata.

Differential Diagnosis Many of the stigmata cited may be seen in *fetal alcohol syndrome* (small for gestational age, postnatal growth delay, slow mental development, congenital heart anomalies, cleft lip and/or palate, abnormal palmar creases, hypoplasia of nails and phalanges). The question has been raised concerning common impaired metabolism.

Prenatal Diagnosis We are not aware that this had been done.

Basic Defect and Other Considerations It is conceivable that the increased rate of cleft lip/cleft palate and congenital heart disease and the slightly decreased intelligence seen in these children are caused by environmental factors due to epilepsy in the mother. Genetic factors may also play a role, for there appears to be a higher rate of epilepsy in families in which the proband has cleft lip and/or cleft palate. There is also an increased risk of anomalies observed in the offspring of epileptic fathers. Epileptics themselves appear to have more anomalies than nonepileptics, and it is possible that the seizures themselves, which appear to be more common during the first trimester in pregnancy, may be teratogenic. If hydantoin is really teratogenic, then it is estimated that 1 in 5000 children may have the syndrome. There does not appear to be a sexual predilection.

Prognosis and Treatment The facial clefting and congenital heart disease require surgical intervention. There is considerable doubt regarding the desirability of removing anticonvulsive treatment during pregnancy. Between 30% and 60% of epileptics have more seizures during pregnancy, especially during the first trimester and pregnancy appears to be followed by a permanent deterioration in seizure control in approximately 3% of epileptics.

REFERENCES

Hanson, J.W., and Smith, D.W. The fetal hydantoin syndrome. *J. Pediatr. 87:* 285–290, 1975.

Hill, R.M. Fetal malformations and antiepileptic drugs. *Am. J. Dis. Child. 130:* 923–925, 1976.

Stumpf, D.A. and Frost, M. Seizures, anticonvulsants and pregnancy. *Am. J. Dis. Child. 132:* 746–748, 1978.

- **hypoplasia of nails and digits**
- **short nose**
- **anteverted nares**
- **eye anomalies**

Fetal Hydantoin Syndrome

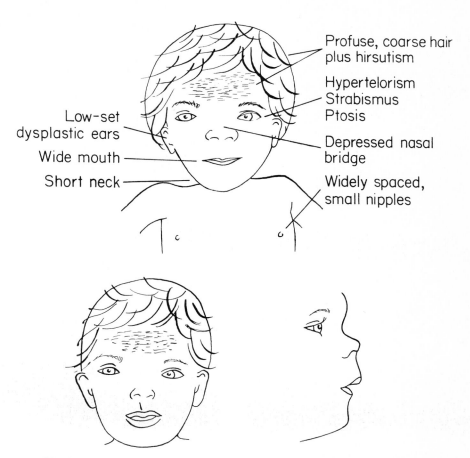

Profuse, coarse hair plus hirsutism

Hypertelorism
Strabismus
Ptosis

Depressed nasal bridge

Widely spaced, small nipples

Low-set dysplastic ears

Wide mouth

Short neck

Similar facies with repair of cleft lip–another infant with anteverted nares and depressed nasal bridge

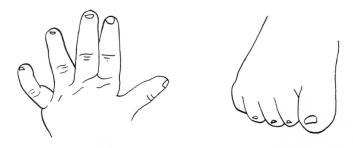

Hypoplasia of nails and terminal digits

7. FETAL RUBELLA SYNDROME

Clinical Features Depending on various factors, infection of the fetus with rubella virus may eventuate in spontaneous abortion, stillbirth, or various congenital abnormalities. Low birth weight, hepatosplenomegaly, purpura, jaundice, and bone lesions are transitory. Not uncommonly a relatively subtle corneal clouding may be observed and the anterior fontanel is large and bulging. Interstitial pneumonitis, meningoencephalitis, hepatitis, pancreatitis, and myocarditis are also transient. Permanent stigmata include congenital heart disease (patent ductus arteriosus, systemic and pulmonary arterial stenosis, multivalvular sclerosis, VSD, or anomalies of the aortic arch), sensorineural hearing loss which varies in degree and may be unilateral, cataract which is unilateral about half the time, microcephaly, microphthalmia, retinopathy, high myopia, and glaucoma. Psychomotor retardation or typical spastic cerebral palsy may eventuate. Delayed stigmata include autism, systemic hypertension, diabetes mellitus (20%), thyroid disease, precocious puberty, bile duct atresia, and cirrhosis.

Specific Diagnosis During the neonatal period there is commonly hemolytic or hypoplastic anemia, thrombocytopenia, elevated protein levels and pleocytosis in the cerebrospinal fluid, and elevated serum IgM. However, only about 20% have high levels of IgM (greater than 20 mg/d1) in cord blood at birth. During the first few months of life this may increase to almost 50%. For diagnostic purposes, an infant's titer should be at least four times higher than the mother's. Rubella virus may be isolated from a pharyngeal swab, cerebrospinal fluid, blood, urine, bone marrow, liver, cataractous lens, and if "otitis" is present, from the middle ear. Specific rubella IgM antibody or other rubella antibodies, after one year of age, is diagnostic. The rubella hemagglutination inhibition antibody test is the most sensitive and least expensive of the antibody tests. Radiographically there may be transient structural alterations in the metaphyseal portions of the long bones.

Differential Diagnosis The clinical manifestations of severe *fetal cytomegalovirus infection* may closely resemble those of fetal rubella syndrome: jaundice, purpura, pneumonitis, encephalomyelopathy, and deafness. Infants with *toxoplasmosis* exhibit hepatosplenomegaly, jaundice, encephalitis, retinopathy, and mental retardation.

Prenatal Diagnosis It should be assumed that the infant is infected if the mother has the disease during the first or second trimester of pregnancy. Although difficult, the virus is recoverable from the amniotic fluid.

Basic Defect and Other Considerations Infection of the conceptus follows decidual infection during maternal viremia prior to the 16th week of gestation. The viremia occurs about one week prior to the maternal rash. At the cellular level, the virus inhibits mitosis and produces inflammation which eventuates in loss of critical cells during organogenesis and in chronic inflammation of various organs. About 50% are affected if infection occurs during the first month of gestation, compared with 5–10% at 20 weeks. Cataracts occur only if the mother is infected from day 26 to 57 of pregnancy; after that the lens bud is pinched off and thus isolated. Patent ductus arteriosus occurs principally from days 25 to 62; stenosis of the pulmonary artery or pulmonary stenosis from days 30 to 71; and VSD from days 31 to 93. Retinopathy or chorioretinitis and hearing loss occur from days 16–131. Mental retardation is most common from days 26 to 45.

Prognosis and Treatment The best treatment is primary prevention by rubella vaccination of all children. Because of the varied anomalies, the services of a variety of specialists are needed. Surgical correction of the patent ductus arteriosus during infancy is indicated. Removal of bilateral cataracts is usually delayed until approximately one year of age. Congenital glaucoma should be corrected immediately following birth. Hearing aids and/or auditory training should be provided as soon as significant hearing loss is ascertained. Prognosis depends on the time at which the mother was infected. Approximately one-third of those who exhibit purpura die during the first year of life. The overall mortality is approximately 10 to 20% during the first year. For those surviving infancy, most have a normal life span but shed virus for a year or more. During early infancy the most common causes of death are congestive heart failure and infection.

REFERENCES

Hardy, J.B. Clinical and developmental aspects of congenital rubella. *Arch. Otolaryngol. 98:* 230–236, 1973.

Rosenberg, H.S., Oppenheimer, E.H., and Esterly, J.R. Congenital rubella syndrome: the late effects and their relation to early lesions. *Persp. Pediat. Pathol. 9:* 183–202, 1981.

Ueda, K., Nishida, Y., Oshima, K. et al. Congenital rubella syndrome: correlation of gestational age at time of maternal rubella with type of defect. *J. Pediatr. 94:* 763–765, 1979.

Fetal Rubella Syndrome

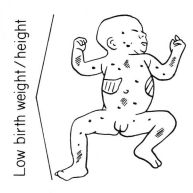

Low birth weight/height

Petechiae, ecchymoses, hepato-splenomegaly, hearing loss and congenital heart disease may be present at birth

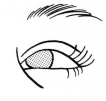

Eye anomalies at birth may include unilateral or bilateral cataracts, glaucoma, microphthalmia, strabismus, nystagmus and iris hypoplasia

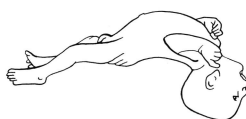

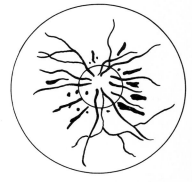

Streaks of black and white (depigmentation) near the disc

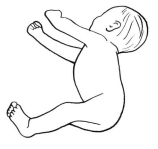

Severe hypotonia or hypertonia may be present

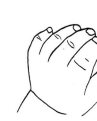

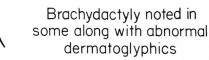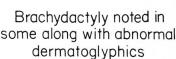

Brachydactyly noted in some along with abnormal dermatoglyphics

Radiolucent areas in long bones– distal femur and proximal tibia

8. FETAL SYPHILIS SYNDROME

Clinical Features The clinical features are similar to those of acquired syphilis. The only lesion never present is the chancre, since the causative agent enters by means of the maternal–fetal circulation. Cutaneous lesions are usually evident at birth. As in the adult, they may be macular, papular, vesiculobullous, eczematous, circinate or annular, or combinations thereof. Occasionally the lesions may be circumoral or circumanal where, due to inflammation, they result in circumferential cracks (rhagades). Palmar or plantar maculopapular lesions are rather common. In the perianal region, flat condylomas may be seen and mucous patches may occur orally. Involvement of the nasal mucosa produces seropurulent and/or hemorrhagic rhinitis (snuffles). Anemia, hepatosplenomegaly, and jaundice are common. Pneumonitis (pneumonia alba) is relatively uncommon except in cases of massive infection. With time, interstitial keratitis and gummatous changes of various organs may be observed. Saddle-nose is such a lesion. Involvement of the teeth produces crenated (mulberry) permanent first molars and so-called Hutchinson incisors, which are narrower at the incisal edge than at the cervix of the tooth. Sensorineural hearing loss and vestibular dysfunction may also occur. In the current penicillin era, the infant may be marasmic with nonspecific signs and symptoms mimicking sepsis, blood group incompatibility, or disease due to TORCH agents.

Specific Diagnosis Radiographic lesions include osteochondritis of long bones. Occasionally the small bones in the hands and feet exhibit this process. Extension of this process may result in diffuse periostitis. When it involves the tibia it produces saber-shin. Clinical diagnosis is most rapidly effected by means of identification of *Treponema pallidum* by dark-field examination of moist skin lesions, mucosal lesions, or mucopurulent nasal discharge. Serologic identification may be difficult in the infant's cord blood or sera due to the presence of nontreponemal maternal antibodies which may be transferred to the fetus. Fetally produced antibodies are contained in the M globulin fraction (as opposed to the G maternal globulin fraction). Infant levels should be at least fourfold those of the maternal serum (FTA-ABS [IgM] test). However, false negative results have been obtained in as high as 35% in delayed onset disease and serial VDRL tests on serum must be done to look for changing titer.

Differential Diagnosis Conditions to be ruled out include a vast array of disorders. For congenital hepatosplenomegaly with or without jaundice one must include all causes of elevated direct or indirect bilirubin, especially the intrauterine infections (*cytomegalic inclusion disease, rubella, herpes simplex infections, coxsackievirus B infections,* etc.), *toxoplasmosis, neonatal hepatitis, disorders of the biliary tract* and a host of *metabolic disorders.*

Prenatal Diagnosis It should be assumed that the infant is infected if the mother has the active disease and the infant is greater than 16 weeks in utero.

Basic Defect and Other Consideration The cause is the spirochete, *Treponema pallidum*, which enters the fetal circulation. While they may enter during the first trimester, severe damage does not occur until after the 16th week of gestation because hosts are not able to respond immunologically with inflammation and tissue reaction earlier in fetal life. Since the organism can invade any tissue, manifestations and protean late manifestations are thought to be due to hypersensitivity which causes swelling of endothelial cells with resultant gummatous necrosis. Although its true incidence is not known, it is believed to occur in fewer than 0.05% of live births.

Prognosis and Treatment Affected children may be aborted or stillborn. Prior to penicillin, mortality in congenital syphilis was about 50%. Now it is less than 2%. While most affected infants exhibit the stigmata immediately, there are others that seem to have deferred manifestation of symptoms. Prognosis depends on treatment of the infected mother and the stage of pregnancy at which the infection occurred. If therapy is initiated prior to the second year of life, prognosis is excellent and permanent sequelae are very uncommon. Prevention and treatment are effective with penicillin as soon as possible following exposure. Both penicillin and erythromycin cross the placenta and thus may be effectively employed for in utero infections. Aqueous penicillin G usually at 50,000 units/kg/day is administered to the newborn child for 10 or more days.

REFERENCES

Fiumara, N.J. Syphilis in newborn children. *Clin. Obstet. Gynecol. 18:* 183–189, 1975.

Kaufman, R.E., Olansky, D.C., and Wiesner, P.J. The FTA:ABS (IgM) test for neonatal congenital syphilis: a critical review. *J. Am. Vener. Dis. Assoc. 1:* 79–84, 1974.

Oppenheimer, E.H. and Dahms, B.B. Congenital syphilis in the fetus and neonate. *Persp. Pediat. Pathol. 6:* 115–138, 1981.

Fetal Syphilis Syndrome

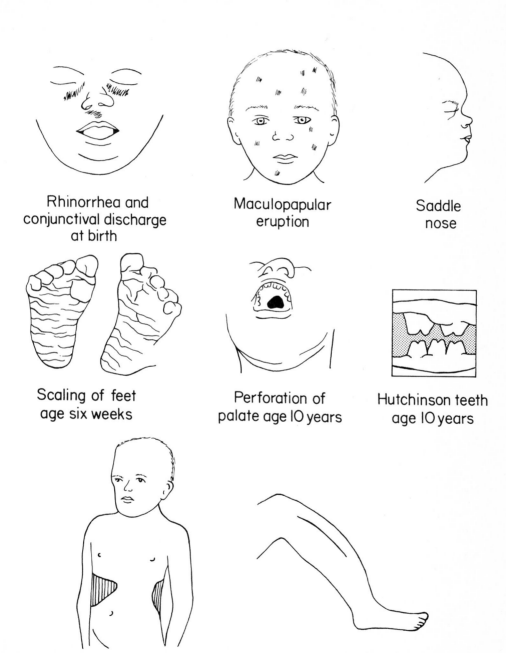

Rhinorrhea and conjunctival discharge at birth

Maculopapular eruption

Saddle nose

Scaling of feet age six weeks

Perforation of palate age 10 years

Hutchinson teeth age 10 years

Syphilitic facies, brachycephaly, frontal bossing, saddle nose, hepatosplenomegaly and saber tibia at age 10 years

9. FETAL TOXOPLASMOSIS SYNDROME

Clinical Features The spectrum of findings is protean, ranging from a stillborn child to a clinically healthy but infected infant. Only 10–20% of infants with serologically proven infection appear clinically ill. Prematurity is common. Among those with severe infection, over 80% exhibit mental retardation and seizures. Opisthotonus may be observed. Other findings include hydrocephaly (sometimes progressive) or microcephaly in about 25%. Impaired sight due to unilateral or bilateral chorioretinitis with microphthalmia occurs in over 75% of the severely affected. The chorioretinitis has a tendency to recur, eventuating in blindness and/or secondary glaucoma but occasionally it may not have its onset until adult life. Microphthalmia, glaucoma, and cystic atrophy are less frequent findings. Psychomotor disturbances are common. Hepatosplenomegaly, jaundice, purpura, a maculopapular skin rash, pneumonitis and carditis may be seen for several weeks following birth. Some children who appear healthy at birth later exhibit seizures, recurrent retinochoroiditis, mental retardation, or hearing loss.

Specific Diagnosis Although high titers for toxoplasma antibodies in the serum of mother and infant are suggestive, they are not diagnostic since they may represent latent acquired toxoplasmosis with the antibodies being transferred to the infant, since about 35% of female adults have positive titers. The uninfected infant with passively transplacentally acquired antibodies will exhibit falling titers approximately by 50% per month. In contrast, in the infected infant, titers rise in serial samples. Elevated IgM globulins and specific toxoplasma IgM antibodies can be demonstrated in the serum of infants 4–8 months of age by means of fluorescent antibody tests. The parasite may also be isolated from spinal or ventricular fluid. Tissue obtained by biopsy or at the time of autopsy may also be employed for isolating the parasite by intraperitoneal inoculation of mice or guinea pigs. Blood platelets may be diminished. The spinal fluid is often yellowish and there is mononuclear pleocytosis and elevated protein. Radiographic studies of the skull show focal cerebral calcifications in about 30%, especially in the periventricular and basal ganglia areas, which enlarge with age.

Differential Diagnosis Hepatosplenomegaly, jaundice, and neonatal petechiae may occur in infants with *fetal rubella, syphilis, herpes virus* and *cytomegalovirus infections* as well as *erythroblastosis fetalis*. Microcephaly, chorioretinitis and microphthalmia and neurologic problems may occur in *rubella* and *cytomegalovirus infections* and intracranial calcifications in *herpes virus* and *cytomegalovirus infections*.

Prenatal Diagnosis Not currently available.

Basic Defect and Other Considerations The etiology is transplacental transmission of the protozoa, *Toxoplasma gondii* to the fetus from a mother initially infected while the child is in utero. Toxoplasmosis acquired prior to the pregnancy is *not* transmitted to the fetus. Proliferation of the organism eventuates in granulomatous inflammation and necrosis of fetal tissues, especially the brain. In the United States, about 6 women per 1000 acquire toxoplasmosis during pregnancy and 1 newborn per 1000 is infected. Congenital toxoplasmosis does not recur in subsequent pregnancies. There is considerable evidence to suggest that the infection occurs in the mother by ingestion of rare meat or exposure to cat feces or soil contaminated by them. After the cat has become infected, it excretes oocytes for one to two weeks after the infectious meal. The oocytes remain infective in soil or water for weeks or months.

Prognosis and Treatment The disorder is lethal within the first month of life in less than 10% of the cases. Another 10% exhibit severe mental retardation. Approximately 25% suffer ocular problems, but perhaps 60% escape with either no or minimal problems. Various agents such as sulphadiazine and pyrimethamine have been utilized, but their efficacy is doubtful.

REFERENCES

Desmonts, G. and Couvreur, J. Congenital toxoplasmosis: a prospective study of 378 pregnancies. *N. Engl. J. Med. 290:* 1110–1116, 1974.

Dische, M.R. and Gooch, W.M. III. Congenital toxoplasmosis. *Persp. Pediat. Pathol. 6:* 83–113, 1981.

Kimball, A.C., Kean, B.H., and Fuchs, F. Congenital toxoplasmosis: a prospective study of 4,048 obstetric patients. *Am. J. Obstet. Gynecol. 111:* 211–218, 1971.

- choreoretinitis
- maculopapular skin rash
- intracranial calcifications
- microphthalmia

Fetal Toxoplasmosis Syndrome

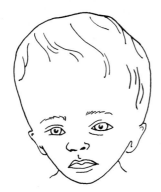

Obstructive
hydrocephalus

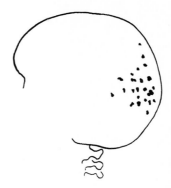

Intracranial
calcifications

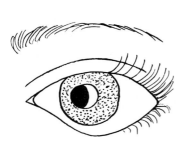

Cataract with
retrolental mass

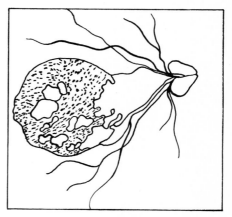

Chorioretinitis at the
macula and involving
the disk

10. FETAL TRIMETHADIONE, PARAMETHADIONE, AND PRIMIDONE SYNDROMES

Clinical Features The clinical features of fetal trimethadione and paramethadione syndromes will be grouped. Although over 50 cases have been reported, only a small fraction of these represent ones in which only one or both of these agents have been used for petit mal seizures. The findings found in at least half the affected children include intrauterine growth retardation, short stature, small head circumference, developmental delay and/or mental retardation, speech impairment, malformed pinnae, and possibly congenital heart disease (VSD>PDA>ASD). In 25 to 50% of the cases, the following have been reported: conductive hearing loss, V-shaped eyebrows, epicanthal folds, depressed broad nasal bridge, small nose with anteverted nostrils, cleft lip and/or cleft palate, hypospadias. Present in 10 to 15% of the cases were palmar simian creases, inguinal or umbilical hernia, and tracheoesophageal fistula, synophrys, and ocular hypertelorism. An extremely limited number of case reports is available concerning primidone embryopathy. Findings have included mild postnatal growth deficiency, microcephaly, jitteriness, hairy forehead, thick nasal root with anteverted nares, ocular hypertelorism, eyelid ptosis, micrognathia, hypoplastic fingernails, and various cardiovascular anomalies such as coarctation of the aorta, tubular hypoplasia of the aortic arch isthmus, ventricular septal defect, pulmonic stenosis, tetralogy of Fallot, pulmonary artery hypertension, and biventricular hypertrophy. Two children we have recently seen had coarctation of the aorta.

Specific Diagnosis Diagnosis is clinical and in large part based on a history of the use of one of the three abovementioned drugs.

Differential Diagnosis *Fetal hydantoin syndrome, fetal alcohol syndrome, Noonan syndrome,* and a number of *fetal infections* must be excluded.

Prenatal Diagnosis We are not aware that this has been done.

Basic Defect and Other Considerations It is difficult knowing the basic defect because the biochemistry is not understood. These particular embryopathies are uncommon for two reasons: petit mal seizures are rather uncommon during childbearing years, and these agents have largely been replaced by more efficacious ones. Nevertheless, over 50 case reports have been published.

Prognosis and Treatment In the case of trimethadione and paramethadione embryopathy, in approximately 25% of the cases, there is a history of spontaneous abortion among women who have been on one of these drugs during their pregnancy and early infant death has been recorded in over one-third of the cases. The embryopathy does not appear to be dosage related. Treatment tends to be supportive but when indicated the congenital heart condition should be corrected.

REFERENCES

Feldman, G.L., Weaver, D.D., and Lovrien, E.W. The fetal trimethadione syndrome. *Am. J. Dis. Child. 131:* 1389–1392, 1977.

Rating, D., Nau, H., Jäger-Roman, E. et al. Teratogenic and pharmacokinetic studies of primidone during pregnancy and in the offspring of epileptic women. *Acta Paediat. Scand. 71:* 301–311, 1982.

Rosen, R.C. and Lightner, E.S. Phenotypic malformations in association with maternal trimethadione therapy. *J. Pediatr. 92:* 240–244, 1978.

- **small head**
- **malformed ears**
- **V-shaped eyebrows**
- **small nose / anteverted nares**

Fetal Trimethadione, Paramethadione, and Primidone Syndromes

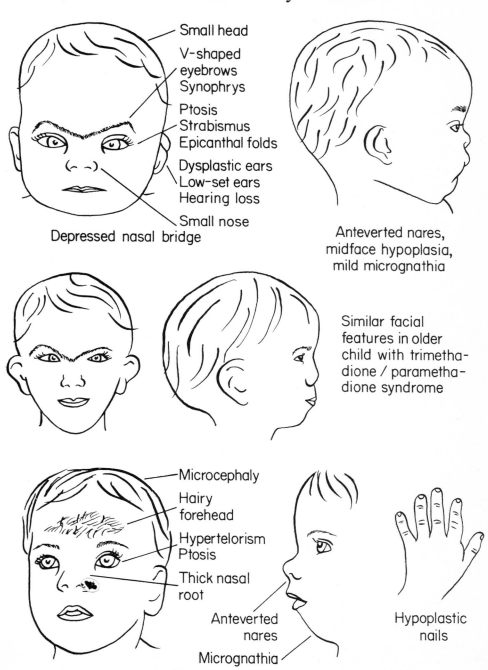

Small head

V-shaped eyebrows Synophrys

Ptosis
Strabismus
Epicanthal folds

Dysplastic ears
Low-set ears
Hearing loss

Small nose

Depressed nasal bridge

Anteverted nares, midface hypoplasia, mild micrognathia

Similar facial features in older child with trimethadione / paramethadione syndrome

Microcephaly

Hairy forehead

Hypertelorism
Ptosis

Thick nasal root

Anteverted nares

Micrognathia

Hypoplastic nails

Child with primidone syndrome

11. PERINATAL HERPES SIMPLEX VIRUS INFECTION

Clinical features Signs of herpes simplex virus (HSV) infection during the first few days of life include cutaneous or conjunctival vesicles, fever, jaundice, seizures, tachypnea, and hydrops. This is followed by poor feeding, cyanosis, and respiratory distress. Approximately 60% of infected infants are premature. Approximately the same number develop meningoencephalitis. Among those who survive, porencephaly, hydranencephaly, and multiple cystic lesions of the brain may be noted. Conjunctivitis is nearly always followed by loss of vision with corneal clouding, cataract formation, iritis, uveitis, and chorioretinitis (20%). Any part of the skin may be involved with vesicles that recede and heal in 7–10 days, but recurrent symptoms may occur for the first two years of life. In the disseminated disease, skin vesicles are absent in 65% of HSV-2 and 50% of HSV-1. HSV infection in utero may possibly be teratogenic (microcephaly, microphthalmia, mental and somatic retardation, abnormal digits, retinal dysplasia, intracranial calcifications) and definitely appears to be associated with an increased spontaneous abortion rate.

Specific Diagnosis Smears from vesicles using Giemsa or Papanicolaou stains often show multinucleated cells or ones with glassy nuclei. HSV can be isolated during life or postmortem. Tissues most often yielding positive culture are liver and brain. At autopsy, liver and adrenal necrosis is a constant feature, inflammatory cell infiltration being practically nonexistent in areas of necrosis. In contrast, inflammation is marked in skin, eye, esophagus, and brain. Inclusions and coagulation necrosis are also marked. Inclusion bodies are not identified in the necrotic areas, but are plentiful in adjacent viable tissues. Inclusions are of two types (a) homogeneous dark pink, occupying most of the nucleoplasm and displacing the nucleus, and (b) small, variable in shape, and occupying the center of the nucleus. Both HSV-1 and HSV-2 are easily cultured and grown in as little as 2–3 days in ordinary viral culture media. On chick chorioallantoic membrane, cultures of pock-lesions of HSV-1 are smaller than those of HSV-2. Ultrastructural study may be carried out.

Differential Diagnosis The cutaneous and mucosal lesions are usually so specific that there is no differential diagnosis. In the acute disseminated form or with herpetic meningoencephalitis without mucocutaneous lesions, one should exclude *aseptic or septic meningitis* and various other neonatal infections (*cytomegalovirus infection, toxoplasmosis,* etc.).

Prenatal Diagnosis Not yet possible.

Basic Defect and Other Considerations The etiologic agent is the herpes simplex virus. HSV-2 is found in 80%, HSV-1 in 20%. Chorioretinitis appears to be associated with HSV-2. In most cases, the infant contracts the disease from the mother's genital tract. However, the endometrium or ovary may be involved without obvious cervical, vaginal, or vulvar lesions. HSV can be recovered from the genitalia in approximately 1% of all gravid women at some time during pregnancy; however, approximately half the women stop shedding virus by the time of delivery. The male having intercourse with the mother late in pregnancy may transmit the organism to the birth canal. Rarely, HSV infection can develop from contact with either parent, nurse, or other person with herpes labialis or herpetic whitlow. The frequency of clinical HSV infection among neonates, 1 per 7500 births, appears to be related to socioeconomic status, with 1 per 3500 in lower income groups to 1 per 30,000 births in higher economic classes. Both sexes are equally affected. Twins appear to be three times as frequently affected. No cases of neonatal HSV infection have been reported in subsequent sibs born to the same mother.

Prognosis and Treatment Neonatal infection with HSV follows a relatively benign course in about 20%. About 50% develop disseminated disease within the first week of life and die after 6–7 days. Of the remainder, about 25–30% exhibit visual, motor, or mental defects regardless of viral strain. Immediate cause of death is respiratory distress and/or failure. Other complications such as cerebral edema, massive intraabdominal hemorrhage, or esophageal stenosis have been noted. There seems to be significant predisposition to sepsis with other organisms, especially cytomegalovirus. Adenine arabinoside and the new agent, acyclovir, appear to offer promising results if started early. If one or both parents are known to be infected with the virus, birth by Caesarean section should be considered.

REFERENCES

Nahmias, A.J. and Roizman, B. Infection with herpes simplex viruses 1 and 2. *N. Engl. J. Med. 289:* 667–674, 719–725, 781–789, 1973.

Singer, D.B. Pathology of neonatal herpes simplex virus infection. *Persp. Pediatr. Pathol. 7:* 243–278, 1981.

Torphy, D.E., Ray, C.G., McAlister, R. et al. Herpes simplex virus infection in infants: a spectrum of disease. *J. Pediatr. 76:* 405–408, 1970.

- **cutaneous vesicles**
- **jaundice**
- **CNS malformations**
- **eye infections**

Perinatal Herpes Simplex Virus Infection

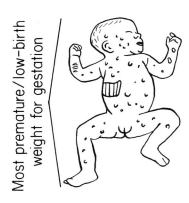

Most premature/low-birth weight for gestation

Vesicles and petechiae, hepatomegaly with jaundice in some

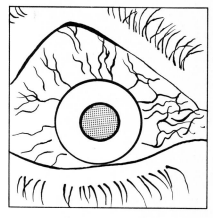

Conjunctivitis and cataract formation

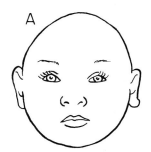

A

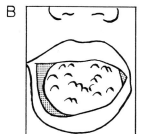

B

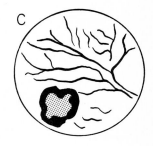

C

A) microcephaly, microphthalmia, B) herpetic stomatitis of tongue, C) area of chorioretinitis

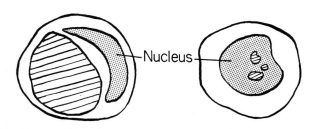

—Nucleus—

Large inclusion body and small ones in center of nucleus

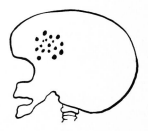

Intracranial calcifications

12. WARFARIN EMBRYOPATHY

Clinical Features Coumarin-related vitamin-K antagonists have been employed for years for treatment of thrombophlebitis and thromboembolic disease. Patients having cardiac valvular prostheses are similarly protected. Warfarin, dicoumarol, and various indan-1,3-diones (diphenadione) are known to cross the placenta and at times produce fetal hemorrhage. However, it was not until approximately 1975 that a well-defined Warfarin syndrome was delineated. Exposure from the sixth to ninth weeks may result in nasal hypoplasia, chondrodysplasia punctata, and possibly retardation, while second- and third-trimester exposure may result in retardation, microcephaly, and/or optic atrophy.

Specific Diagnosis The nose is hypoplastic; the bridge is depressed and the nostrils anteverted. A deep groove between the nasal wing and nasal tip is often present, secondary to cartilage hypoplasia. The nares and air passages are small, resulting in neonatal respiratory distress in half the cases, with true choanal atresia in about 15%. Stippled epiphyses are present in virtually all cases. They may not be evident after the first year. The stipplings primarily involve the axial skeleton at the proximal femora and in the calcanei.

Differential Diagnosis Fetal Warfarin syndrome is easily distinguished from the *recessive rhizomelic and dominant Conradi type of chondrodysplasia punctata* where stippling takes entirely different patterns, but which share nasal hypoplasia as a hallmark. Birth weight is less than the 10th percentile for gestational age in about 40%. While there may be catch-up growth in weight and height, the nose usually remains small. Significant developmental retardation has been found in over 30%. Blindness, optic atrophy, and microphthalmia have been observed in about 15%. Half have variable degrees of hypoplasia of the extremities, being more often mild (shortened fingers and dystrophic nails). Other sequelae are death (about 20%), scoliosis (about 15%), profound hearing loss (10%), congenital heart disease (10%), seizures (5%). The CNS changes have been quite variable: agenesis of the corpus callosum, Dandy-Walker malformation, midline cerebellar atrophy and ventral midline dysplasia, optic atrophy. On follow-up of those with CNS findings, all were mentally retarded and about 25% have seizures. There does not appear to be a critical period of exposure for CNS complications.

Prenatal Diagnosis Fetoscopy may possibly be used to detect nasal hypoplasia in a highly suspected pregnancy.

Basic Defect and Other Considerations The pathogenesis of Warfarin embryopathy is not known. Coumarin derivatives are anticoagulants via inhibition of post-translational carboxylation of coagulative proteins. Vitamin K forms gamma-carboxyglutamyl residues from glutamyl residues, so that many proteins may bind calcium. Such proteins, the so-called osteocalcins, have been found in bone. Inhibition of such proteins during a critical embryologic period of ossification may possibly explain the stigmata of Warfarin embryopathy, that is, nasal hypoplasia and stippled epiphyses. Fetal hemorrhage results from competitive inhibition of vitamin K, effecting decreased synthesis of clotting factors II, VII, IX, and X. Of over 400 cases in which the mothers have taken coumarin derivatives during gestation, only about 4% manifest typical Warfarin embryopathy, but nearly 20% have various fetal complications such as spontaneous abortion, stillbirth, prematurity, CNS abnormalities, and/or fetal hemorrhage.

Prognosis and Treatment As indicated earlier, the chance of having Warfarin embryopathy is on the order of 5%. However, of those having the disorder, the nose remains small and mental retardation has been observed in about 30%. Congenital eye problems occur in about 15% and almost 50% have dystrophic fingernails. Treatment is supportive.

REFERENCES

Hall, J.G., Pauli, R.M., and Wilson, K.M. Maternal and fetal sequelae of anticoagulation during pregnancy. *Am. J. Med. 68:* 122–140, 1980.

Pauli, R.M., Madden, J.D., Kranzler, K.J., et al. Warfarin therapy initiated during pregnancy and phenotypic chondrodysplasia punctata. *J. Pediatr. 88:* 506–508, 1976.

Warkany, J. Warfarin embryopathy. *Teratology 14:* 205–209, 1976.

M.R. [+ / some]

- hypoplastic nose
- anteverted nares
- eye anomalies
- hypoplastic digits

Warfarin Embryopathy

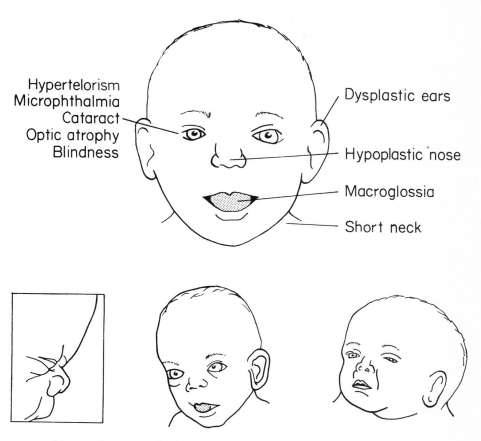

Hypertelorism
Microphthalmia
Cataract
Optic atrophy
Blindness

Dysplastic ears

Hypoplastic nose

Macroglossia

Short neck

Note characteristic hypoplastic nose with deformed
nasal cartilage and anteverted nares

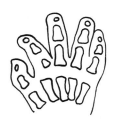

Hypoplasia of terminal phalanges
and proximal phalanx of
index finger

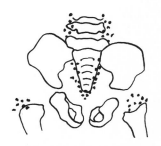

Stippling of epiphyses
lumbosacral area and
trochanters of femurs

B. Developmental Defects

13. ABDOMINAL MUSCLE DEFICIENCY
(prune-belly syndrome)

Clinical Features The abdominal muscular deficiency syndrome consists of a triad of congenital defects including aplasia of the musculature of the lower and medial abdominal wall, anomalies of the urinary tract, and bilateral cryptorchidism. Due to the resultant large thin-walled flaccid abdomen, which is replete with creases, the disorder has been called the "prune-belly" or later in childhood "pot-belly" syndrome. The viscera can easily be palpated and peristalsis is obvious. The weakness of the abdominal musculature is patchy and differs in degree and location from patient to patient. The anomalies of the urinary tract include dilation of the bladder, which may be fixed to the umbilicus, or patent urachus may be noted and the ureter may be grossly dilated (hydroureter). The prostatic urethra is usually enlarged and there are varied and grotesque kidney forms which tend to be hydronephrotic and/or dysplastic. Many patients exhibit obstruction to the bladder outlet. The testes are intraabdominal. Approximately 40% have talipes equinovarus, usually bilateral. Those with the most severe urinary tract anomalies appear to most often have talipes. Hip dysplasia is not uncommon. Thirty percent have intestinal abnormalities (most often malrotation of the bowel) and 30% have cardiac defects but without consistent type.

Specific Diagnosis Diagnosis is based on clinical findings, but microscopic studies of the abdominal wall and ureter show a deficiency of muscle. The prostate shows a reduced number of tubules and the kidneys exhibit a marked degree of renal dysplasia: embryonic tubules, cartilage, cysts, and a reduction in the number of glomeruli. Changes in the testes are those normally associated with cryptorchidism. Intraabdominal calcifications within the gastrointestinal or genitourinary tracts attributed to secondary effects of stasis may be seen in some affected infants. Cinecystourethography may be carried out.

Differential Diagnosis At initial glance, one may consider *congenital ascites*, but findings are so characteristic that the disorder ordinarily is not confused with other disorders. However, children with *uremia due to severe congenital urethral valvular obstruction* may have a distended abdomen with flabby musculature. Lower rectus muscles are present, however, in these children.

Prenatal Diagnosis Elevated α-fetroprotein levels have been found in the maternal serum and in the amniotic fluid in some cases. Sonography may detect the enlarged bladder, oligohydramnios, and ascites. Radiodense material has also been injected into the bladder showing megacystis.

Basic Defect, Genetics, and Other Considerations It is likely that the disorder results from a localized defect in the embryonic mesoderm which gives rise to the abdominal musculature, the renal parenchyma, the urinary tract musculature, and possibly the gubernaculum testis. The frequency of the disorder has been estimated to be about 1 per 50,000 births. It occurs predominantly in males. Multiple cases of the full syndrome in families have rarely been reported and there is no clear genetic pattern. Perhaps no more than 5% of patients are female and in those cases all are mildly affected without severe urinary tract involvements. At least 300 cases have been reported. In cases where identical twins have been observed, there has been a general lack of concordance.

Prognosis and Treatment Prognosis depends on the degree of renal insufficiency and/or complications arising from urine output. About 20% are either stillborn or die within a month, 50% succumbing within two years to uremia and/or urinary infection. However, we have seen the condition in a 54-year-old male with chronic renal failure. Pulmonary infections are frequent due to inability to have a normal forceful cough. The diaphragm is flattened and the lower ribs flared outward. Treatment is essentially supportive, involving abdominal binding which improves bowel function and respiration.

REFERENCES

Ives, E.J. The abdominal muscle deficiency triad syndrome—experience with ten cases. *Birth Defects 10(4):* 127–135, 1974.

Riccardi, V.M. and Grum, C.M. The prune-belly anomaly: heterogeneity and superficial X-linkage mimicry. *J. Med. Genet. 14:* 266–270, 1977.

Williams, D.I. and Burkholder, G.V. The prune belly syndrome. *J. Urol. 98:* 244–251, 1967.

- protuberant abdomen
- flaccid abdominal wall
- absent abdominal muscles
- genitourinary anomalies

Abdominal Muscle Deficiency
[prune-belly syndrome]

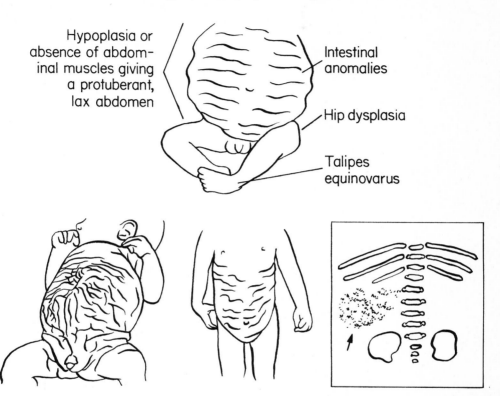

Hypoplasia or absence of abdominal muscles giving a protuberant, lax abdomen

Intestinal anomalies

Hip dysplasia

Talipes equinovarus

Degrees of abdominal muscle hypoplasia- calcifications within the colon (arrow)

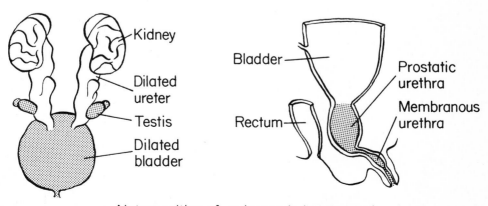

Kidney

Dilated ureter

Testis

Dilated bladder

Bladder

Prostatic urethra

Membranous urethra

Rectum

Note position of undescended testes and dilated prostatic and membranous urethra

14. ANENCEPHALY

Clinical Features The most extreme example of neural tube defect (NTD) is *craniorachischisis* (total dysraphism) in which both the brain and spinal cord are completely open. This anomaly is essentially limited to aborted embryos and fetuses. Anencephaly has been classified into two major types: *holoacrania,* in which the defect extends through the foramen mangum, and *meroacrania,* in which the foramen magnum is not included in the opening. The cranial vault is absent; only the basal portion of the frontal, parietal, and occipital bones are present. The CNS shows varied pathology depending on the extent of the lesion in the neurocranium and the gestational age. The cerebral hemispheres and cerebellum may be rudimentary or absent. The remaining cerebral tissue is distorted and mixed with an angiomatous stroma. The angioneural tissues are covered by a membrane. Due to small orbits, the eyeballs protrude. There are variable alterations in the facial skeleton and the hard palate is usually malformed. Cleft palate and facial duplication may be noted in some cases. A number of anencephalics have spinal retroflexion. Malformations of the limbs, thoracic cage, abdominal wall, gastrointestinal tract, and genitourinary system are relatively frequent in anencephaly. There appears to be an increased incidence of spina bifida occulta, pilonidal cysts, and/or scoliosis in parents of NTD index cases.

Specific Diagnosis Microscopic examination of the cranial tissue shows islands of ependyma, choroid plexus, and connective tissue interspersed with thin-walled vascular channels. Fragments of glial fibers and cells as well as occasional neurons are found. The brainstem, though grossly distorted, is present in about 25% of cases, but the pyramidal tracts are absent. Vascular proliferative changes and colobomas may be present in the retina, the chamber angles are malformed, and commonly there is hypoplasia of the proximal optic nerve. The eyes not uncommonly do not have a central connection. Virtually every bone in the skull is abnormal. The heart, lungs, kidneys, and especially the adrenals are hypoplastic, while the thymus is usually enlarged. The anterior lobe of the pituitary gland is nearly always present and in about 25% of those cases some posterior lobe is also found.

Differential Diagnosis The clinical features are so characteristic that anencephaly cannot be confused with other disorders. Various causes of elevated α-fetoprotein (AFP) are discussed under Prenatal Diagnosis.

Prenatal Diagnosis Maternal hydramnios frequently arouses suspicion. Maternal serum screening for elevated AFP with follow-up amniotic fluid testing around the 15th week of pregnancy and ultrasonography should be diagnostic in about 90% of the cases. However, elevated AFP levels are not specific for neural tube defects; for example, they may also be elevated in fetal death, twins, omphalocele, gastroschisis, intestinal atresia, congenital nephrosis, misdated pregnancies, Meckel syndrome, etc. Acetylcholinesterase should be used as an adjunctive test.

Basic Defect, Genetics, and Other Considerations Craniorachischisis represents an earlier failure of neurulation involving either the neural plate, neural folds, or first fusion of the neural folds, all of which occur between the 17th and 23rd day. Anencephaly, a somewhat later defect, is estimated to occur from the 23rd to the 26th day and results from failure in closure of the anterior neuropore. The question has been raised whether anencephaly and myelomeningocele can be caused by reopening of a closed neural tube due to increased intralumenal pressure. The disorder appears to be multifactorial. Prevalence figures vary with geographic location, racial and ethnic background, sex, and socioeconomic status. Both nutritional factors and hyperthermia have been suggested as etiologic factors. In the United States, the frequency has been estimated to be approximately 1 in 1000 live births. In selected areas of Ireland and Wales, the incidence has been reported as high as 5 to 7 per 1000 live births. NTD is especially low in blacks, Ashkenazi Jews, and Orientals. There appears to be an approximately 5% chance of recurrence of a neural tube defect (anencephaly, myelomeningocele) in subsequent pregnancies. The risk after two affected offspring rises to 20–25%. There is a sexual predilection of 2F:1M.

Prognosis and Treatment The disorder is lethal, the child being either stillborn or extremely shortlived. Vitamin supplements taken during subsequent pregnancies appear to be preventive.

REFERENCES

Crandall, B.F., Lebherz, T.B., and Freihube, R. Neural tube defects: maternal serum and prenatal diagnosis. *Pediatr. Clin. N. Am. 25:* 619–629, 1978.

Milunsky, A. and Alpert, E. Prenatal diagnosis of neural tube defects. *Obstet, Gynecol. 48:* 1–5, 6–12, 1976; *49:* 532–536, 1977; *55:* 60–66, 1980.

Pietrzyk, J.J. Neural tube malformations: complex segregation analysis and recurrence risk. *Am. J. Med. Genet. 7:* 293–300, 1980.

- **absent cranial vault**
- **protruding eyes**
- **facial anomalies**
- **multiple malformations**

Anencephaly

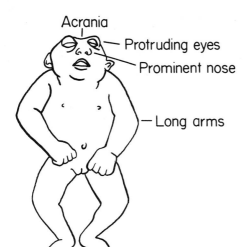

Acrania
— Protruding eyes
— Prominent nose

—Long arms

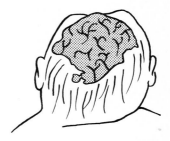

Absence of skull bones with
exposure of part of brain

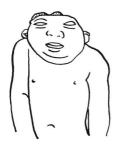 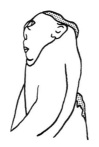 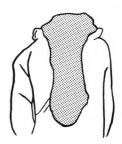

Severe form with extensive cleft in vertebral
column and malformation of spinal cord

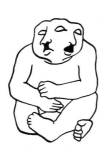 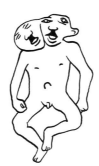 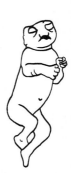

Anencephaly associated with duplication of
facial parts and cleft lip palate

15. ARTHROGRYPOSIS
(congenital contractures)

Clinical Features When evaluating a child with multiple congenital contractures it is important to note the range of motion both active and passive, positioning of limbs, amount of muscle and connective tissue mass, bony structures, neurologic status, and the presence of other congenital anomalies. The more common associated congenital malformations may include the following: midline facial hemangiomas, limited range of motion of the jaw, high-arched palate, cleft palate, submucous palatal cleft, chest wall anomalies, scoliosis, covered meningomyelocele, skin dimples over involved joints, scalp defects, amniotic bands on limbs, dysplastic nails, muscular imbalance, short digits, syndactyly, and pterygia. Other findings that have been described are facial asymmetry, flat nasal bridge, micrognathia, multiple eye anomalies, congenital heart disorders, craniosynostosis, microcephaly, altered dermatoglyphics, various skeletal and visceral anomalies, cryptorchidism, and hypoplasia of the external genitalia in both males and females. In an effort to group the physical findings in a child with multiple congenital contractures three categories have been suggested: (1) conditions in which only the limbs are involved, (2) those in which there appears to be significant CNS dysfunction, and (3) those where several organ systems are affected.

Specific Diagnosis Laboratory studies in most cases are not helpful in making a diagnosis. However, when multiple systems are involved chromosome studies should be done; viral cultures when an infectious agent is suspected; a muscle biopsy if myopathy is considered; and radiographs when bony anomalies are present. The most common and nongenetic type of arthrogryposis is *amyoplasia* characterized by specific positioning in the newborn, talipes equinovarus, extended elbows, flexed wrists, and internally rotated shoulders, hemangioma of the glabella, normal intelligence, and lack of other major congenital malformations. *Distal arthrogryposis* appears to be the most common inherited type of congenital contractures. It is characterized by distal involvement of limbs with overlapping fingers and clenched fist in the newborn, which then open out with use, leaving residual ulnar deviation of fingers in the adult. Foot involvement may be either an equinovarus or a calcaneovalgus deformity. Of interest is an *X-linked recessive type* of arthrogryposis which resolves spontaneously.

Differential Diagnosis Arthrogryposis should be differentiated from conditions which present with pterygium such as the *multiple pterygium* and *popliteal pterygium* syndromes. *Camptodactyly* may be an isolated finding or part of the physical features observed in a number of genetic syndromes. Mothers with *myotonic dystrophy, myasthenia gravis,* and even *multiple sclerosis* have been known to give birth to children with congenital contractures.

Prenatal Diagnosis This has been attempted in a number of cases using real time ultrasound to observe intrauterine movement. However, decreased movement may not be obvious by the 20–24th week of intrauterine development in familial arthrogryposis.

Basic Defect, Genetics, and Other Considerations Although the basic mechanism is not usually known, the major causes of arthrogryposis can be divided into four groups: (1) an intrauterine muscular alteration (dystrophy, aplasia, or myopathy); (2) intrauterine neuropathy (alteration in function, innervation, loss of cells, or CNS malformation); (3) connective tissue abnormality with alteration in development of tendons, bone, cartilage, and joint tissue; and (4) mechanical factors (oligohydramnios, amniotic bands, uterine myomata, twins, etc.).

One infant in 3000 to 4000 live births has multiple congenital contractures. The risk of having a second affected child for parents with one arthrogrypotic baby who dies under one month of age without a specific diagnosis is relatively high: in the range of 10–15%. If no diagnosis can be made, the empiric recurrence risk for another child with multiple congenital contractures is 5%.

Prognosis and Treatment Those with CNS findings may have mental retardation with a shortened life span. Infants with only contractures of the limbs due to the deformational processes have a very good prognosis, while those due to malformational processes do well, but often are left with residual contractures. Early and vigorous physical therapy combined with proper orthopedic and surgical intervention when indicated are the main components of treatment.

REFERENCES

Hall, J.G. An approach to congenital contractures (arthrogryposis). *Pediatr. Ann. 10:* 249–257, 1981.

Hall, J.G., Reed, S.D., and Green, G. The distal arthrogryposes: delineation of new entities — review and nosologic discussion. *Am. J. Med. Genet. 11:* 185–239, 1982.

Hall, J.G., Reed, S.D., Scott, C.W., et al. Three distinct types of X-linked arthrogryposis seen in 6 families. *Clin. Genet. 21:* 81–97, 1982.

- joint contractures
- skin dimples
- muscle / connective tissue alterations
- CNS / other anomalies

Arthrogryposis
[congenital contractures]

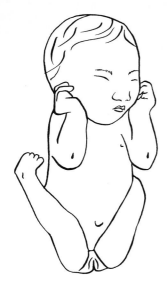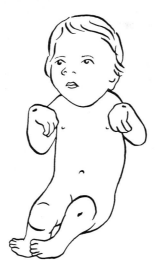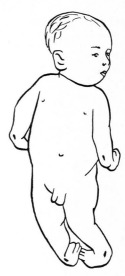

Symmetrical contractures of the limbs, skin dimples, micrognathia, flat facies and popliteal pterygia middle infant

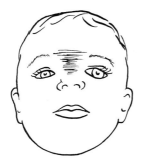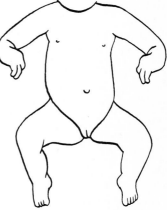

Amyoplasia with round face, midline hemangioma, short nose, decrease in muscle mass, straight elbows, flexion of wrists and knees

Autosomal dominant distal form—contractures and ulnar deviation of fingers and talipes equinovarus

16. CLOVERLEAF SKULL

Clinical Features Cloverleaf skull is a sign rather than a specific disorder. It may be an isolated anomaly or may occur in association with bony ankylosis of the limbs, thanatophoric dysplasia, or a variety of craniosynostotic disorders such as Crouzon syndrome, Apert syndrome, Carpenter syndrome, and Pfeiffer syndrome. Rarely, it may be iatrogenic. While cloverleaf skull is classically, as the name implies, one exhibiting trilobular configuration, it varies from relatively mild to severe and in some cases may be asymmetric. In severe examples, the ears are displaced downward, facing the shoulders. Maxillary hypoplasia and relative mandibular prognathism are frequently encountered. The nasal bridge is depressed and the nose may be beak-like. Severe proptosis, ocular hypertelorism, and antimongoloid obliquity are commonly observed. The eyelids may fail to close, leading to corneal ulceration and clouding. Hydrocephalus and psychomotor and mental retardation have been noted. Natal teeth have been observed in several cases as well as oblique facial clefts. Various other findings have been reported, many of which may be adventitious. These have included: iris coloboma, obstructed nasolacrimal duct, absent external auditory canals, patent ductus arteriosus, atrial septal defect, bicuspid aortic valve, and omphalocele.

Specific Diagnosis Diagnosis depends on whether the finding is isolated or whether it is associated with a known disorder as indicated above. Considering only the skull, roentgenographically there is trilobular contour with marked convolutional impressions and a thin distorted vault producing a honeycombed appearance. Synostosis of the coronal, lambdoidal, and metopic sutures may occur with bulging of the cerebrum through an open sagittal suture and, in some cases, through open squamosal sutures. The squamosal and sagittal sutures may be closed in some cases. Synostosis and shortening of the cranial base is often seen. The posterior cranial fossa is small. The maxillary sphenoid and ethmoid bones are often underdeveloped and malformed and the orbits shallow. In a number of cases, there are bony ankyloses of elbows, subluxation of radial heads, subluxation of hips, thoracic and/or cervical spina bifida, split xiphoid, fixed flexed fingers, and webbed third and fourth toes. For diagnostic aspects of the associated syndromes, see below.

Differential Diagnosis The anomaly is so characteristic that discussion of differential diagnosis is really limited to patterns of defects that may occur with cloverleaf skull.

Prenatal Diagnosis Theoretically, if moderate to severe in degree, it should be possible by ultrasonography or fetoscopy.

Basic Defect, Genetics, and Other Considerations Over 100 cases have been reported. There is no sex predilection. Nearly all have been sporadic. Familial cases would be those associated with other syndromes. It is interesting that thanatophoric dysplasia, normally nongenetic, when associated with cloverleaf skull, appears to have autosomal recessive inheritance.

Prognosis and Treatment Prognosis for life span depends on the associated condition (thanatophoric dysplasia is congenitally lethal, etc.). In some cases, life is threatened by increased intracranial pressure due to hydrocephalus. The group with skeletal changes other than thanatophoric dysplasia usually live for several months, while those with the various craniosynostotic syndromes appear to have much earlier death than expected for the conditions, in many cases succumbing in months or in a few years. Occasionally, mild cloverleaf skull is self-resolving.

REFERENCES

Eaton, A.P., Sommer, A., and Sayers, M.P. The Kleeblattschädel anomaly. *Birth Defects 11(2):* 238–246, 1975.

Iannaccone, G. and Gerlini, G. The so-called "cloverleaf skull syndrome." *Pediatr. Radiol. 2:* 175–183, 1974.

Partington, M.W., Gonzales-Crussi, F., Khakee, S.F. et al. Cloverleaf skull and thanatophoric dwarfism. Report of four cases, two in the same sibship. *Arch. Dis. Child. 46:* 656–664, 1971.

- **trilobular skull**
- **beak-like nose**
- **low set ears**
- **eye anomalies**

Cloverleaf Skull

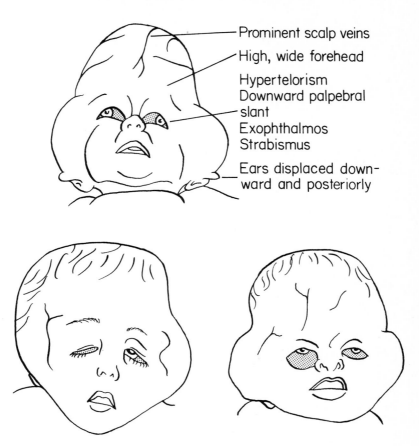

Prominent scalp veins

High, wide forehead

Hypertelorism
Downward palpebral slant
Exophthalmos
Strabismus

Ears displaced downward and posteriorly

Varying degrees of skull deformity with facial alterations—note subluxation of eyeballs

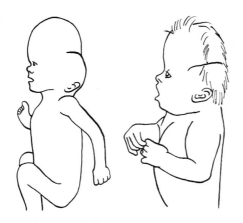

Lateral view—commonly ankylosis of elbows

17. CRANIOSYNOSTOSIS

Clinical Features The shape of the skull may be significantly deformed by premature fusion of sutures. If the sagittal suture fuses prematurely, the skull is long (*dolichocephalic* or *scaphocephalic*). When the coronal suture is bilaterally involved, the skull is short (*brachycephalic*). If a unilateral coronal suture or lambdoidal suture fuses prematurely, this may eventuate in skewed cranium (*plagiocephaly*). If the metopic suture closes too early, the skull has an anterior triangular form (*trigonocephaly*). Premature fusion of all sutures results in high or pointed skull (*oxycephalic* or *turricephalic*). Sagittal synostosis is most common, representing about 55–60%, while coronal synostosis is less frequent (20–30%). Metopic and lambdoidal synostosis or other sutural combinations are infrequent. Mental retardation is noted in about 25% of those with bilateral coronal synostosis, but in less than 10% with sagittal synostosis. Associated anomalies are much more common with coronal synostosis than with sagittal synostosis; however congenital heart defects (5%) are observed with about equal frequency in both types. In some families, some members may have bilateral coronal synostosis while others have unilateral coronal synostosis. Cohen listed 57 craniosynostosis syndromes as well as 22 conditions with secondary or occasional craniosynostosis.

Specific Diagnosis There is lack of movement of the calvarial bones in infancy and palpable ridging. In addition to skull radiographs, one may wish to establish a cephalic index (maximum head width/maximum head length × 100 = mean 70–80) to observe any change in the index.

Differential Diagnosis One must exclude *cranial molding*. This usually improves with time, while craniosynostosis becomes progressively marked. As noted above, it is mandatory to exclude the plethora of *craniosynostotic syndromes* by the presence of other physical findings. In addition there are a number of other disorders such as *rickets of various types, spherocytosis,* and *hypophosphatasia* which can produce a deformed skull.

Prenatal Diagnosis The disorder has been diagnosed late in pregnancy by means of radiography in which fused sutures were detected. Ultrasonography may show an unusually shaped head, the biparietal diameter being severely reduced in sagittal synostosis.

Basic Defect, Genetics, and Other Considerations Most cases of isolated craniosynostosis have an unknown basic defect. The incidence is probably between 0.4 and 1 per 1000 live births. Males are more often affected with sagittal synostosis, while females more frequently have coronal synostosis. While most cases of isolated craniosynostosis are sporadic with multifactorial inheritance, it may be due to a single gene. Both autosomal dominant and autosomal recessive inheritance have been reported, the former being more common with penetrance being complete or very high. It has been estimated that 8% of cases of coronal synostosis and 2% of sagittal synostosis are familial. In the case of isolated sagittal synostosis, the risk of recurrence is about 1–2%. If a parent and child have craniosynostosis or if two sibs are affected with the parents being normal, the risk may approach Mendelian expectations.

Prognosis and Treatment There may be social problems arising from having an unusual head shape, but there is little evidence that there are associated problems due to increased intracranial pressure as was once believed. Early neurosurgical intervention is indicated for removal of the involved suture or sutures. Some neurosurgeons use a plastic sheeting to prevent reunion.

REFERENCES

Barrett, J., Brooksbank, M., and Simpson, D. Scaphocephaly: aesthetic and psycho-social considerations. *Develop. Med. Child. Neurol. 23:* 183–191, 1981.

Cohen, M.M., Jr. Craniosynostosis and syndromes with craniosynostosis: incidence, genetics, penetrance, variability, and new syndrome updating. *Birth Defects 15 (5B):* 13–63, 1979.

Hunter, A.G.W. and Rudd, N.L. Craniosynostosis. *Teratology 14:* 185–193, 1976; *15:* 301–310, 1977.

- abnormal shape skull
- ridging of skull
- premature fusion of sutures
- other anomalies

Craniosynostosis

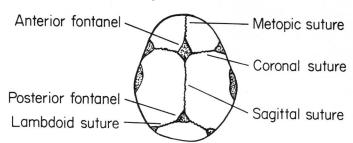

Anterior fontanel — Metopic suture

Coronal suture

Posterior fontanel
Lambdoid suture

Sagittal suture

NORMOCEPHALY

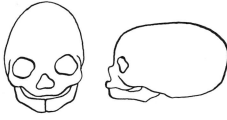

BRACHYCEPHALY

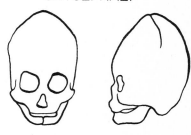

Premature closure (p.c.)
of coronal sutures

DOLICHOCEPHALY

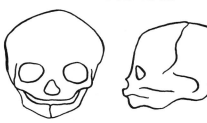

p.c. of sagittal suture

OXYCEPHALY

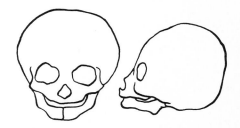

p.c. of all sutures

PLAGIOCEPHALY

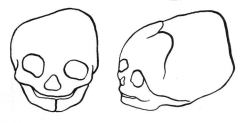

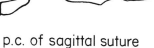

p.c. of one coronal or
lambdoidal suture

TRIGONOCEPHALY

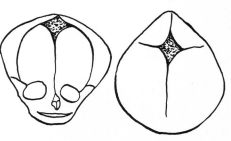

p.c. of metopic suture

18. CYSTIC HYGROMA

Clinical Features Cystic hygroma (lymphangioma) is present at birth in about 55% of cases, with the remainder nearly always becoming apparent by the second year of life. Some grow rapidly, especially following hemorrhage into the cystic spaces (about 15%), or in the case of secondary infection (about 15%), while others enlarge slowly. Pain occurs only in the presence of infection. At least 50% of the cases affect the lateral (3L:2R) cervical region. Perhaps 10% are bilateral. In the cervical area, it occurs most frequently in the posterior triangle of the neck, occupying the supraclavicular fossa. Less commonly it is in the anterior upper portion of the neck in the submandibular and submental triangles. The skin overlying the mass may be thinned by the underlying tumor. If sufficiently superficial, it has a bluish hue. Larger lesions possess ill-defined borders and characteristically are multilobulated, irregular, and compressible. Extension, especially in congenital examples, may involve the axilla, mediastinum, or oral cavity (tongue, oral floor, buccal mucosa, oropharynx). Difficulty with respiration, stridor, and cyanotic attacks occur in about 20% of cases. Dysphagia is found in less than 10%. The mass is fluctuant, varying in size from 2.5 to 15 cm. Similar examples occur in the groin and retroperitoneal regions.

Specific Diagnosis The gross specimen is composed of intact and collapsed cysts of various sizes (cavernous, capillary). The cysts are lined by a single layer of flat endothelial cells. The cyst content is clear or cloudy yellow fluid which contains cholesterol crystals. Supporting stroma consists of varying amounts of collagenous connective tissue, nodules of lymphoid tissue, occasional vestiges of striated muscle, iron pigment, and fetal fat. The lymphangioma may be seen to dissect the muscle bundles and surround nerves and blood vessels. Large loculations have been demonstrated by aspiration and injection of opaque material. Radiographic studies of extensive lesions may exhibit lateral displacement of the trachea and encroachment upon the airway or extension manifested by widening of the upper part of the mediastinum.

Differential Diagnosis This disorder should be differentiated from *branchial cleft cyst, dermoid cyst, tuberculous adenitis, malignant neoplasm with cystic degeneration,* and *lipoma.*

Prenatal Diagnosis With recently refined ultrasonography, prenatal diagnosis may be possible. Extreme examples have been associated with elevated α-fetoprotein levels.

Basic Defect, Genetics, and Other Considerations The most common sites of occurrence correspond to the anatomic locations of the primitive lymph sacs. There are two theories regarding origin: one suggests that the tumors arise from sequestrations of the primitive embryonic lymph sacs. Subsequent irregular growth and canalization leads to cyst formation. The enlargement of the cysts results in the accumulation of lymph. The other theory postulates that cystic hygroma arises from lymphatic endothelium which sends out buds that later canalize and form cysts. Various theories are discussed by Ward and co-workers. The most common location for cystic hygroma is in the neck where the primitive jugular lymphatic sac is located. Since these are the larger of the group, the greater incidence of cervical lesions is understandable. Cystic hygroma is not considered to have a genetic etiology.

Prognosis and Treatment Respiratory obstruction is a common problem due to displacement of the trachea or enlarged tongue size, but mortality does not exceed 3%. A tracheostomy may be necessary. Those with a cavernous pattern are more difficult to remove and hence recur more frequently. Secondary infection occurs in about 15%; this commonly led to septicemia and death in the preantibiotic era. While numerous therapeutic modalities have been employed (aspiration, incision and drainage, sclerosing agents, and radiotherapy), only surgical extirpation has been of value. Extensive initial excision of as much involved tissue as possible with protection of nerves, vessels, etc. is required. Any cyst not surgically removed should be unroofed. Repeated partial excisions may be required through childhood. Spontaneous regression occurs in about 2%.

REFERENCES

Broomhead, I.W. Cystic hygroma of the neck. *Br. J. Plast. Surg. 17:* 225–244, 1964.

Ninh, T.N. and Ninh, T.X. Cystic hygroma in children: a report of 126 cases. *J. Pediatr. Surg. 9:* 191–196, 1974.

Ward, P.H., Perry, P.F., and Downey, W. Surgical approach to cystic hygroma of the neck. *Arch. Otolaryngol. 91:* 508–514, 1970.

Cystic Hygroma

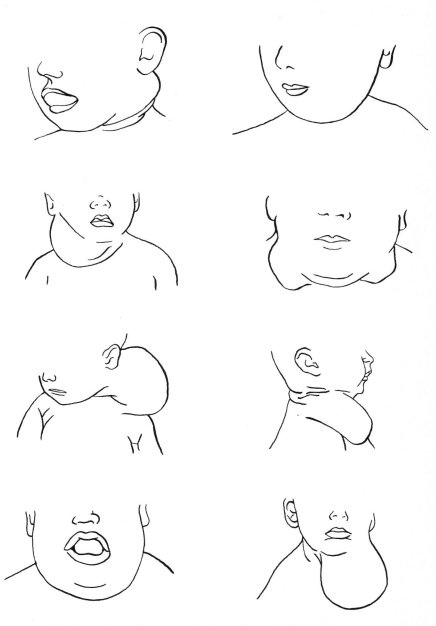

Various locations and size of cystic hygroma,
bottom ones show extension into floor of mouth
and enlargement due to hemorrhage into hygroma

19. DiGEORGE MALFORMATION COMPLEX

Clinical Features The disorder is nonspecific, occurring in several forms and syndromes. Signs and symptoms depend on the degree of suppression of development of the thymus and parathyroid glands and cardiovascular abnormalities. Within the first few days of life, most affected infants present with cyanosis, cardiac murmur, tachycardia, or tachypnea. After the first week, about half these patients exhibit tetanic signs and seizures. Among those that survive past the first month, there is increased susceptibility to infection, purulent rhinorrhea, abscesses, maculopapular rashes, and recurrent pneumonitis due to various acid-fast, viral, and *Pneumocystis carinii* infections. There is also a tendency to develop oral candidosis. About 60% have a characteristic facies (perhaps this combination should be called DiGeorge Syndrome). There is a lateral displacement of inner canthi, short downward-slanting palpebral fissures, anteverted nostrils, short philtrum, various pinnal deformities, cupid-bow mouth, and micrognathia. The pinnae may be small, posteriorly rotated, and malformed with atretic auditory canals. Nearly all have congenital cardiovascular anomalies (interrupted or double aortic arch 35%, aberrant right subclavian artery 35%, and membranous VSD 50%). There is no correlation beteen the degree of thymus and parathyroid hypoplasia and the type of congenital cardiac defect. Less common features include hydronephrosis and urinary tract infections with or without nephrocalcinosis, cleft lip or palate, esophageal atresia, diaphragmatic abnormalities, malformed stapes, and mild psychomotor retardation.

Specific Diagnosis Both radiographically and on autopsy, about half exhibit agenesis of the thymus, the other half hypoplasia. Cell-mediated immunity is decreased, manifested by absent or delayed homograft rejection, decreased T-cells, failure to induce delayed hypersensitivity to dinitrochlorobenzene, impaired proliferative response to mitogens such as diminished or absent response of cultured lymphocytes to PHA, allogenic cells, or antilymphocyte serum. Microscopic examination of lymph nodes shows decreased cells in deep cortical areas, but well developed germinal centers. Some patients exhibit lymphopenia. Parathyroid glands may be absent, but less often 1, 2, 3, or even all are present. Serum calcium is often decreased and serum phosphate increased. If serum calcium is low, signs of tetany can usually be elicited (Trousseau and Chvostek signs). Immunoglobulin levels and antibody responses are normal.

Differential Diagnosis The DiGeorge malformation complex may be seen in associations described below and in the *CHARGE* (congenital *C*oloboma of iris and/or choroid and optic nerve, *H*eart anomalies, *A*tresia of choanae, mental and somatic *R*etardation, *G*enital hypoplasia in males, *E*ar anomalies and/or deafness) complex.

Basic Defect, Genetics, and Other Considerations There is variable failure of development of structures derived from the third and fourth pharyngeal pouches. From pouch III the thymus and inferior parathyroid glands develop. From IV, the superior parathyroid glands are derived. Absence of the left and right fourth branchial arches accounts for interrupted aortic arch and aberrant right subclavian artery, respectively. It is likely that the primary effect is vascular. The complex may occur in association with holoprosencephaly and occasionally arhinencephaly. It has also occurred in maternal half-sibs of opposite sex and in siblings. Most cases, however, are isolated. Its precise frequency is not known, but it has been found in about 3% of children dying of congenital heart disease.

Prognosis and Treatment There is failure to thrive and death within a month in most cases. The severe cardiac anomalies are responsible for death within the first week, infection for those that survive for several months. Neonatal seizures associated with the hypocalcemic tetany are responsible for neurologic impairment. Therapy consists of isolation, fetal thymic transplants in those cases with complete agenesis of the thymus, as well as calcium, parathormone, and vitamin D supplements. In those cases where there is some thymus, transplant rejection is common.

REFERENCES

Carey, J.C. Spectrum of the DiGeorge "syndrome." *J. Pediatr. 96:* 955–956, 1980.

Conley, M.E., Beckwith, J.B., Mancer, J.F.K. et al. The spectrum of the DiGeorge syndrome. *J. Pediatr. 94:* 883–890, 1979.

Robinson, H.B., Jr. DiGeorge's or the III–IV pharyngeal pouch syndrome: pathology and a theory of pathogenesis. *Persp. Pediatr. Pathol. 2:* 173–206, 1975.

- **increased infections**
- **congenital heart disease**
- **tetanic signs**
- **altered facies**

DiGeorge Malformation Complex

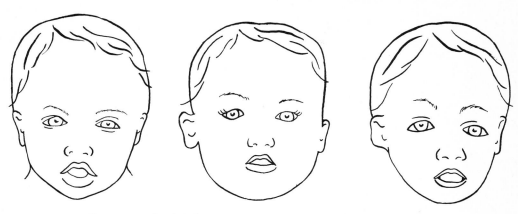

Common facial features include lateral displacement of inner canthi, short downward slanting palpebral fissures, anteverted nares, short philtrum, cupid-bow mouth, small dysplastic ears and micrognathia

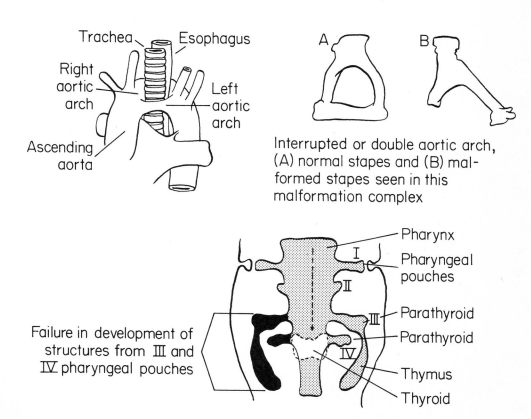

Trachea Esophagus

Right aortic arch

Left aortic arch

Ascending aorta

A B

Interrupted or double aortic arch, (A) normal stapes and (B) malformed stapes seen in this malformation complex

Pharynx

Pharyngeal pouches

I

II

III Parathyroid

Parathyroid

IV

Thymus

Thyroid

Failure in development of structures from III and IV pharyngeal pouches

20. ENCEPHALOCELE

Clinical Features When brain tissue is herniated through a defect in the cranium, the term *encephalocele* is employed. When prolapse involves only the meninges, the term *meningocele* is used. Encephaloceles are ordinarily classified into site: occipital (75%), parietal (10%), or anterior (15%), with the anterior ones further being divided into those that are visible (sincipital) and those that are not (basal). Because encephalocele is a symptom, one must consider the characteristics of specific syndromes in which encephalocele may be a component. The cerebral and skull defects are extremely variable. With *occipital encephalocele,* the foramen magnum and posterior arch of the atlas may be included. If the encephalocele is large, one often finds associated microcephaly. If herniation of the cerebral hemisphere occurs, the encephalocele is often asymmetric. Occipital encephalocele may be seen in association with iniencephaly apertus (enlarged foramen magnum, retroflexion of head onto spine, spina bifida of several vertebrae, natal death). Apart from its unusual appearance, an occipital meningocele may be asymptomatic. However, if the ventricular system is involved, hydrocephalus may occur. Some exhibit involvement of various cranial nerves, seizures, muscle weakness, etc. *Anterior encephalocele* is characterized by swelling at the base of the nose which may progress in size and may be solid or cystic or both. There may be microcranium and/or hydrocephaly associated, and very frequently ocular hypertelorism. There may be problems with vision, breathing, and feeding. With frontoethmoidal encephalocele it has been estimated that approximately 25% are mentally retarded. Cleft palate may be associated with intranasal encephalocele. Pulsating exophthalmos is also suggestive of anterior encephalocele.

Specific Diagnosis Transillumination and CT scan are employed to determine the nature of the contents of the sac and associated brain anomalies. Isotope cisternography, ventriculography, and rarely angiography may also be employed.

Differential Diagnosis One must exclude *herniation of the brain through the anterior fontanel, enlarged metopic suture,* and *congenital subgaleal (dermoid) cyst* with frontoethmoidal encephalocele. For its presence in specific syndromes see below.

Prenatal Diagnosis Alpha-fetoprotein is commonly elevated. Ultrasonography may also be employed in diagnosis.

Basic Defect, Genetics, and Other Considerations Pathogenesis is not understood. The frequency of encephalocele has ranged in various surveys from 1 per 2000 to 1 per 5000 live births, making it less common than myelomeningocele. The anterior variety may be more common in Africa, Thailand, and India. Anterior basal encephalocele is extremely rare, possibly 1 per 35,000 live births. There is a definite female predilection for occipital encephalocele, but not for the anterior form. Although most encephaloceles are sporadic, occipital examples may be associated with several single gene disorders such as *Meckel syndrome, dyssegmental dwarfism, Knobloch syndrome* (severe myopia, retinal detachment), *Warburg syndrome* (lissencephaly, cataracts, hydrocephaly, retinal abnormalities), *cryptophthalmos* and *von Voss syndrome* (agenesis corpus callosum, hypoplastic olives and pyramids of medulla, phocomelia, and thrombocytopenia). Anterior encephalocele may occur with *frontonasal dysplasia.* Numerous small encephaloceles occur in conjunction with *amniotic band disruption syndrome.*

Prognosis and Treatment For all encephaloceles, disability and mortality depend on size and contents of the sac. With occipital meningocele, mortality is approximately 30% if hydrocephaly is present, and about 2% if it is not. For encephaloceles in general, if hydrocephaly is present, mortality rises to about 60%. However, with massive occipital encephalocele with microcephaly, mortality is essentially 100%. Among those who survive, about half appear to have normal intelligence while the other half have both mental and physical disability (paralysis, blindness, hydrocephaly, seizures, growth retardation, ataxia). If cranial venous sinuses are opened, hemorrhage or air embolism may result. Removal of CSF from a lateral ventricle may aid in decompression of the sac. Most patients with parietal encephaloceles have associated brain malformation, and about 40% are mentally retarded to varying degrees.

REFERENCES

Cohen, M.M., Jr. and Lemire, R.J. Syndromes with cephaloceles. *Teratology 25:* 161–172, 1982.

Harverson, G., Bailey, I.C., and Kiryabwire, J.W.M. The radiological diagnosis of anterior encephaloceles. *Clin. Radiol. 25:* 317–322, 1974.

McLaurin, R.L. Parietal cephaloceles. *Neurology (Minneap.) 14:* 764–772, 1964.

• **herniation of brain through skull**

Encephalocele

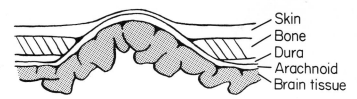

Encephalocele–herniation of brain
tissue through a defect in the cranium

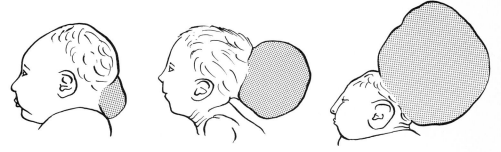

Degrees of occipital encephaloceles

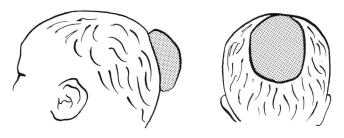

Posterior parietal encephalocele

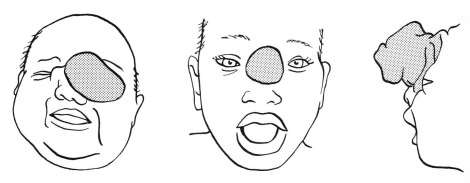

Degrees of anterior encephaloceles

21. EPIDERMAL NEVUS SYNDROME

Clinical Features The disorder has been reported under several names: organoid nevus phakomatosis, linear sebaceous nevus syndrome, encephalocraniocutaneous lipomatosis, etc. It consists of linear epidermal verrucous nevus, seizures, and moderate to severe mental retardation. Commonly there are extensive unilateral, rarely bilateral orange-tan verrucous lesions in whites and black in blacks which extend from the crown of the scalp to the nose or lip. In most cases, the nevus occurs on the head with a special predilection for the sutural areas of the scalp, around the ear, temple, and forehead, stopping at the midline. The involved scalp area is usually bald. A lipodermoid of the entire lateral bulbar subconjunctiva, ptosis of the eyelid, colobomas of the choroid, iris or upper eyelid; and nystagmus have been observed. Occasionally, corneal opacity or vascularization of the cornea or unilateral oculomotor palsy has been reported. Nearly all have mental retardation. Frequent focal (ipsilateral), myoclonic, or generalized seizures appear during the first few years of life; occasionally there is hemiplegia. The ventricles often are enlarged with cortical atrophy. Porencephaly and communicating hydrocephalus have been described as well as cerebral angiomas or vascular malformations. Several have exhibited asymmetry of the skull, calvarial defects, and premature closure of the sphenofrontal suture. By extension, the nevus may involve the upper lip and hard palate. The deciduous and permanent teeth in the involved area are frequently hypoplastic, resembling teeth having odontodysplasia. There may be an associated increase in neoplasia, especially Wilms tumor.

Specific Diagnosis Diagnosis is largely clinical. Microscopically, the lesions constitute a form of epithelial dysplasia, a component of which may occasionally be sebaceous glands. The latter impart a yellowish-brown appearance and a greasy consistency to the verrucous plaque. The dermoid of eye consists of a mixture of lacrimal gland, vascular, nervous and adipose tissue, smooth muscle, cartilage, and even bone. A host of variable primary bone defects have been reviewed by Solomon and Esterly. Patients have had lytic defects of the ribs, clavicles or humerus or tibia, while others have exhibited generalized osteomalacia with a rachitic appearance and a renal tubular defect with nonspecific aminoaciduria.

Differential Diagnosis In large series of patients with *isolated sebaceous nevus,* there have been neither mental deficiency nor convulsions. *Isolated nevus unius lateris, neurofibromatosis, Sturge-Weber syndrome, tuberous sclerosis, cerebriform cranial nevus* and *bathing-trunk nevus,* and *lichen striatus* should all be considered.

Prenatal Diagnosis Theoretically, fetoscopy with a skin biopsy, if possible, may be helpful in making a diagnosis when skin lesions are severe. Brain malformations could be detected using ultrasound but such findings would not be diagnostic.

Basic Defect, Genetics, and Other Considerations The basic defect is not known, although clinical findings suggest early embryonic alterations involving cell differentiation, division, and migration. All cases have been sporadic with no special sexual or racial predilection.

Prognosis and Treatment Prognosis is poor. Several children have died soon after birth from secondary infection or during seizures. There is failure to thrive, poor growth and development, mental retardation, and severe seizure activity in those that survive. Therapy consists of anticonvulsant medication and possibly surgical removal of the lesions for cosmetic reasons if deemed feasible.

REFERENCES

Chalhub, E.G., Volpe, J.J., and Gado, M.H. Linear sebaceous nevus syndrome associated with porencephaly and nonfunctioning major cerebral venous sinuses. *Neurology 25:* 857–860, 1975.

Solomon, L.M. and Esterly, N.B.: Epidermal and other congenital organoid nevi. *Curr. Prob. Pediatr. 6:* 3–45, 1975.

Wilkes, S.R., Campbell, R.J., and Waller, R.R. Ocular malformation in association with ipsilateral facial nevus of Jadassohn. *Am. J. Ophthalmol. 92:* 344–352, 1981.

- linear verrucous nevus about scalp and face
- eye anomalies
- CNS malformations with seizures

Epidermal Nevus Syndrome

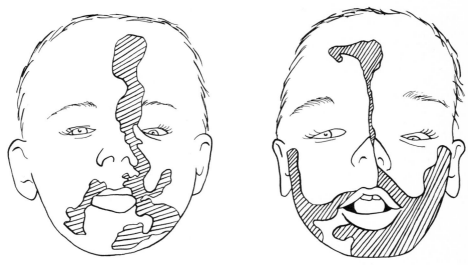

Linear nevus extending from forehead to chin,
note downward slant of palpebral fissures

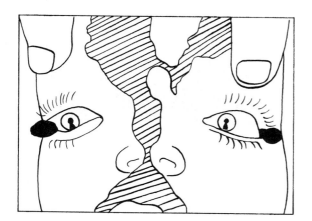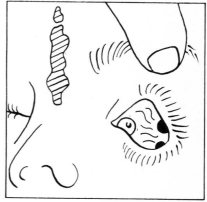

Eye findings include dermoid or lipodermoid
tumors of the conjunctiva, ptosis, strabismus,
nystagmus, microphthalmia, colobomas and
vascularization of the cornea

22. FACIAL CLEFTS, USUAL AND UNUSUAL

Clinical Features *Cleft lip with or without cleft palate* CL(P) and *isolated cleft palate* (CP) are not rare anomalies. Isolated CL may be unilateral or bilateral (ca. 20%) and when unilateral the cleft is more commonly on the left side (ca. 70%). CL(P) is more common in males (about 2:1). About 85% of cases of bilateral CL and 70% of unilateral CL are associated with CP. CL is not always complete (extending into the nostril). In about 10%, the cleft is associated with skin bridges. Isolated CP is a different disorder from CL(P). A 2:1 F/M ratio is seen in complete cleft of hard and soft palate. The ratio changes to about 1:1 for clefts of the soft palate only. Cleft uvula appears to be an incomplete form of CP. *Submucous CP* refers to imperfect muscular union across the velum, but an intact mucosal surface. There is the deficiency or notch in the bone in the posterior edge of the hard palate and often there is cleft uvula. *Lateral facial cleft* is a relatively unusual type. It runs from the corner of the mouth toward the tragus of the ear, although its course is variable. *Oblique facial cleft* is extremely rare. It is bilateral in about 25%. There have been attempts to define two types: (a) naso-ocular cleft, extending from nostril to lower eyelid border with possible extension to temporal region (along line of closure of nasolacrimal groove), and (b) oro-ocular cleft—extending from eye to lip. This last may be further subdivided into medial orocanthal type and lateral orocanthal type. *Median cleft of mandible* is extremely rare.

Specific Diagnosis In most cases this is quite evident. However in some cases of submucous palatal cleft a light source introduced into the nasal cavity may demonstrate the cleft more clearly.

Differential Diagnosis One must be extremely careful to exclude the more than 200 facial cleft syndromes, since genetic counseling may be vastly different.

Prenatal Diagnosis This has been accomplished by ultrasound techniques and in some instances by fetoscopy.

Basic Defect, Genetics, and Other Considerations The basic defect in CL is failure of closure of the primary palate, i.e. fusion between the median nasal process and maxillary process does not occur. CP is due to failure of closure of the secondary palate, i.e. the two palatine processes in the midline do not fuse. The soft palate and uvula do not form by fusion but by posterior extension from bilateral sites. Lateral facial cleft probably results from incomplete invasion of ectomesenchyme between the maxillary and mandibular parts of the first arch. The oblique facial cleft results from failure of covering of the nasolacrimal groove by ectomesenchyme. The naso-ocular form represents failure of fusion of median nasal, lateral nasal, and maxillary processes, while the median orocanthal type represents failure of the fused nasal processes to unite with the maxillary processes. A number of bizarre clefts cannot be explained embryologically but probably represent tears in the ectomesenchyme. Others claim association with amniotic bands. The frequency of the usual facial clefts depends on racial background. Among whites the usual facial clefts occur approximately 1 per 600; among blacks, perhaps 1 per 3000; in Orientals, about 1 in 350; and in various Amerindian groups from 1 in 150 to 1 in 250. There is approximately one case of lateral facial cleft for every 350 cases of common facial clefts. The oblique facial cleft is probably even rarer. Risks of recurrence for CP and CL(P) range from 2 to 5%, if both parents are normal. If two children are affected or if the cleft is bilateral, the risk is somewhat enhanced (4–10%). It is not known whether one is dealing with multifactorial inheritance or with a single gene with incomplete penetrance.

Prognosis and Treatment Closure of the lip is usually done within the first few weeks of life, while palatal closure is delayed until 18 months to two and one half years.

REFERENCES

Boo-Chai, K. The transverse facial cleft: its repair. *Br. J. Plast. Surg.* 22: 119–124, 1969.

Boo-Chai, K. The oblique facial cleft: a report of two cases and a review of 41 cases. *Br. J. Plast. Surg.* 23: 352–359, 1970.

Lynch, H.T. and Kimberling, W.J. Genetic counseling in cleft lip and cleft palate. *Plast. Reconstr. Surg.* 68: 800–815, 1981.

Facial Clefts, Usual and Unusual

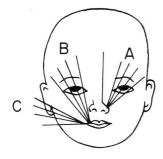

Paths of oblique and
transverse clefts

A–Oblique clefts involving
   lip and nostril
B–Oblique clefts lateral to
   philtrum not involving nostril
C–Transverse clefts

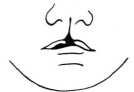

Median cleft from
upper lip to nose

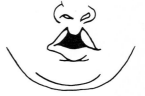

Bilateral cleft
lip incomplete

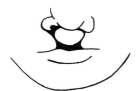

Bilateral cleft
lip complete

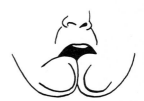

Clefting of mandible
lower lip and tongue

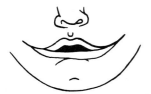

Bilateral transverse
facial cleft

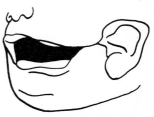

Unilateral cleft
extending to ear

23. HEMIHYPERTROPHY

Clinical Features Hemihypertrophy appears to be a nonspecific sign which may be observed in association with a variety of different disorders. The enlarged area may vary from a single digit or single limb or unilateral facial enlargement to involvement of half of the body. While it is usually segmental and unilateral, it may be crossed. Further, while it may be limited to a single system (muscular, vascular, skeletal, nervous), most frequently it involves multiple systems. Asymmetry is usually evident at birth but may become accentuated with age, especially at puberty. In total hemihypertrophy, the right side is more often involved. The skin is thickened in the affected area; it exhibits excessive secretion of sebaceous and sweat glands, hypertrichosis on the affected side, and polythelia. A medusa-like complex on the lower abdomen is sometimes observed. Occasionally bones in the involved area appear to be enlarged and increased bone age has been reported. Various skeletal manifestations include macrodactyly, syndactyly, polydactyly, etc. Occasionally there is unilateral enlargement of a cerebral hemisphere and mental retardation has been observed in about 15%. Of special interest is the association with various neoplasms such as adrenal cortical carcinoma, nephroblastoma, hepatoblastoma, as well as adrenal adenoma, adrenal neuroblastoma, and undifferentiated sarcoma of the lung. Medullary sponge kidney has been reported in several cases. In cases in which the hemihypertrophy is largely restricted to the head there is usually unilateral macroglossia, the fungiform papillae on that side being hypertrophic. The lips, palate, maxilla, mandible, and dentition (especially the permanent) are all enlarged. On the affected side there may be premature exfoliation of deciduous teeth with early eruption of permanent teeth.

Specific Diagnosis Diagnosis is made on clinical grounds, essentially by exclusion of a large number of other disorders.

Differential Diagnosis Body asymmetry may occur with *arteriovenous aneurysm, congenital lymphedema, neurofibromatosis, Russell-Silver syndrome, McCune-Albright syndrome, Beckwith-Wiedemann syndrome,* and especially *Klippel-Trenaunay-Weber syndrome.*

Prenatal Diagnosis Theoretically possible by ultrasonography or fetoscopy if enlargement is marked.

Basic Defect, Genetics, and Other Considerations Hemihypertrophy is not a disorder *sui generis,* but a nonspecific sign which may be observed in a variety of different disorders. Although almost all instances appear to be sporadic, there have been reports of familial instances. However, this does not appear to be due to a single gene and these cases are not well documented. In total hemihypertrophy males are more frequently affected. The frequency of the disorder is about 1 per 15,000 live births.

Prognosis and Treatment Life span may be decreased due to associated congenital anomalies (neoplasia, renal dysplasia). Nonprogressive mental retardation occurs in about 15%. Leg length asymmetry may require orthopedic procedures. Periodic examination is required to exclude the occurrence of neoplasia. Plastic surgical procedures may be required for esthetic correction of facial enlargement.

REFERENCES

Fraumeni, J.F. and Miller, R.W. Adrenocortical neoplasms with hemihypertrophy, brain tumors, and other disorders. *J. Pediatr. 70:* 129–138, 1967.

Kirks, D.R. and Shackelford, G.D. Idiopathic hemihypertrophy with associated ipsilateral benign nephromegaly. *Radiology 115:* 145–148, 1975.

Parker, D.A. and Skalko, R.G. Congenital asymmetry: report of 10 cases with associated developmental abnormalities. *Pediatrics 44:* 584–589, 1969.

• unilateral enlarge-
ment of parts
of body

Hemihypertrophy

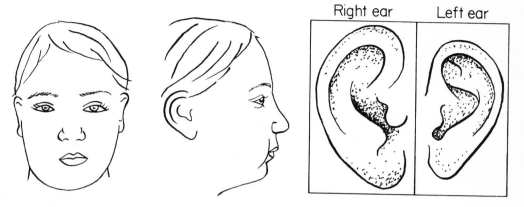

Right ear   Left ear

Hypertrophy of right side of face and right ear

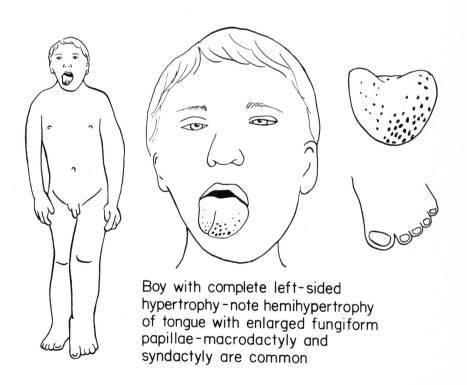

Boy with complete left-sided
hypertrophy – note hemihypertrophy
of tongue with enlarged fungiform
papillae – macrodactyly and
syndactyly are common

24. HOLOPROSENCEPHALY

Clinical Features Holoprosencephaly is a malformation complex which is associated with several distinct facies: in *cyclopia,* the most extreme variant, a single median eye-globe with varying degrees of doubling of the intrinsic ocular structures is associated with arhinia and usually with proboscis formation. Rarely, there is absent proboscis with or without mandible. In *ethmocephaly,* there are two separate hypoteloric eyes associated with arhinia and usually with proboscis formation. *Cebocephaly* is characterized by ocular hypotelorism and a single blind-ended nostril nose. In *premaxillary agenesis* there is ocular hypotelorism, flat boneless nose, and a median pseudocleft of the upper lip. There are less severe forms of facial dysmorphia characterized by ocular hypotelorism and defects of the upper lip and/or nose. Combinations with anencephaly have been noted. Not uncommonly these children have some degree of microcephaly. Abnormal gestation is rather common, about 40% of the mothers having first trimester bleeding. About 25% have required Caesarean section. Polyhydramnios is relatively common. General clinical findings include seizures, failure to thrive, apneic episodes, deafness. In those with milder forms, spasticity and athetoid movements are common.

Specific Diagnosis Cyclopia, ethmocephaly, cebocephaly, and premaxillary agenesis are associated with alobar holoprosencephaly; that is, the forebrain is monoventricular, i.e. without corpus callosum or septum pellucidum. The diencephalon and telencephalon are uncleft and there is an absence of olfactory bulbs and tracts and no interhemispheric fissure. Less severe facial dysmorphias are associated with less severe anomalies of brain development: semilobar holoprosencephaly is characterized by rudimentary cerebral lobes and occasionally a posterior interhemispheric fissure. In lobar examples, the brain lobes are well formed and the interhemispheric fissure is complete. EEG changes are bizarre, ranging from various abnormal waves to asynchrony to multifocal spikes. CT scanning is clearly indicated in cases of ocular hypotelorism.

Differential Diagnosis Holoprosencephaly may occur with *trisomy 13, 18p−, 13q−, triploidy,* and other *chromosomal disorders;* however, other noncraniofacial signs are present. *Meckel syndrome* should be excluded.

Prenatal Diagnosis Theoretically, prenatal diagnosis is possible using ultrasonography and fetoscopy.

Basic Defect, Genetics, and Other Considerations The basic defect is impaired sagittal cleavage of the forebrain into cerebral hemispheres, transversely into the telencephalon and diencephalon, and horizontally into olfactory and optic bulbs. Holoprosencephaly in all forms occurs with a frequency of about 1 per 15,000 births. Among conceptuses from spontaneous abortion, the frequency may be as high as 1 in 250. For the alobar forms, there appears to be a 3:1 female predilection. No sex preference was noted in lobar examples. Etiology is heterogeneous. All forms have been associated with trisomy 13, 18p−, and triploidy. The 13q− syndrome has been noted with semilobar or lobar holoprosencephaly, but most have had normal karyotype. There are many examples of sibs affected with like or unlike forms of holoprosencephaly, suggesting autosomal recessive inheritance of some cases. There may be a mild dominant form. However, most examples are isolated.

Prognosis and Treatment Those with alobar holoprosencephaly do not survive infancy, while those with semilobar or lobar forms live into childhood but exhibit moderate to severe mental retardation. The degree of facial involvement usually, but not always, predicts the extent of brain malformation.

REFERENCES

Cohen, M.M., Jr., Jirasek, J.E., Guzman, R.T. et al. Holoprosencephaly and facial dysmorphia: nosology, etiology and pathogenesis. *Birth Defects 7(7):* 125–135, 1971.

Lazjuk, G.I., Lurie, I.W., and Nedzved, M.K. Further studies on the genetic heterogeneity of cebocephaly. *J. Med. Genet. 13:* 314–318, 1976.

Roach, E., DeMyer, W.E., Palmer, K. et al. Holoprosencephaly: birth data, genetic and demographic analysis of 30 families. *Birth Defects 11(2):* 294–301, 1975.

- severe hypotelorism
- nasal anomalies
- eye anomalies

Holoprosencephaly

Cyclopia

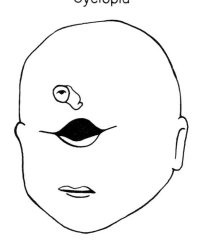

Central eye, proboscis
with single opening

Ethmocephaly

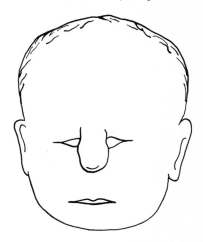

Separate eye orbits,
proboscis above eye

Cebocephaly

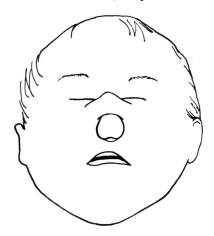

Microphthalmia, hypotelorism,
single-nostril nose

Premaxillary agenesis

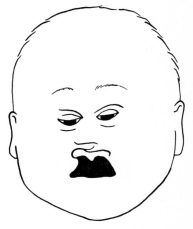

Hypotelorism, oblique
palpebral fissures, absent
nasal bones and cartilage,
agenesis of philtrum

25. HYDROCEPHALY

Clinical Features Hydrocephaly is heterogeneous. *Internal hydrocephalus* implies increased fluid within ventricles, *external hydrocephalus,* increased fluid in the subdural space. The latter may be associated with normal or even small cranium. If there is no obstruction within the ventricular system or spinal canal, the condition is *communicating hydrocephalus;* if free passage is impeded, it is *obstructed hydrocephalus.* About 80% of obstructed hydrocephalus infants have associated spina bifida cystica. The enlarged cranium may be detected at birth ("obstetric hydrocephaly"—about 33%) or, more frequently, during the first four months of life ("infantile hydrocephaly"—about 50%). In obstetric hydrocephaly, breech presentation occurs in over 30%, head circumference may exceed 50 cm, there is associated hydramnios in 10%, and spina bifida cystica in about 35%.

Specific Diagnosis If hydrocephaly has thinned the cerebral cortex to 1 cm or less, transillumination is positive. While CT scan shows ventricular enlargement, the site at which the obstruction is present cannot be determined. Pneumoencephalography or isotope ventriculography may be employed to determine whether the obstruction of the air is within or outside the enlarged ventricles.

Differential Diagnosis One must exclude *macrocephaly* due to enlarged brain or abnormal head form (*cerebral gigantism*). Various *chondrodystrophies* may be associated with hydrocephaly. Hydrocephaly may be secondary to infections (*toxoplasmosis,* rarely *CMV,* etc.), *subarachnoid or intraventricular hemorrhage,* or rarely *brain tumor.* Hydrocephalus may be associated with a legion of syndromes (*basal cell nevus syndrome, linear epidermoid nevus syndrome, Warburg syndrome,* etc.). Occasionally the head looks larger due to a small face (*Russell-Silver syndrome*). While adducted thumbs have been suggested as a hallmark of the *X-linked aqueductal stenotic form,* we do not believe that the sign has any specificity.

Prenatal Diagnosis In obstetric hydrocephaly, prenatal diagnosis may be possible by ultrasonography.

Basic Defect, Genetics, and Other Considerations All hydrocephalus is due to diminished absorption of cerebrospinal fluid. It is produced in normal amounts (except in the rare case of choroid plexus papilloma) and cannot be absorbed, thus accumulating proximal to the block. About 75–90% have prenatal etiology. Among those not having a specific genetic etiology are the following types: aqueductal stenosis (35%) communicating hydrocephalus (35%), Dandy-Walker malformation (10%), and miscellaneous malformations (20%). Hydrocephaly may be secondary to spina bifida or to various postnatal causes (10%): infection, hemorrhage, cyst, or tumor. Possibly as many as 25% of males with aqueductal stenosis have the X-linked recessive hydrocephaly. However, the empirical recurrence risk of a sporadic case of aqueductal stenotic hydrocephaly is about 4.5%. Conversely, however, only about 2% of patients with uncomplicated hydrocephaly have the X-linked form. The recurrence risk for the other forms is no greater than 1%. The slight male predilection reflects the aqueductal stenotic form. Overall frequency has ranged from 1 per 500 to 1 per 1500 births.

Prognosis and Treatment Those with true congenital hydrocephaly causing dystocia are often stillborn (45%), sacrificed at birth to save the mother, or die soon following birth (25%). Only about 5% survive to leave the hospital and live long enough for corrective surgery. Among unoperated infantile cases, about 50% die and 50% spontaneously arrest. Among arrested cases, almost 50% have normal IQ, 25% are retarded but educable, and 25% are severely retarded. Therapy consists of shunting of the cerebrospinal fluid (CSF) from the ventricles to the heart or abdominal cavity. It should be noted that mantle thickness before or after shunting, although correlated with subsequent intellectual performance, is not always a reliable indicator. Shunt blockage or shunt infection occurs in 25% or more. Recent modes of therapy include head wrapping until sutures fuse (which promotes absorption of CSF) and possible use of acetozolamide and furosemide which inhibit CSF production.

REFERENCES

Burton, B.K. Recurrence risks for congenital hydrocephalus. *Clin. Genet. 16: 47–53, 1979.*
Raimondi, A. and Soare, P. Intellectual development in shunted hydrocephalic children. *Am. J. Dis. Child. 127:* 664–671, 1974.

Shurtleff, D.B., Foltz, E.U., and Loeser, J.D. Hydrocephalus: a definition of its progression and relationship to intellectual function, diagnosis and complications. *Am. J. Dis. Child. 125:* 688–693, 1973.

- **enlarged head**
- **prominent scalp veins**
- **large open sutures and fontanelles**

Hydrocephaly

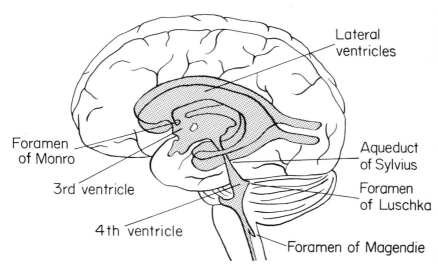

Sites of possible obstruction in ventricular system of the brain

Lateral ventricles

Foramen of Monro

3rd ventricle

4th ventricle

Aqueduct of Sylvius

Foramen of Luschka

Foramen of Magendie

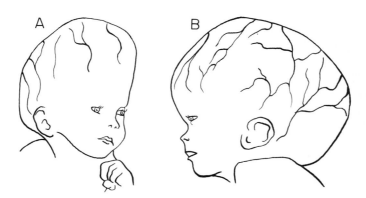

Hydrocephaly due to A) X–linked aqueductal stenosis, B) Dandy–Walker malformation (atresia of foramens of Luschka and Magendie)–physical appearance not diagnostic

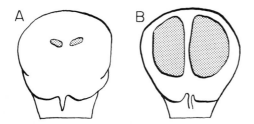

A) normal lateral ventricular size in an infant, B) dilated lateral ventricles in an infant with hydrocephaly

26. HYPOGLOSSIA-HYPODACTYLIA SPECTRUM

Clinical Features Among the several disorders of oromandibular limb hypogenesis, specific boundaries are blurred. These will be briefly discussed under the following categories: hypoglossia-hypodactylia syndrome, glossopalatine ankylosis syndrome, Charlie M. syndrome, Hanhart syndrome, and Moebius syndrome. *Hypoglossia-hypodactylia syndrome* is characterized by small mandible and small tongue. Variability is marked. Mandibular incisors may be absent with concomitant atrophy of associated alveolar ridge. Fusion of the anterior alveolar processes and cleft palate have been reported in several cases. Limb anomalies are extremely variable, ranging from hemimelia of all four limbs to involvement of both limbs on the same side to oligodactyly, syndactyly, or adactyly. Speech is usually good and patients often have normal intelligence. *Glossopalatine ankylosis* refers to attachment of the anterior tongue (of normal size) to the hard palate or maxillary alveolar ridge. Similar dental and limb anomalies may occur. *Hanhart syndrome* refers to extreme micrognathia, normal tongue size, hypodontia or delayed eruption, and various limb anomalies as noted above. *Charlie M. syndrome* is characterized by ocular hypertelorism, facial palsy, absent or conically crowned incisors, cleft palate, and variable degrees of hypodactyly. *Moebius syndrome* consists of VI–VII usually bilateral cranial nerve palsies and occasionally other cranial nerves (III, V, IX, XII), reductive limb anomalies (30%), Poland anomaly complex (15%), and mild mental retardation (10%). The mask-like facies is characteristic. In addition there may be eyelid ptosis, nystagmus, strabismus, or epicanthus. Some patients may be unable to close their eyes either during sleep or while awake. The angles of the mouth droop, allowing saliva to escape. Unilateral tongue hypoplasia is frequent, but occasionally there is bilateral involvement.

Poor palatal mobility, inefficient sucking and swallowing, coarse voice, and speech impairment are often noted.

Specific Diagnosis Diagnosis is based solely on clinical findings.

Differential Diagnosis There is considerable overlap between these syndromes. Limb defects have the same range of variability in all five variants discussed above and similar limb defects may be observed in the *Poland complex, amniotic band disruption complex,* and *autosomal recessive acheiropody.* Intraoral mucosal bands may be seen in the *popliteal pterygium syndrome* and the *van der Woude syndrome.* Isolated facial palsy may result from *birth trauma.*

Prenatal Diagnosis Not likely to be made; however, severe limb anomalies could be recognized using ultrasonography or fetoscopy.

Basic Defect, Genetics, and Other Considerations The etiology of this group of conditions is unknown. All of the disorders save Moebius syndrome are rare. Since virtually all cases are sporadic and since clinical features, especially limb anomalies, are remarkably variable, etiologic heterogeneity is likely. Whether they represent separate and distinct entities or simply a spectrum of a single disorder is not known. In cases of Moebius syndrome, postmortem studies have shown nuclear agenesis.

Prognosis and Treatment Normal life span is expected in all forms of the spectrum. Mild mental retardation occurs in up to 10–15%. Orthopedic surgical correction and prosthetic appliances should be employed as needed. In the neonatal period, tube feeding may be necessary.

REFERENCES

Cohen, M.M., Jr. Nosologic and genetic considerations in the aglossy-adactyly syndrome. *Birth Defects* 7(7): 237–240, 1971.

Herrmann, J., Pallister, P.D., Gilbert, E.F. et al. Nosologic studies in the Hanhart and the Möbius syndrome. *Europ. J. Pediatr.* 122: 19–55, 1976.

Kaplan, P., Cummings, C., and Fraser, F.C. A "community" of face-limb malformation syndromes. *J. Pediatr.* 89: 241–247, 1976.

- **hypodactyly**
- **micrognathia**
- **hypoglossia**
- **eye anomalies**

Hypoglossia-Hypodactylia Spectrum

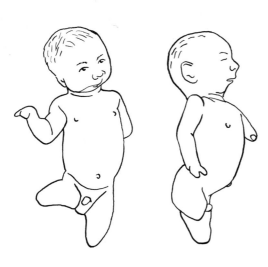

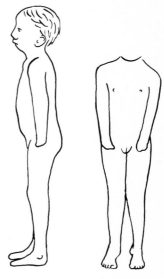

Severe hypodactylia, micro-gnathia and hypoglossia

Hanhart syndrome with limb anomalies, micro-gnathia and hypodontia

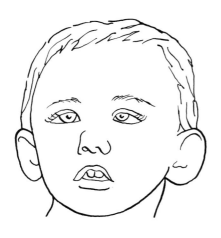

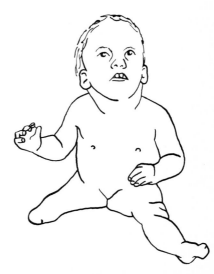

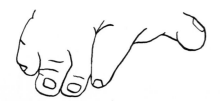

Moebius syndrome - lack of facial expression, ptosis, strabismus, protruding ears, limb anomalies, hypoplastic fingers and nails

27. KARTAGENER SYNDROME
(immotile cilia syndrome)

Clinical Features Kartagener syndrome classically consists of a combination of thick mucoid nasal secretions since infancy with pansinusitis, partial or complete situs inversus (mirror-image dextrocardia, totally reversed abdominal organs, and lower position of the right testicle), chronic serous otitis media, and bronchiectasis. The frontal sinuses are often absent or hypoplastic. Tachypnea, chest retraction, and rales in affected infants are common features. The expression of the syndrome is variable. Some patients may have one, two, or all of the signs.

Specific Diagnosis Thick mucoid rhinorrhea, recurrent respiratory infections, and chronic bronchitis become manifest during the first year of life in over 90%. They persist to adulthood. Pansinusitis usually dates from childhood. The thick nasal secretion may be associated with anosmia and nasal polyps with resultant mouth breathing and nasal speech. Most patients have chronic serous otitis media which may result in secondary conductive hearing loss. By the third year of life, bronchiectasis which is usually tubular initially but becomes saccular, may be complicated by respiratory distress, pneumonia, and atelectasia of the lower lobes. Occasionally there are accompanying asthma, hemoptysis and acrocyanosis, and clubbing of the fingers. Situs inversus, present in about 50% of cases, is usually not recognized for many years. If the situs inversus is incomplete, dextrocardia or other cardiac anomalies may be present. Adult males may be sterile, due to immotile spermatozoa. Electron microscopy of cross sections of cilia obtained by biopsy of nasal epithelium may be employed to establish diagnosis.

Differential Diagnosis The disorder should be differentiated from *isolated dextrocardia, isolated bronchiectasis,* or *isolated sinusitis.* Some patients have been erroneously thought to be suffering from *cystic fibrosis* because of the thick tenacious bronchial secretions, nasal polyposis, chronic sinusitis, and bronchiectasis.

Prenatal Diagnosis This is not currently available.

Basic Defect, Genetics, and Other Considerations The primary anomaly in respiratory epithelium and sperm consists of abnormalities of number, orientation, and structure of the filament complex (9 peripheral and 2 central microtubular doublets) of cilia, i.e. absence of dynein arms and randomly oriented cilia. Dynein arms are protein structures with ATP activity which form temporary bridges between adjacent microtubular doublets to produce ciliary movement. This apparently is not a constant finding, however, and may be found in normal individuals. The immotile or abnormally motile respiratory epithelial cilia result in mucus retention which produces blockage of the paranasal sinuses, eustachian tube, and lobes of the lung, which in turn become easily infected. The immotile sperm tails result in sterility. Possibly during early embryonic life, ciliary beats in the growing embryo determine the type of laterality. In the absence of ciliary beats, laterality may be random, thus effecting the situs inversus in about half the affected cases. The disorder has autosomal recessive inheritance. Its frequency appears to be approximately 1 in 50,000 in the United States, 1 in 20,000 in Japan, and 1 in 120,000 in Israel.

Prognosis and Treatment Life expectancy is essentially normal. Although most patients reach adult life, pulmonary function tests demonstrate ventilatory obstruction in all patients. If severe, this can constrain vigorous physical activity. Serial bronchograms are helpful in the bronchiectasis. Chronic cough and constant rhinorrhea bother the patients, although they are generally not aware of their difficulty in ability to hear or to smell. As indicated earlier, infertility is not uncommonly encountered in the male. Antibiotic therapy is almost constantly required. Especially in the infant, the use of aerosols, postural drainage, and decongestants are needed several times daily. Segmental resection or lobectomy of the lungs is performed in about 30% of the patients.

REFERENCES

Afzelius, B.A. The immotile-cilia syndrome and other ciliary diseases. *Internat. Rev. Exp. Path.* 19: 2–43, 1979.

Rott, H.D. Kartagener's syndrome and the syndrome of immotile cilia. *Human Genetics* 46: 249–261, 1979.

Veerman, A.J.P., van Delden, L., Feenstra, L. et al. The immotile cilia syndrome: phase contrast light microscopy, scanning and transmission electron microscopy. *Pediatrics* 65: 698–702, 1980.

- sinusitis
- partial or complete situs inversus
- serous otitis media
- bronchiectasis

Kartagener Syndrome
[immotile cilia syndrome]

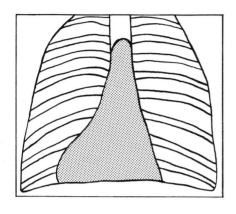

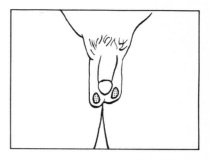

Dextrocardia as part of situs inversus-lower position of right testicle

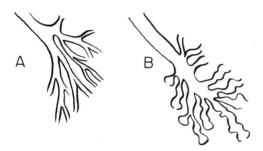

(A) normal left lower bronchus,
(B) bronchiectasis in Kartagener syndrome

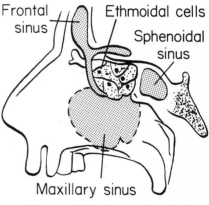

Frontal sinus   Ethmoidal cells

Sphenoidal sinus

Maxillary sinus

Sites of possible sinusitis

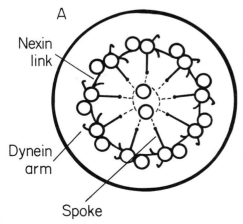

A

Nexin link

Dynein arm

Spoke

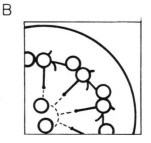

B

(A) cross-section of sperm tail, dynein arms responsible for motility (B) defective dynein arms in Kartagener syndrome

28. KLIPPEL-FEIL ANOMALY

Clinical Features The term Klippel-Feil anomaly should refer to massive fusion of cervical vertebrae with painless limitation of head movement, shortness of the neck, and low posterior hairline due to cervical vertebral abbreviation. Unfortunately, the term has been loosely used to refer to any form of cervical vertebral fusion. A particularly severe form is iniencephaly. The head appears to sit directly upon the thorax without an interposing neck. The trapezius muscles flare, extending from the mastoid areas to the shoulders. In some individuals there may be facial asymmetry, one eye being situated lower than the other. Scoliosis and/or Sprengel deformity have been noted in approximately one-third of the cases. Various associated neurologic disturbances such as spasticity or hyperreflexia, bimanual synkinesis or mirror movements, syringomyelia or syringobulbia, hemiplegia, paraplegia, quadriplegia, etc. have been noted. Convergent strabismus is relatively common. Approximately one-third of the patients manifest deafness due to abnormality of development of the inner ear, but these may be examples of Wildervanck syndrome (see Differential Diagnosis). Congenital heart disease, usually ventricular septal defect, is occasionally noted. Unilateral renal agenesis is the most common urogenital finding in this disorder. Cleft palate occurs in 5–10% of the cases.

Specific Diagnosis Diagnosis is essentially clinical. However, roentgenographically several or occasionally all cervical vertebrae are fused into a solid mass. This may extend to involve some upper thoracic vertebrae. Scoliosis, cervical ribs, and Sprengel deformity have all been described. Less common findings include spina bifida occulta, fusion of atlas with occipital bone, cleft vertebrae, and hemivertebrae.

Differential Diagnosis The flaring trapezius muscles may give the patient an appearance of having pterygium colli. Thus one must exclude *Turner syndrome, Noonan syndrome, multiple pterygium syndrome, craniocarpotarsal dysplasia,* and various other disorders that manifest cervical pterygia. *Wildervanck syndrome or cervicooculoacoustic syndrome* (Klippel-Feil anomaly, profound hearing loss, abducens paralysis, and retraction of the bulb) may possibly be a variant. Most of these patients are female. Isolated fusion of the second and third cervical vertebrae appears to be inherited as an autosomal dominant trait. *Spondylothoracic dysplasia* in which the head appears to sit upon the shoulders is a genetic heterogeneity consisting of dominant and recessive forms. The entire vertebral column is involved in fusions, hemivertebrae, scoliosis, etc. Klippel-Feil anomaly has also been reported in association with conductive hearing loss and absent vagina and uterus, as well as in association with unilateral renal agenesis, vaginal agenesis and bicornuate uterus; whether this is the same disorder as that noted above is not known.

Prenatal Diagnosis To the best of our knowledge this has never been accomplished.

Basic Defect, Genetics, and Other Considerations It has been suggested by many authors that the condition arises from faulty segmentation of the mesodermal somites somewhere between the third and seventeenth week in utero. Virtually all cases are sporadic. There have been a few reports of familial occurence. There is a sex predilection: over 65% of cases of massive cervical vertebral fusion occur in females. The frequency of the disorder has been estimated to be approximately 1 per 35,000 individuals.

Prognosis and Treatment The disorder is not progressive. No attempt is made to resolve the cervical fusion. The restriction of abduction of the eye can be partly or completely corrected by temporal transplantation of the superior and inferior recti combined with resection of the internal rectus.

REFERENCES

Gunderson, C.H., Greenspan, R.H., Glaser, G.H. et al. The Klippel-Feil syndrome: genetic and clinical reevaluation of cervical fusion. *Medicine 46:* 491–512, 1967.

Moore, W.B., Matthews, T.J., and Rabinowitz, R. Genitourinary anomalies associated with Klippel-Feil syndrome. *J. Bone Joint Surg. 57A:* 355–357, 1975.

Mosberg, W.H. Jr. The Klippel-Feil syndrome: etiology and treatment of neurologic signs. *J. Nerv. Ment. Dis. 117:* 479–491, 1953.

- **limited head movement**
- **short neck**
- **low posterior hairline**

Klippel-Feil Anomaly

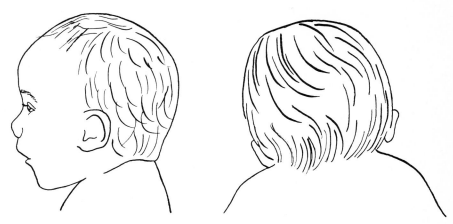

Infant with short neck, head tilt, neck
immobility and low posterior hair line

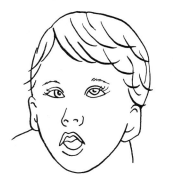 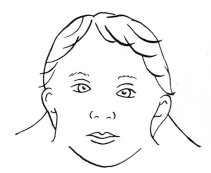

Head appears to be directly on thorax, strabismus,
distorted facies and low-set ears

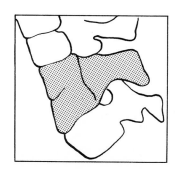

Fusion of cervical
vertebrae

69

29. KLIPPEL-TRENAUNAY-WEBER SYNDROME

Clinical Features Although the original description defined the syndrome as consisting of unilateral extremity enlargement with cutaneous and subcutaneous hemangiomas, varicosities, phlebectasia, and occasionally arteriovenous fistula, the syndrome has been expanded to include almost every conceivable body area so that it includes lymphangiomatous anomalies, macrodactyly, syndactyly, polydactyly, oligodactyly, and abdominal hemangiomas. Occasionally more than one limb is involved and the enlargement does not necessarily involve the area exhibiting hemangiomatous involvement. Craniofacial involvement, albeit rare, when present, is similar to that seen in the Sturge-Weber anomaly, both in degree of variability and distribution of angiomatous occurrence. Where there is such cutaneous involvement, patients may exhibit mental retardation. Occasionally there may be unilateral bony overgrowth of the jaws.

Specific Diagnosis Unilateral hypertrophy is the most frequent finding and is usually noted at birth but may occur at any age and progresssively increase in degree. Circumference and/or length are usually increased, but occasionally only the proximal or distal limb segment may be disproportionately large. In most instances a visible vascular abnormality is present in the hypertrophied area. Varicosities, phlebectasia, nevus flammeus or port wine mark, and vascular masses predominate, but other hemangiomatous lesions have been described. They vary in size, the larger vascular masses causing a generalized bleeding diathesis of the Kasabach-Merritt variety, due to pooling of blood platelets. Lymphangiectasia can result in marked limb swelling with recurrent cellulitis. Extremities or digits may be massive or digits may be of unequal length. Cutaneous vascular lesions are most frequently present over the lower limbs, although the buttocks or lower back, flank, or lateral chest may be involved. There may be pigmented streaks or spots. Visceral involvement consists of hemangiomatous lesions of the gastrointestinal and urinary tracts, rarely the mesentery or pleura. Generalized nonspecific visceromegaly may involve the kidney and abdominal lymphangiectasia and protein-losing enteropathy secondary to the lymphangiectasia have been reported. Enlargement of the genitalia with secondary ambiguity has been reported as well as lipodystrophy of the upper extremities.

Differential Diagnosis *Neurofibromatosis* must be excluded, since limb hypertrophy and skin hemangiomas may be associated with the disorder. Cafe-au-lait spots do not occur in the KTW syndrome. *Beckwith-Wiedemann syndrome* may be associated with hemihypertrophy and skin hemangiomas. *Maffucci syndrome* with frequent limb hypertrophy and vascular lesions must also be differentiated. *Hemihypertrophy* has been reported with vascular anomalies of the skin.

Prenatal Diagnosis This has been accomplished by ultrasonography. Fetoscopy could be used to possibly visualize the skin lesion and limb anomalies.

Basic Defect, Genetics, and Other Considerations The etiology is unknown. Virtually all cases have been sporadic.

Prognosis and Treatment Most patients do reasonably well. Surgical intervention is required in cases of severe disproportionate growth which may necessitate epiphyseal fusion or removal of a gigantic digit. In those cases with gigantic extremities with clotting difficulties, amputation may be required. Ulcers and chronic skin problems are not uncommon. Surgical correction of arteriovenous aneurysms is always required.

REFERENCES

Hatjis, C.G., Philip, A.G., Anderson, G.G. et al. The in utero ultrasonographic appearance of Klippel-Trénaunay-Weber syndrome. *Am. J. Obstet. Gynecol. 139:* 972–974, 1981.

Kuffer, F.R., Starzynski, T.E., Girolami, A. et al. Klippel-Trenaunay syndrome, visceral angiomatosis and thrombocytopenia. *J. Pediat. Surg. 3:* 65–72, 1968.

Lindenauer, S.M. The Klippel-Trenaunay syndrome: varicosity, hypertrophy, and hemangioma with no arteriovenous fistula. *Ann Surg. 162:* 303–314, 1965.

- **unilateral hyper-trophy of tissues and / or bone**
- **vascular anomalies**

Klippel-Trenaunay-Weber Syndrome

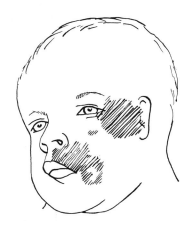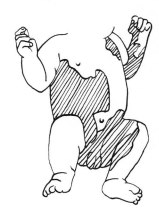

Nevus flammeus involving facial area supplied by second branch
of trigeminal nerve and also other parts of the body

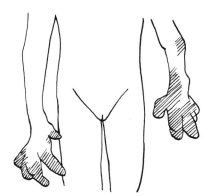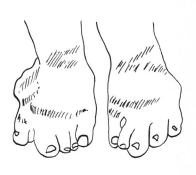

Gigantism with malformed hands and toes

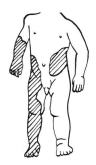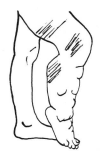

Hemangiomatous involvement
may not coincide with hypertrophy

Varicose veins, hemangiomas
and hypertrophy of leg

30. MICROCEPHALY

Clinical Features Microcephaly is a sign, rarely a disorder. It includes those with single gene, gross chromosomal, and environmentally caused disorders as well as a large number of children having small heads of unknown genesis. By definition, the infant has a head circumference smaller than 3 SD (standard deviations) for age and sex. In extreme cases, microcephaly may be clinically evident in the newborn (receding forehead, flat occiput, small or closed fontanels). Commonly the frontal scalp hair exhibits an upsweep. Somatic growth is generally retarded. Walking and speech and mental development are variably delayed and some patients also exhibit strabismus, seizures, and spasticity. Infants having true hereditary microcephaly rarely have anomalies other than craniofacial. They have a mean IQ of 35 (range 10–67). As the child grows, the small size of the cranium becomes accentuated. The forehead recedes, the scalp hair becomes thick and rough and commonly there is redundant scalp. The ears and nose appear large. Personality is extremely variable and vacillating (cheerful, moody, excitable, aggressive, etc.).

Specific Diagnosis Microcephaly is diagnosed by measurement. One should beware of being erroneously impressed by abnormal head form, overriding sutures, and various craniosynostoses. The clinician must perform serial measurement. Radiographically, the anterior fontanel is prematurely closed (normal range 7–19 months). A further caveat is necessary: a small head is *not* always associated with mental retardation. Family history, karyotype, TORCH titers, and metabolic screening should be carried out to exclude various etiologic factors. Pneumoencephalographic studies show prenatal brain damage in 90%.

Differential Diagnosis See section on Basic Defect, Genetics, and Other Considerations.

Prenatal Diagnosis Ultrasound studies may be of use in prenatal diagnosis of this condition.

Basic Defect, Genetics, and Other Considerations Microcephaly is etiologically heterogeneous. Environmental factors include prenatal radiation (< 17 weeks), various prenatal infections (*rubella, CMV, toxoplasmosis,* and possibly *syphilis*), and several teratogens (*alcohol, trimethadione,* possibly *hydantoin,* and *methyl mercury*). *Children of phenylketonuric women are* microcephalic. Microcephaly may also be a component of a host of *chromosomal trisomies, partial trisomies,* and *deletions,* as well as syndromes of known and unknown etiology (*deLange, Rubinstein-Taybi, Langer-Giedion,* etc.). *Seckel bird-headed dwarfism* is a rare, presumably autosomal recessive disorder characterized by microcephaly, small facies, low birth weight, severe growth retardation, mild mental retardation, and a small cerebrum with simplified convolutional pattern. So-called true hereditary microcephaly (no other anomalies) appears to have autosomal recessive inheritance. Heterozygotes may have some decreased intelligence. Frequency of microcephaly is about 1 per 10,000. Genetic microcephaly ranges between 20–35% (1 per 30,000–50,000 live births) in the general population. This of course excludes population isolates where the frequency can reach 1 per 2,000 births. Among the severely retarded, about 5% have primary microcephaly. One-fourth of these have affected relatives.

Prognosis and Treatment While true microcephalics often live a normal life span, others die early because of associated congenital anomalies or infectious disorders. Treatment is supportive.

REFERENCES

Daniel, W.L. A genetic and biochemical investigation of primary microcephaly. *Am J. Ment. Defic. 75:* 653–662, 1971.

Majewski, F. and Goecke, T. Studies of microcephalic primordial dwarfism: approach to a delineation of the Seckel syndrome. *Am. J. Med. Genet. 12:* 7–21, 1982.

Qazi, Q.H. and Reed, T.E. A problem in diagnosis of primary versus secondary microcephaly. *Clin. Genet. 4:* 46–52, 1973.

- **small head**
- **receding forehead**
- **large ears and nose**

Microcephaly

TRUE HEREDITARY MICROCEPHALY

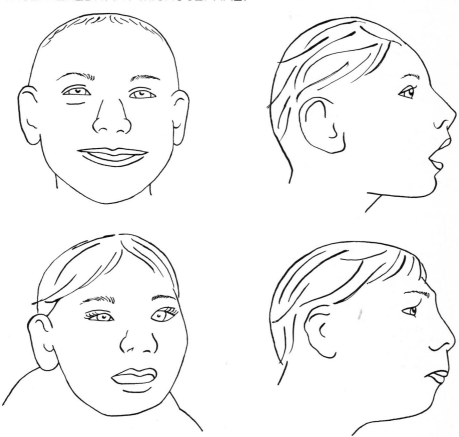

Normal size face with microcephaly, sloping forehead, prominent nose, flat occiput and large, protruding ears

SECKEL BIRD-HEADED DWARFISM

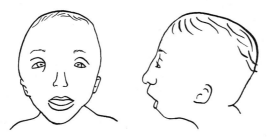

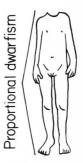

Proportional dwarfism

Microcephaly, narrow face, prominent eyes, low-set lobeless ears, beak-like nose and micrognathia

Slender build

31. POLAND ANOMALY

Clinical Features The Poland anomaly or developmental field defect is clinically variable. It consists of unilateral absence of the sternal and costal portions of the pectoralis major muscle, and symbrachydactyly of the hand on the ipsilateral side. In its full expression there are hypoplasia of the skin and subcutaneous tissues of the anterior chest, absence or hypoplasia and upward displacement of the nipple and breast, pectoral and axillary hypotrichosis, absence of the sternocostal portion of the pectoralis major, absence of the pectoralis minor (one-third as often), absence of portions of costal cartilages two, three, and four or three, four, and five; absence of the middle phalanges of all the fingers or fusion of the middle and distal phalanges with webbing between the proximal phalanges. There is no bony synostosis. The hand on the ipsilateral side is usually smaller than that on the unaffected side. The thumb is often normal. Occasionally other muscles about the shoulder girdle have been deficient, and Sprengel deformity has been noted in some cases.

Specific Diagnosis The diagnosis is a clinical one. The condition has occurred without defects of the hand, without costal defects, and without recognizable defects of other muscles of the shoulder girdle. However, the virtually constant features are anomalies of the nipple, of the subcutaneous tissues, and of the pectoralis major and minor. Webbing of the axilla is not uncommon. Moebius syndrome exhibiting paralysis of the sixth and seventh cranial nerves may be associated with, among other defects, the hand and chest wall features of Poland anomaly in approximately 15% of cases.

Differential Diagnosis The disorder is so characteristic that discussion of differential diagnosis is not relevant.

Prenatal Diagnosis When the limb and chest deformities are severe, ultrasound studies and possibly fetoscopy could be used to diagnosis this condition.

Basic Defect, Genetics, and Other Considerations The disorder is not hereditary. The primary defect appears to be a local one in mesoderm in the quadrant from the pectoral area to the distal upper limb. It has been estimated that approximately 10% of patients with syndactyly of the hand have the Poland anomaly. Approximately 75% of patients with Poland anomaly are male and in about 70% the right side is involved. Most cases have been sporadic. Various estimates concerning its frequency have ranged from 1 in 7000 to 1 in 100,000. However, this may not reflect the true frequency if the hand anomalies are mild. There have been several familial examples, most involving parent and child. But the recurrence rate is considerably less than 1%.

Prognosis and Treatment The chest abnormalities are not treated. Correction of syndactyly may be carried out if function may be improved.

REFERENCES

Gorlin, R.J. Risk of recurrence in usually nongenetic malformation syndromes. *Birth Defects 15(5C):* 181–188, 1979.
Ireland, D.C.R., Takayama, N., and Flatt, A.E. Poland's syndrome. A review of 43 cases. *J. Bone Joint Surg. 58A:* 52–58, 1976.

Mace, J.W., Kaplan, J.M., Shanenberger, J.E. et al. Poland's syndrome. Report of 7 cases and review of the literature. *Clin. Pediatr. 11:* 98–102, 1972.

- **unilateral hypo-plasia of anterior chest wall**
- **hypoplasia / absent nipple**
- **symbrachydactyly**

Poland Anomaly

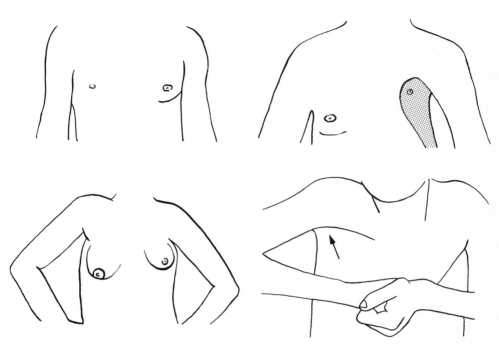

Unilateral absence or hypoplasia of the pectoralis minor and sternal portion of pectoralis major (arrow), absence or hypoplasia of nipple and areola

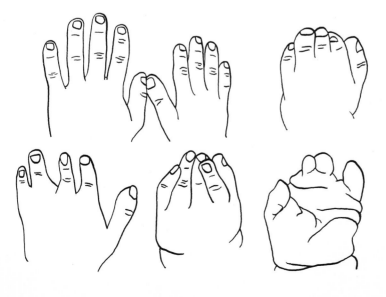

Ipsilateral hand deformities with small hand, brachydactyly, syndactyly and terminal symphalangism

32. RENAL AGENESIS—BILATERAL
(Potter syndrome)

Clinical Features There is a distinct facies that is associated with bilateral renal agenesis. The so-called Potter facies resulting from oligohydramnios is characterized by redundant dehydrated skin, ocular hypertelorism, a prominent fold arising at the inner canthus and extending laterally to the outer canthus, a squashed nose, micrognathia, and large ears with deficient and flattened pinnae. There may be either oligohydramnios or total absence of amniotic fluid. Amnion nodosum is common. Labor is often premature. Birth weight is disproportionately low and breech delivery is common. Genital organ abnormalities occur such as absence of the vas deferens and seminal vesicles or agenesis of the uterus and upper vagina. Lung hypoplasia is severe. Gastrointestinal malformations include anal atresia, absent sigmoid and rectum, esophageal and duodenal atresia. Club foot is the most common skeletal malformation. An extreme form of limb anomaly is sirenomelia.

Specific Diagnosis Potter syndrome is ordinarily classified as having three degrees of severity: *Type A*—limited to the lower ducts (bilateral agenesis of kidneys and ureters with absence of uterus and vagina but normal fallopian tubes in females and absent vas deferens and seminal vesicles in males); *Type B*—the same anomalies as Type A but includes hindgut and cloacal membrane derivatives (imperforate anus with atresia of hindgut with or without rectovesical or retrovaginal fistula and with variable genital abnormalities such as hypoplasia of phallus and/or scrotum in males and enlarged phallic tubercle with formation of male urethra in females); and *Type C,* with the anomalies seen in Types A and B but includes the entire caudal end of the embryo, resulting in sirenomelia.

Differential Diagnosis While there are several syndromes which may be associated with renal hypoplasia (*branchio-oto-renal syndrome, Winter syndrome,* etc.), the phenotype is so distinctive that Potter syndrome should be easily recognized. Anatomically, one must rule out cases of *renal adysplasia* in which kidney remnants are present. This disorder, possibly having autosomal dominant inheritance, has milder expression in females (unilateral renal adysplasia) than in males (bilateral renal adysplasia). Potter syndrome is seen also in *7q+ syndrome* and in *XYY syndrome.*

Prenatal Diagnosis Conceivably ultrasonography may be employed with sufficient accuracy to prenatally diagnose bilateral renal agenesis between 16 and 20 weeks of gestation. Maternal serum α-fetoprotein has been elevated in some cases but normal in others.

Basic Defect, Genetics, and Other Considerations The disorder is due to oligohydramnios which in turn reflects the primary defect of bilateral renal agenesis. There is no evidence to indicate that Potter syndrome has a simple pattern of inheritance but there are families in which affected sibs have been reported. Males are approximately three times as frequently affected as females. The frequency of Potter syndrome is approximately 1 per 10,000 births. The recurrence risk is probably about 1% but may be as high as 3% if the propositus is severely affected. Pattern of recurrence suggests multifactorial inheritance. There have been twin pregnancies in which one fetus had bilateral renal agenesis while the other did not. In such cases, the usual stigmata of Potter syndrome were absent because there was no oligohydramnios. There is some evidence that bilateral renal agenesis and unilateral renal agenesis may occur in the same sibship. An increased rate of anencephaly-myelomeningocele in sibs of infants with Potter syndrome is seen.

Prognosis and Treatment Approximately 40% of these infants are stillborn. Most of those born alive die within the first four to five hours of life. There is pulmonary hypoplasia due to compression of the chest from lack of amniotic fluid which results in death due to asphyxia. In the rare case that survives for a day or two, death results from renal failure. The prognosis is inevitably fatal and there is no treatment.

REFERENCES

Buchta, E.M., Viseskul, C., Gilbert, E.F. et al. Familial bilateral renal agenesis and hereditary renal adysplasia. *Z. Kinderheilk. 115:* 111–129, 1973.

Cain, D.R., Griggs, D., Lackey, D.A. et al. Familial renal agenesis and total dysplasia. *Am. J. Dis. Child. 128:* 377–380, 1974.

Carter, C.O., Evans, K., and Pescia, G. A family study of renal agenesis. *J. Med. Genet. 16:* 176–188, 1979.

- **wrinkled facies**
- **skin fold under eye**
- **flat nose**
- **dysplastic low-set ears**

Renal Agenesis—Bilateral
[Potter syndrome]

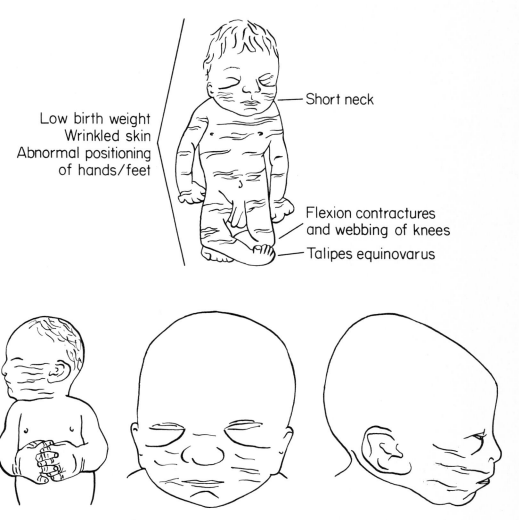

Short neck

Low birth weight
Wrinkled skin
Abnormal positioning
of hands/feet

Flexion contractures
and webbing of knees

Talipes equinovarus

Large wrinkled hands, skin fold from inner canthus to
upper cheek, blunt nose, crease on chin, large, low-set
ears posteriorly rotated and wrinkled facial skin

33. ROBIN ANOMALY

Clinical Features The Robin anomaly consists of micrognathia, glossoptosis, and cleft palate. It should be recognized that this triad is not a specific disorder but can be seen in association with various conditions. The facies is striking at birth. The mandible is small and symmetrically receded. Congenital murmurs and/or heart disease have been observed in 15–25% of those patients who die in early infancy. Necropsy has revealed a wide variety of congenital heart disorders (atrial septal defect, patent ductus arteriosus, ventricular septal defect, etc.). Ocular findings are common, especially esotropia and congenital glaucoma. It has been established that about 20% of patients exhibit severe mental retardation, but it is not known whether this is primary or secondary to asphyxia. The palatal defect may vary widely from cleft uvula to clefting which involves two-thirds of the hard palate and is horseshoe in shape. The majority of patients have a defect of intermediate degree. In this disorder, cleft lip does not occur in combination with cleft palate. The small mandible achieves catch-up growth by four to six years of age, although the angle is always somewhat abnormal. Difficulty in the inspiratory phase of respiration is apparent, with periodic cyanotic attacks, labored breathing, and recession of the sternum and ribs. This becomes especially apparent when the child is in supine position. The respiratory difficulty is usually evident at birth, although it may not be severe for the first week. Only rarely is its initiation delayed until the first month.

Specific Diagnosis Diagnosis is entirely clinical. If it is syndromally associated, diagnosis will depend on identification of the specific disorder. Cohen has listed a large number of associated syndromes (see below). About one-third of cases are associated with other anomalies which do not constitute a recognizable syndrome.

Differential Diagnosis The condition most commonly associated with the Robin anomaly is *Stickler syndrome,* which may account for as much as 30% of the cases; but it can be seen with *cerebrocostomandibular syndrome, campomelic dysplasia, spondyloepiphyseal dysplasia congenita, diastrophic dysplasia, femoral hypoplasia, fetal alcohol syndrome, fetal hydantoin syndrome, fetal trimethadione syndrome,* etc. The difficulty in nursing, the choking fits, and the cyanotic bouts may also suggest *tracheoesophageal fistula.*

Prenatal Diagnosis There is no currently available method for diagnosing the condition prenatally.

Basic Defect, Genetics, and Other Considerations Pathogenesis is probably based on arrested development, the primary defect lying in hypoplasia of the mandible preventing the normal descent of the tongue between the palatal shelves. While many of the conditions with which the Robin anomaly is associated are single gene disorders, when it is not associated with any of these conditions, Robin anomaly does not appear to have single gene inheritance; it may be multifactorial.

Prevention and Treatment Immediate airway maintenance is critical. This may be accomplished in mild cases by keeping the infant prone with the head pulley-suspended in a stockinette cap. In more severe cases, the tongue tip may be temporarily sutured to the lower lip or anterior mandible. Tracheotomy may rarely be required. As indicated earlier, the mandible exhibits catch-up growth. The cleft palate is repaired at 18–36 months.

REFERENCES

Cohen, M.M., Jr. The Robin anomaly—its nonspecificity in associated syndromes. *J. Oral Surg. 34:* 587–593, 1976.

Hanson, J. and Smith, D.W. U-shaped palatal defect in the Robin anomaly: developmental and clinical relevance. *J. Pediatr. 87:* 30–33, 1975.

Randall, P., Krogman, W., and Jahins, S. Pierre Robin and the syndrome that bears his name. *Cleft Palate J. 2:* 237–246, 1965.

- **micrognathia**
- **glossoptosis**
- **U-shaped cleft palate**

Robin Anomaly

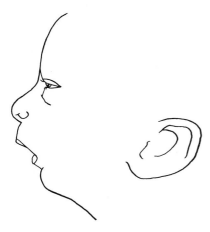

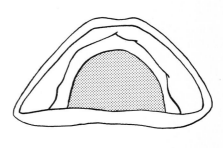

Severe micrognathia and
low-set dysplastic ear

U-shaped cleft palate

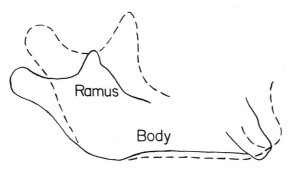

Normal mandible broken line, Robin solid line–
note difference in height of ramus, length of
body and inclination of ramus to body

34. SPINAL CORD ANOMALIES

Clinical Features Spina bifida (SB) is a form of neural tube defect (NTD) in which the spinal column is open. There are several forms or degrees of severity. One of the most severe types, *anencephaly,* is discussed on p. 40. *Encephalocele,* a somewhat analogous disorder, is reviewed on p. 52. *Spina bifida occulta* (SBO), the least severe, refers to a defect in a single vertebral arch (usually lumbosacral). It may be apparent only on a radiograph and is usually not noticeable on the surface except for the presence of a small tuft of hair or skin dimple which may be present over the affected area. The spinal cord and nerves are usually normal and there are no neurological symptoms. A *meningocele* refers to a defect in more than one or two vertebrae, the meninges extending into a sac covered with skin. *Myelomeningocele* indicates a defect which contains not only the meninges but also the spinal cord and nerves. Commonly myelomeningocele is associated with displacement caudally of the medulla and part of the cerebellum into the spinal canal which leads to obstruction and consequent hydrocephaly, and with descent of the upper cervical nerve roots from the intervertebral foramina toward the spinal cord. This is known as the *Arnold-Chiari malformation.* The most common site is lumbosacral, less often cervical. *Rachischisis* implies almost complete failure of fusion, widely exposing the nervous tissue which at times shows considerable overgrowth but becomes necrotic either shortly before birth or almost immediately postnatally.

Specific Diagnosis Diagnosis is based on clinical appearance, neurologic deficits, transillumination, and radiographic evidence. Lower motor neuron type loss with absent reflexes, loss of sphincter control, and segmental sensory loss is typical of myelomeningocele in the lumbosacral area. The higher the lesion and the greater its extent, the greater the deficit.

Differential Diagnosis Since an elevated α-fetoprotein level is a crucial finding in the prenatal diagnosis of spinal cord anomalies, it is important to know that raised levels may also be found in *fetal demise, twins, fetal blood contamination, skin defect, tracheo-esophageal fistula, omphalocele, cystic hygroma, encephalocele, congenital nephrosis,* etc.

Prenatal Diagnosis Ultrasonography and, especially, elevated α-fetoprotein levels at 10–15 weeks' gestation are of considerable help in diagnosis of open NTD. However, the small or closed defect may be missed. Acetylcholinesterase assay of the amniotic fluid is an excellent adjunct.

Basic Defect, Genetics, and Other Considerations As with anencephaly, spina bifida results from abnormal closure of the neural tube at about 28 days. Another theory suggests that it results from secondary rupture of a previously closed tube. Various studies have shown that the frequency of NTD varies with time, place, sex, ethnic groups, social class, and maternal age. The isolated malformation appears to exhibit multifactorial inheritance. The risk of recurrence in a family with one affected child is approximately 3–4%. The frequency of all types of NTD is approximately 1 to 2 per 1000 births. In the United States, about 3000–6000 infants are born with NTD each year.

Prognosis and Treatment Rachischisis is not compatible with life. With early treatment of the other types, more than 80–90% survive. No treatment is required for SBO. The meningocele is reduced by the neurosurgeon usually without resultant impairment. Myelomeningocele, depending on size and position, nearly always results in neurologic deficit. Yet, following repair, nearly all such affected children are able to stand in braces and platforms by one or two years of age and even those with high lesions may be taught to ambulate with braces and crutches. Appropriate orthopedic bracing and/or fusion may be required for the kyphosis and scoliosis. Most (70–90%) will develop hydrocephaly. Modern shunt technology or furosemide will allow most to have normal intellect. Ultrasound in infancy and later CT scans should be periodically employed to detect subtle changes. Urinary incontinence, reflux, hydronephrosis, and pyelonephritis formerly led to early death, but reimplantation of ureters, antibiotics, medication to alter bladder and sphincter tone, or artificial sphincters have drastically improved prognosis. Fecal incontinence has been treated successfully by biofeedback, bowel stimulation, and dietary management.

REFERENCES

Hunt, G.M. Spina bifida: implications for 100 children at school. *Develop. Med. Child. Neurol. 23:* 160–172, 1981.

Shurtleff, D.B., Hayden, P.W., Loeser, J.D. et al. Myelodysplasia. Decision for death or disability. *N. Engl. J. Med. 291:* 1005–1011, 1974.

Stein, S.C., Schut, L., and Ames, M.D. Selection for early treatment of myelomeningocele: a retrospective analysis of selection procedures. *Develop. Med. Child. Neurol. 17:* 311–319, 1975.

Spinal Cord Anomalies

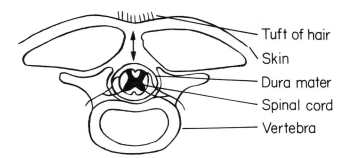

Tuft of hair
Skin
Dura mater
Spinal cord
Vertebra

Spina bifida occulta (arrow shows defect)

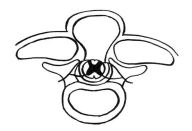

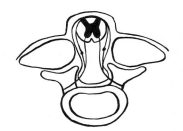

Meningocele

Meningomyelocele

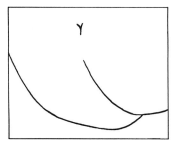

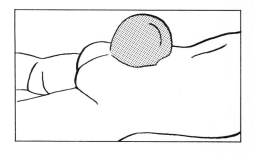

Skin dimple over site of spina bifida

Meningocele-lumbosacral area

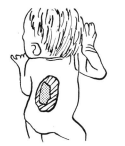

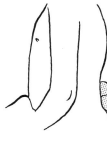

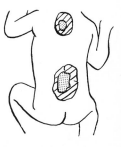

Meningomyelocele-dorsolumbar, lumbar and thoracolumbar

35. STURGE-WEBER ANOMALY

Clinical Features The Sturge-Weber anomaly is characterized by unilateral venous angiomatosis of the leptomeninges, ipsilateral facial angiomatosis, ipsilateral gyriform calcifications of the cerebral cortex, seizures, mental retardation, hemiplegia, and ocular defects. A nevus flammeus lesion occurs on the ipsilateral side of the face in approximately 90% of patients. The nevus may extend onto the neck, chest, and back. Occasionally bilateral facial nevus or no facial nevus may occur. Color varies from pink to purplish red and rarely decreases in intensity with age. The characteristic brain lesion consists of the unilateral thin-walled angioma in the leptomeninges overlying the posterior temporal, posterior parietal, and occipital areas. Occasionally bilateral involvement may be present. Seizures, usually focal, rarely generalized, have been noted in 90% of the cases; the symptoms appear during infancy and occur contralateral to the angiomatosis. Hemiparesis is less frequent. At least 30% of patients exhibit mental deficiency. With extensive cerebral changes, retardation may be pronounced. Choroidal angioma is common, and glaucoma is not an uncommon complication. Any of the various findings associated with the Klippel-Trenaunay-Weber syndrome may be included with the Sturge-Weber anomaly, including macrocephaly. Intraoral angiomatosis occurs most frequently on the buccal mucosa and lips (macrocheilia). The palate is less frequently affected. Tongue involvement may be accompanied by hemihyperplasia. Gingival vascular lesions, when present, may range from mild enlargement to monstrous overgrowth making closure of the mouth impossible.

Specific Diagnosis The diagnosis is essentially a clinical one. Gyriform, double-contoured lines of calcification develop in the underlying cerebral cortex usually after the second year of life. Rarely they may be present at birth. The radiographic appearance is pathognomonic for the disorder. Calcific deposits become stationary, usually by the end of the second decade. Electroencephalographic studies are abnormal, usually revealing unilateral depression of cortical activity.

Differential Diagnosis The relationship between the Sturge-Weber anomaly and the *Klippel-Trenaunay-Weber syndrome* is usually not a problem, though the two may exist concurrently and may well represent the same basic disorder in a different site. Transitory nevus flammeus lesions during the neonatal period are extremely common; however, in many cases they may not be as intense in color as the Sturge-Weber lesion, which tends to be darker and more frequently unilateral in distribution. Although the facial nevus in the Sturge-Weber anomaly varies considerably in extent, dark supraocular involvement should arouse suspicion. The association of macrocephaly and angiomatosis may occur in *disseminated hemiangiomatosis, neurofibromatosis, Beckwith-Wiedemann syndrome, Klippel-Trenaunay-Weber syndrome,* and *cutis marmorata telangiectatica congenita.*

Prenatal Diagnosis There is no technique currently available for prenatal diagnosis of the disorder but if the nevus were extensive, it might be seen on fetoscopy.

Basic Defect, Genetics, and Other Considerations The basic defect is due to a form of embryologic anomaly with secondary sequences. During the sixth week of embryonic development, a vascular plexus develops around the cephalic portion of the neural tube and under the ectoderm destined to become the facial skin. Normally the vascular plexus regresses during the ninth week, but in the Sturge-Weber anomaly it persists, resulting in angiomatosis of the ipsilateral side. Variation in the degree of persistence or regression of the plexus accounts for cases of bilateral involvement and also for cases with unilateral occurrence in which angioma of the leptomeninges occurs in the absence of facial involvement. Perhaps some form of altered vascular dynamics results in precipitation of calcium deposits in the cerebral cortex underlying the angioma, which in turn probably give rise to seizures and mental deficiency. All cases reported to date have been sporadic. There is neither sex nor ethnic predilection.

Prognosis and Treatment Prognosis depends on whether there are seizures and/or mental retardation associated with the disorder. The seizures can be treated by standard anticonvulsive therapy. The nevus flammeus lesions can be covered by various cosmetic pastes.

REFERENCES

Andriola, M. and Stolfi, J. Sturge-Weber syndrome. *Am. J. Dis. Child. 123:* 507–510, 1972.

Chao, D.H.C. Congenital neurocutaneous syndromes of childhood. III. Sturge-Weber disease. *J. Pediatr. 55:* 635–649, 1959.

Peterman, A.F., Hayles, A.B., Dockerty, M.B., et al. Encephalotrigeminal angiomatosis (Sturge-Weber disease): clinical study of 35 cases. *JAMA 167:* 2169–2176, 1958.

M.R. [+ / some]

- unilateral angiomatosis about face, chest, and upper extremity
- seizures
- glaucoma on ipsilateral side

Sturge-Weber Anomaly

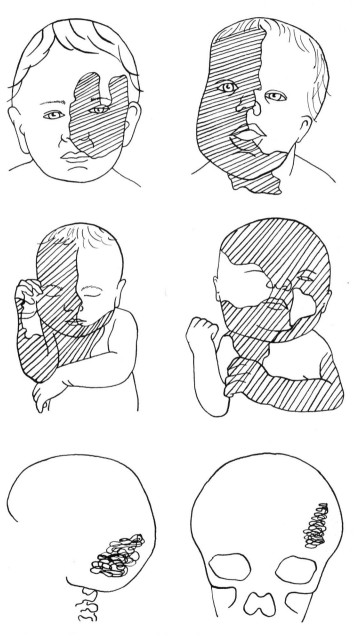

Nevus flammeus mainly unilateral about face
with facial hypertrophy, eye, forehead, upper chest
and extremity—areas of intracranial calcification

36. VATER ASSOCIATION

Clinical Features VATER is an acronym used to describe a group of anomalies that cluster with a greater than random tendency. An expanded version of the anomalies include: V = vertebral or vascular abnormalities; A = anal malformations; TE = tracheoesophageal fistula, esophageal atresia; and R = radial limb or renal anomalies.

Specific Diagnosis Diagnosis is clinical. Usually the tracheoesophageal fistula or the anal malformation will bring the association to mind. Most clinicians are reluctant to employ the term VATER association unless at least three of the components are present. Cardiac malformations occur in approximately 60% of patients. In about two-thirds of this number, the cardiac malformation is ventricular septal defect, with atrial septal defect and tetralogy of Fallot being seen about one-fifth as often as the former. Approximately two out of every three VATER infants have renal anomalies, about 40% having unilateral aplasia. Various other anomalies have been noted such as contractural ureteropelvic obstruction, crossed renal ectopia, or pelvic kidney and horseshoe kidney. Approximately 60% have anal-rectal abnormalities. High (supralevator) imperforate anus is at least twice as common as low (infralevator) imperforate anus. Tracheoesophageal malformations are found in almost 85%. Virtually all of the tracheoesophageal malformations involve esophageal atresia with distal tracheoesophageal fistula. Approximately 60% have either vertebral and/or radial limb abnormalities, none of which require therapy. Among the vertebral anomalies, hemivertebrae and sacral deformity are about equally frequent. Absent radius occurs half as often as either anomalies of the sacrum or hemivertebrae.

Differential Diagnosis Differential diagnosis involves any of the anomalies seen individually or any of the manifold syndromes into which any of the anomalies might individually occur, for example various chromosomal anomalies (+18, 13q−, 4p−, 6q−), the *thrombocytopenia-radial aplasia syndrome,* etc.

Prenatal Diagnosis There is no technique available for the prenatal diagnosis of this condition, but ultrasonography could detect certain components (vertebral, renal, and radial anomalies) of this association.

Basic Defect, Genetics, and Other Considerations The majority of the anomalies found involve defects of septation. Based on the concurrence of anomalies, it has been assumed that an intrauterine event is probably responsible for maldevelopment in multiple organ systems, most likely involving developing mesoderm, the event occurring between the fourth and seventh intrauterine week, that is during differentiation of the various organ systems. Virtually all cases have been sporadic with no recognized teratogen or chromosomal abnormality.

Prognosis and Treatment Overall survival is approximately 75%. Cardiac failure, if it occurs, is usually associated with more complicated lesions and is the most common cause of mortality. Considering the multiplicity of anomalies and the need for operative procedures in almost every patient, it is surprising that catch-up growth occurs and weight-for-height is usually in the range of the 25th percentile by the beginning of the fourth year of life. By five years of age, the majority of infants achieve the 50th percentile in growth. Tracheoesophageal fistula is routinely treated with gastrostomy under local anesthesia shortly after birth, with delayed thoracotomy for definitive repair of the anomaly. Infants with supralevator imperforate anus have a diverting colotomy at the time of placement of the gastrostomy, the delay allowing for treatment of pulmonary complications and permitting initiation of digitalis and diuretic therapy if cardiac failure is present. Gastroesophageal reflux is common following tracheoesophageal repair and fundoplication may be necessary for prevention of aspiration pneumonia. Infants with infralevator imperforate anus should have peroneal anoplasty early in infancy, while pull-through operations for supralevator anal malformations are performed at approximately one year of age. Postcardiac and renal anomalies do not require operation. Antibiotic prophylaxis should be provided to those infants with cardiac lesions during performance of other surgical procedures.

REFERENCES

Greenwood, R.D. and Rosenthal, A. Cardiovascular malformations associated with tracheo-esophageal fistula and esophageal atresia. *Pediatrics 57:* 87–91, 1976.

Kwan, L. and Smith, D.W. The VATER association. *J. Pediatr. 82:* 104–107, 1973.

Weber, T.R., Smith, W., and Grosfeld, J.L. Surgical experience in infants with the VATER association. *J. Pediatr. Surg. 15:* 849–854, 1980.

- vertebral or vascular anomalies
- anal malformation
- T-E fistula / esophageal atresia
- radial or renal anomalies

VATER Association

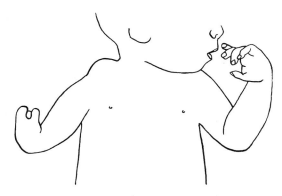

Radial aplasia, ectrodactyly – child has tracheoesophageal fistula

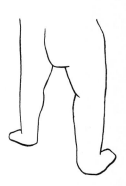

Hypoplasia left leg and absent anal opening

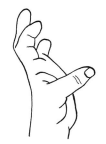 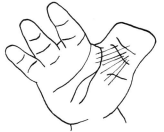 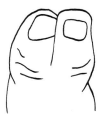 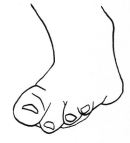

Stiff tapering thumb, syndactyly of thumb, preaxial polydactyly and syndactyly of toes 3–4 with absent 5th toe

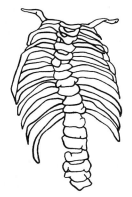

Multiple vertebral and rib anomalies

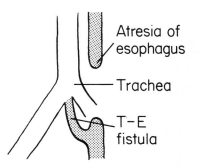

Atresia of esophagus

Trachea

T–E fistula

Most T–E malformations involve esophageal atresia with distal T–E fistula

C. Genetic Syndromes
a. Chromosomal

37. 3q +

Clinical Features Birth is usually spontaneous and at term with birth weight somewhat reduced (mean of 2800 g). In addition to severe mental and somatic retardation and hypotonia, the facies is rather characteristic. The features include microcephaly, plagiocephaly, seizures, persistent lanugo (hypertrichosis), square shaped face, confluent and dense eyebrows (synophrys), long curly eyelashes, congenital glaucoma, mongoloid obliquity of palpebral fissures, ocular hypertelorism, epicanthus, strabismus, lowset or malformed pinnae, broad nasal bridge, short nose with anteverted nostrils, long philtrum, thin and inverted upper lip, prominent maxilla, retracted lower lip, downturned corners of mouth, microretrognathia, short triangular chin, and short or webbed neck. Cleft palate or bifid uvula has been noted in nearly all cases. The cry may be low pitched and growling. Alterations in the digits include retroflexed toes, syndactyly, clinodactyly of fifth fingers, and proximally placed thumbs. The thorax is often deformed. The nipples are often widely separated. The extremities tend to be short and talipes is relatively common. Edema of the hands and feet is occasionally noted at birth. Congenital heart anomalies noted in over 75% of the cases include tetralogy of Fallot and other septal defects. Urogenital malformations observed in 60–70% include renal cortical cyst or duplications, bicornuate uterus, double vagina, cryptorchism. Hearing loss has been reported in several cases.

Specific Diagnosis Skeletal anomalies are not striking. Hemivertebrae have been noted in about 25% of the cases. Phalangeal anomalies have been relatively nonspecific. Simian palmar creases appear to be increased. Increased finger-print arches or low ridge counts are frequent. Galactose-1-phosphate uridyl transferase activity is higher in the red blood cells in these children.

Differential Diagnosis There is considerable clinical similarity with the *deLange syndrome* due to failure to thrive, profound mental retardation, microcephaly, brachycephaly, short nose with anteverted nostrils, long eyelashes, synophrys, etc. Edema of the hands and feet may suggest *Turner* or *Noonan syndrome*.

Prenatal Diagnosis If a parent is a known balanced carrier, amniocentesis should be carried out.

Basic Defect, Genetics, and Other Considerations The basic anomaly is trisomy for part of the long arm of chromosome 3, most often involving segments 3q12→qter. Trisomy for the longer segment 3q12→qter does not appear to be more severe. In most cases there has been a balanced translocation in one of the parents, but pericentric inversion has been found in one of the parents in a few cases. Rarely it is de novo. Trisomy for 3q12→q27 has also been reported. Hypertrichosis appears to be associated with trisomy for the 3q21→q25 segment. Clinically there is no significant difference between dup(3q) and dup(3q)del(3p) syndromes. About 40 cases have been reported.

Prognosis and Treatment Death before 12 months occurs in almost 40%. Most of these have had severe heart or renal anomalies. In those that survive, there is severe somatic and mental retardation. All have repeated seizures and recurrent infections. Treatment is supportive.

REFERENCES

Steinbach, R., Adkins, W.N., Jr., Caspar, H. et al. The dup(3q) syndrome: report of eight cases and review of the literature. *Am. J. Med. Genet. 10:* 159–178, 1981.

Stengel-Rutkowski, S., Murken, J.D., Pilar, V. et al. Partial trisomy 3q. *Eur. J. Pediatr. 130:* 111–125, 1979.

Yunis, E., Quintero, L., Casteñeda, A. et al. Partial trisomy 3q. *Hum. Genet. 48:* 315–320, 1979.

M.R. [+ / all]

- **asymmetric cranio-stenosis**
- **hypertrichosis**
- **square-shaped face**
- **thin, inverted upper lip / retracted lower lip**

3q+

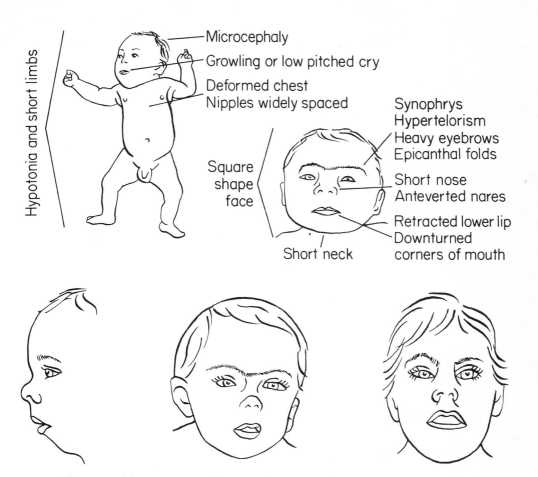

Hypotonia and short limbs

Microcephaly
Growling or low pitched cry
Deformed chest
Nipples widely spaced

Square shape face

Short neck

Synophrys
Hypertelorism
Heavy eyebrows
Epicanthal folds

Short nose
Anteverted nares

Retracted lower lip
Downturned corners of mouth

Micrognathia, anteverted nares, heavy eyebrows, curly lashes, strabismus, upward slant of palpebral fissures and epicanthal folds

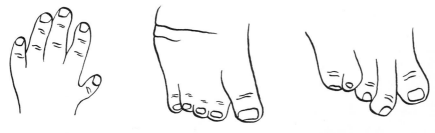

Proximal thumb, retroflexed toes and syndactyly 2-4 and 4-5

89

38. 4p −

Clinical Features This syndrome, also known as the Wolf-Hirschhorn syndrome or del(4p) syndrome, is characterized by very severe psychomotor and growth retardation. The phenotype is reasonably characteristic and does not change with time as in the cri-du-chat syndrome. Because of its rare occurrence, however, the phenotype is less familiar. Nevertheless, clinicians who have seen several patients or clinical photographs of affected infants will often make a presumptive diagnosis before the cytogenetic evidence is available. Despite normal gestation time, birth weight is usually reduced (ca. 2000 g). Fetal activity is diminished and when born the child is characteristically hypotonic. Marked microcephaly and seizures are constant and often there is dolichocephaly. Midline scalp defects have been noted in about 10%. The forehead is high. A wide nasal bridge and ocular hypertelorism are virtually constant features. The eyebrows are somewhat sparse medially. Ptosis of the eyelids, antimongoloid obliquity of the palpebral fissures, and divergent strabismus have been noted in approximately half the cases. Less frequent are coloboma of the iris and corectopia. The ears have narrow external canals and are low-set with adherent lobes. Approximately one-third of the patients have a preauricular dimple or sinus. The philtrum is short and deep and the mouth usually has downturned corners. In over half of the cases there is cleft lip or especially cleft palate and micrognathia.

Specific Diagnosis The facial stigmata often lead to the diagnosis. Congenital heart malformations, most often atrial or ventricular septal defects, and seizures have been noted in about 50%. Cryptorchidism and especially hypospadias are commonly found in affected males and absent uterus and streak gonads have been described. A wide spectrum of renal anomalies has been described. The trunk is long and the limbs are thin. Talipes equinovarus is relatively common. Several patients have exhibited dimpling over the sacrum, shoulders, elbows, and knees. Radiographic findings are not especially striking. The pelvic and carpal bones are late in ossification and pseudoepiphyses are seen in the phalanges and at the base of each metacarpal. Dermatoglyphic changes are also not remarkably altered: single transverse palmar crease has been present in about 25%, dermal ridges are frequently hypoplastic with increased arch patterns. There may be supernumerary flexion creases on the first and second digits.

Differential Diagnosis Occasionally the midline scalp defect and cleft lip and/or cleft palate may cause the clinician to briefly consider *13 trisomy*. However, we believe the phenotype is sufficiently different so that this error should not be made.

Prenatal Diagnosis If one parent is a known balanced translocation carrier, karyotype analysis using amniocentesis should be carried out.

Basic Defect, Genetics, and Other Considerations The basic defect is due to partial deletion of the short arm of chromosome 4, specifically the 4p16 band. In most cases one-third to two-thirds of the short arm is deleted. The deletion may be due to translocation, occurring in perhaps 10–15% of the cases. There have been several examples in which a ring chromosome 4 has been formed, but in over 85% of the cases the deletion is de novo. The oldest known living patient is approximately 30 years of age. This chromosomal state is not found among abortions spontaneously lost within the first trimester of pregnancy. At least 100 case reports have been published. The frequency appears to be about 1 per 50,000 births. There appears to be a 2F:1M sex predilection.

Prognosis and Treatment Mental retardation is severe. At least 35% of the patients die during the first two years of life but some survive to adult life. Treatment is supportive.

REFERENCES

Fryns, J.P., Eggermont, E., Verresen, H. et al. The 4p− syndrome, with a report of two new cases. *Humangenetik 19:* 99–109, 1973.

Johnson, V.P., Mulder, R.D., and Hosen, R. The Wolf-Hirschhorn (4p−) syndrome. *Clin. Genet. 10:* 104–112, 1976.

Lurie, I.W., Lazjuk, G.I., Ussova, Y.I. et al. The Wolf-Hirschhorn syndrome. *Clin. Genet. 17:* 375–384, 1980.

M.R. [+ / all]

4p−

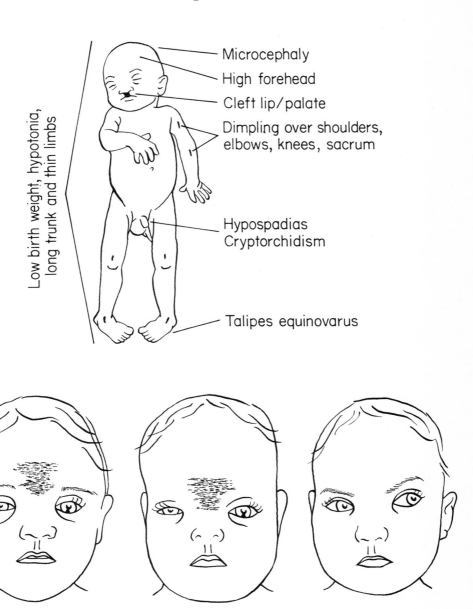

Microcephaly

High forehead

Cleft lip/palate

Dimpling over shoulders, elbows, knees, sacrum

Hypospadias
Cryptorchidism

Talipes equinovarus

Low birth weight, hypotonia, long trunk and thin limbs

Hemangioma on forehead, ptosis, epicanthal folds, hypertelorism, iris coloboma, short, deep philtrum, small downcurved mouth and short neck

39. 4p+

Clinical Features The consistent finding is psychomotor retardation. Noted with a frequency of 50% or more are postnatal growth retardation, microcephaly, prominent glabellar or supraorbital ridge, deep-set eyes, ocular hypertelorism, short (usually large) nose with rounded tip, broad and depressed nasal bridge, apparent macrostomia, pointed or prominent chin, abnormal form and size (usually large) and posterior rotation of pinnae, short neck with low hairline, and micropenis. Puberty is probably delayed. Somewhat less common (25–49%) are neonatal feeding problems, seizures, strabismus which resolves by six months, hypertonia, hypotonia, flexion contractures, scoliosis, clinodactyly of fifth fingers, camptodactyly, abnormal length of fingers, hallux valgus, prominent heels, widely spaced nipples, cryptorchidism, hypoplastic scrotum, hypospadias. Inguinal hernia and congenital heart disease have been noted in about 15%. Various additional eye anomalies seen in 15–20% include microphthalmia, nystagmus, antimongoloid obliquity of palpebral fissures, asymmetry in size of eyes or pupils, synophrys, and long bushy eyebrows. Other less constant facial anomalies include long philtrum, thin lips, and downturned angles of mouth.

Specific Diagnosis Diagnosis is made by chromosome analysis. Dermatoglyphic changes are not very striking. Digital whorls were found to be in excess and there is often a distal t' triradius in the palm. Abnormal electroencephalograms have been noted in over 50%. Radiographic changes are not very striking: digital impressions (35%), small sella (20%), early closure of fontanel (20%), and hypoplasia of mandible (20%), abnormal length of cervical and thoracic vertebral bodies (25%), hypoplasia of single ribs (25%), scoliosis (30%), hypoplastic middle and/or distal phalanges (30%), and delayed bone age (65%).

Differential Diagnosis Probably not easily diagnosed on clinical grounds, since most diagnoses have been arrived at by performing a karyotype on a child with mental retardation and multiple malformations.

Prenatal Diagnosis Possible, since in nearly all cases one of the parents has a balanced chromosomal translocation or other anomaly.

Basic Defect, Genetics, and Other Considerations The basic defect is trisomy for the short arm of chromosome 4. In most cases the trisomy has been for most or all of the short arm. There does not appear to be good correlation between the amount of short arm replication and clinical stigmata. Over 35 cases have been reported. There is no sex predilection. While several mechanisms have been described, about 85% have arisen from a balanced translocation, most involving an acrocentric chromosome (usually 22, 21, or 15), in one of the parents. The risk of transmission to an offspring is about 15% from a parent of either sex. Among normal offspring, about one-half are carriers, as would be expected. The frequency of stillbirths is increased.

Prognosis and Treatment Death has occurred prior to the age of two years in about 25% from infections, respiratory complications,or congenital heart disease. While intelligence quotients have ranged from 20 to 65, about an equal number are only moderately affected.

REFERENCES

Crane, J., Sujansky, E., and Smith, A. 4p trisomy syndrome: report of 4 additional cases and segregation analysis of 21 families with different translocations. *Am. J. Med. Genet. 4:* 219–229, 1979.

Gonzalez, C.H., Sommer, A.M., Meisner, L.F. et al. The trisomy 4p syndrome: case report and review. *Am. J. Med. Genet. 1:* 137–156, 1977.

Qazi, Q.H., Madahar, C., Kanchanapoomi, R. et al. Partial chromosome 4 trisomy. *Clin. Genet. 20:* 179–184, 1981.

- microcephaly
- prominent glabella
- bulbous nose
- pointed chin

4p+

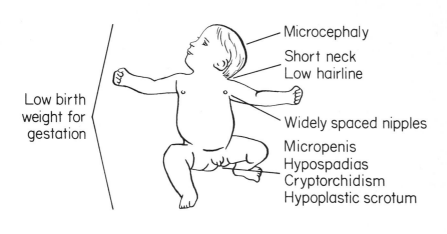

Low birth weight for gestation

Microcephaly
Short neck
Low hairline
Widely spaced nipples
Micropenis
Hypospadias
Cryptorchidism
Hypoplastic scrotum

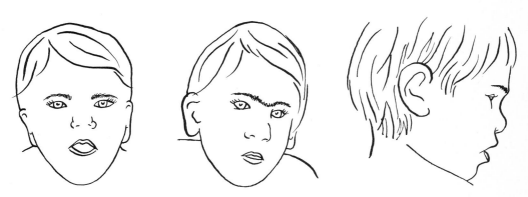

Hypertelorism, synophrys, heavy eyebrows, depressed nasal bridge, bulbous nose, pointed chin, large dysplastic ears, long philtrum, thin lips and short neck with low hairline

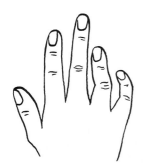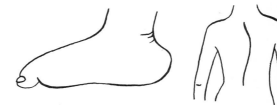

Long fingers, camptodactyly, clinodactyly, prominent heel and scoliosis

40. 4q −

Clinical Features Several reported cases have established the existence of the 4q− syndrome which exhibits a rather characteristic phenotype. While birth weight is normal, mild postnatal growth retardation, microcephaly of variable degree, and mild to moderately severe mental retardation are common features. Craniofacial abnormalities include cranial contour anomalies, lowset posteriorly rotated pinnae with malformed helices, usually a depressed nasal bridge with an abbreviated nose having anteverted nostrils and short septum, and micrognathia. Cleft palate, with or without cleft lip, is common as is ocular hypertelorism, epicanthal folds, and laterally displaced inner canthi. Originally stressed but with a frequency of less than 30% are antimongoloid obliquity of the palpebral fissures and oropharyngeal hypotonia, cardiac defects, especially ASD and VSD, limited extension at the elbow, clinodactyly of the fifth finger, transverse palmar crease, and displacement of toes. Various anomalies have occurred with a frequency of 25% or less. These have included low-set posteriorly rotated ears and various digital-skeletal anomalies including proximally implanted thumbs, camptodactyly, short distal phalanx of the fifth finger, absence of fourth metacarpal, dislocated hips, and talipes equinovarus. Electroencephalographic abnormalities and seizures have not been common findings.

Specific Diagnosis Diagnosis is made on karyotype. There are no specific radiographic findings.

Differential Diagnosis Most diagnoses arrived at by doing karyotypes on children with mental retardation and multiple malformations.

Prenatal Diagnosis Possible in approximately 10% of the cases in which one parent is a known balanced translocation carrier.

Basic Defect, Genetics, and Other Considerations The basic defect is due to partial deletion of the long arm of chromosome 4, specifically the terminal segment from 4q31→qter. A few cases of interstitial deletion of the long arm of 4 have been reported having rather variable phenotypes. Although it has been inferred that 4q33→qter has a milder phenotype, our experience would not support this finding.

Prognosis and Treatment About 70% of the patients have died within the first two years of life from congenital heart disease or oropharyngeal incoordination with resultant pneumonia. Those that survive exhibit moderate to severe mental retardation and mild growth retardation. Treatment is supportive.

REFERENCES

Frias, J.L., Nelson, R.M., and Ray, S.L. Deletion of the long arm of chromosome 4: a clinically identifiable syndrome? *Birth Defects 14(6C):* 355–358, 1978.

Mitchell, J.A., Packman, S., Loughman, W.D. et al.

Deletions of different segments of the long arm of chromosome 4. *Am. J. Med. Genet. 8:* 73–89, 1981.

Townes, P.L., White, M., DiMarzo, S.V. The 4q-syndrome. *Am. J. Dis. Child. 133:* 383–385, 1979.

- **abnormal head shape**
- **short nose /
  anteverted nares**
- **low set,
  dysplastic ears**
- **micrognathia**

4q−

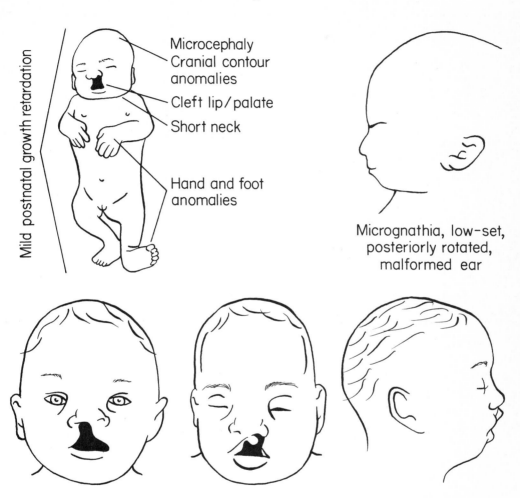

Mild postnatal growth retardation

Microcephaly
Cranial contour
anomalies
Cleft lip/palate
Short neck

Hand and foot
anomalies

Micrognathia, low-set,
posteriorly rotated,
malformed ear

Cleft lip/palate, epicanthal folds, hypertelorism, depressed
nasal bridge, anteverted nares and micrognathia

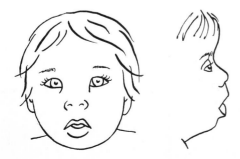

Hypertelorism, epicanthal folds,
depressed nasal bridge,
anteverted nares and micrognathia

41. 4q+

Clinical Features In addition to the severe psychomotor retardation which has been evident in most cases, cardiac and genitourinary anomalies are frequent. Birth weight has been low in about half the cases. Microcephaly with sloping forehead is common. The facies is somewhat variable for the most frequently observed features include epicanthal folds, bushy eyebrows, hypertelorism, strabismus, narrow palpebral fissures, antimongoloid obliquity of palpebral fissures, large or prominent nasal bridge, straight nasofrontal angle, short philtrum with protruding lateral margins, downturned corners of the mouth, a horizontal dimple beneath the lower lip, microretrognathia, pointed chin; low-set, posteriorly rotated, or malformed pinnae with prominent anthelix and hypoplastic tragus; and short neck. Hyper- or hypotonia has been noted in over 60% and umbilical or inguinal hernia in about 30%. Cardiovascular anomalies noted in about one-half the cases have included tetralogy of Fallot and various venous-return anomalies. Genitourinary anomalies seen in about half the patients include horseshoe kidney, renal hypoplasia, urethrovesicular reflux with or without hydronephrosis. Cryptorchidism is a constant feature. The hands may have unusual form and the feet are often malformed with rockerbottom heels.

Specific Diagnosis Diagnosis is established by chromosome karyotype. Radiographic changes include microcephaly, wide cranial sutures, variable rib anomalies (short first rib, deficient rib, extra rib), various thumb abnormalities (bifurcated thumb, absent thumb, bifurcated index finger, digitalization of thumb). The most common dermatoglyphic alteration is simian creases.

Differential Diagnosis This disorder does not resemble other conditions. Most diagnoses are arrived at by doing karyotype of child with severe mental retardation with multiple malformations.

Prenatal Diagnosis This can be done if one of the parents is carrying a balanced translocation.

Basic Defect, Genetics, and Other Considerations The condition is due to trisomy for part of the long arm of chromosome 4. In 90% of the cases, one of the parents had a balanced translocation. These have ranged from 4q21→qter to 4q32→qter. A clear correlation between karyotype and phenotype cannot be established. When accompanied by a partial monosomy, the phenotype of the monosomy may prevail.

Prognosis and Treatment Prognosis is poor due to marked psychomotor retardation. Neonatal mortality of about 30% occurs in those with more severe cardiac or renal anomalies. Treatment is supportive.

REFERENCES

Cervenka, J., Djavadi, G.R., and Gorlin, R.J. Partial trisomy 4q syndrome: case report and review. *Hum. Genet. 34:* 1–7, 1976.

Sparkes, R.S., Francke, U., Muller, H. et al. Partial 4q duplication due to inherited der(20),t(4;20) (q25;q13) mat. *Ann. Génét. 20:* 31–35, 1977.

Stella, M., Bonfante, A., Ronconi, G. et al. Partial trisomy 4q: two cases with a familial translocation t(4;18)(q27;q23). *Hum. Genet. 47:* 245–251, 1979.

M.R. [+ / all]

- **microcephaly**
- **narrow palpebral fissures**
- **large nasal bridge**
- **short philtrum**

4q+

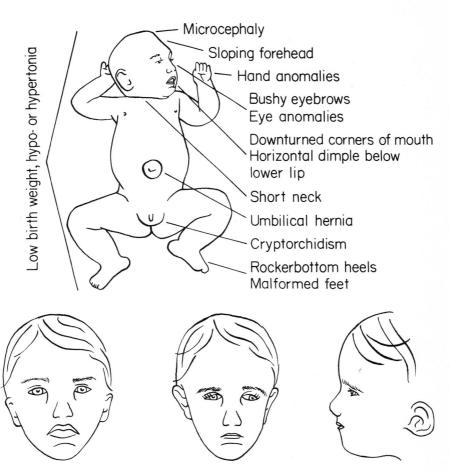

Low birth weight, hypo- or hypertonia

Microcephaly
Sloping forehead
Hand anomalies
Bushy eyebrows
Eye anomalies
Downturned corners of mouth
Horizontal dimple below lower lip
Short neck
Umbilical hernia
Cryptorchidism
Rockerbottom heels
Malformed feet

Epicanthal folds, bushy eyebrows, downward slant of palpebral fissures, strabismus, short philtrum, downward corners of mouth, horizontal dimple, low-set, malformed ears

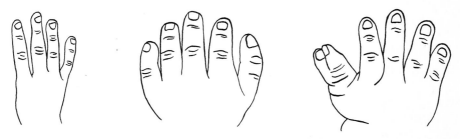

Absent, digitalization and bifurcated thumb anomalies

42. 5p −

Clinical Features This syndrome, often referred to as the cri-du-chat syndrome, is characterized by a high, shrill cry similar to that of a cat. However, the cry is not pathognomonic, since it has been reported in other chromosomal disorders, nor is it present in all patients with this disorder. The child exhibits microcephaly, ocular hypertelorism, a round face, and marked somatic and mental retardation. There is usually muscular hypotonia, various congenital defects of the heart and genitourinary tract, and severe respiratory and feeding problems. The hallmarks noted at birth change with age so that it is rather difficult to make the diagnosis once infancy is past, for the cry disappears and the facies is no longer round. Most patients will then blend into the group of institutionalized severely mentally retarded individuals, if routine karyotyping has not been carried out.

Specific Diagnosis During infancy, microcephaly, round facies, antimongoloid obliquity of palpebral fissures, mild ocular hypertelorism, epicanthal folds, posteriorly rotated pinnae, preauricular tags, prominent nasal bridge, and micrognathia characterize the face. With time, the face becomes asymmetric and the plumpness is lost. The cat-cry usually disappears or changes pitch. The facial bones begin to change in relative growth and the hypertelorism and micrognathia are not as apparent. Malocclusion is common, especially overjet. The hair becomes prematurely gray. Hypotonia, so marked in infancy, disappears and the reflexes become hyperactive. The gait becomes shuffling. Radiographic changes are usually not marked, consisting most often of large frontal sinuses, scoliosis, and small wings of the ilia. Simian palmar creases have been noted in about 30%.

Differential Diagnosis Most diagnoses are arrived at by doing karyotype of child with severe mental retardation and multiple malformations.

Prenatal Diagnosis Possible if one parent is a known balanced translocation carrier.

Basic Defect, Genetics, and Other Considerations The basic defect is due to a partial deletion which may be either terminal or interstitial, of the short arm of chromosome 5 in the area of p14 to p15.1. This may result from either a de novo deletion of the short arm, including at least the p15.1 band (c. 85%), unbalanced translocation inherited from a parental carrier (c. 15%), or rarely due to ring formation with deletion of the proximate distal ends of the chromosome. The greater the deletion, the lower the intelligence, height, and weight. The precise frequency of this syndrome is not known, but it has been estimated to be about 1 in 50,000 births and that approximately 1% of institutionalized mentally retarded patients have this disorder.

Prognosis and Treatment Prognosis is not good. The patients are severely retarded and there is a reduced life span. The oldest known patient is now approximately 60 years of age. Treatment is supportive.

REFERENCES

Breg, W., Steele, M., Miller, O. et al. The cri-du-chat in adolescents and adults, clinical findings in 13 older patients with partial deletion of the short arm of chromosome No. 5 (5p−). *J. Pediatr. 77:* 782–791, 1970.

Gordon, R.R. and Cooke, P. Facial appearance in the cri-du-chat syndrome. *Develop. Med. Child. Neurol. 10:* 69–76, 1968.

Niebuhr, E. The cri-du-chat syndrome. *Hum. Genet. 42:* 143–152, 1978; 44: 227–275, 1978.

- **cat-like cry**
- **microcephaly**
- **round face**
- **hypertelorism**

5p−

Hypotonia, low birth weight

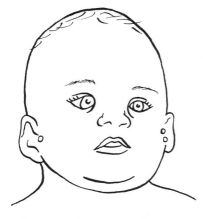

In infancy cords fail to approximate
posteriorly, producing a cat-like cry

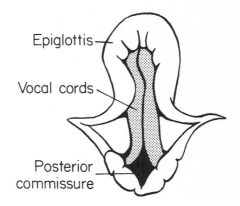

Epiglottis

Vocal cords

Posterior
commissure

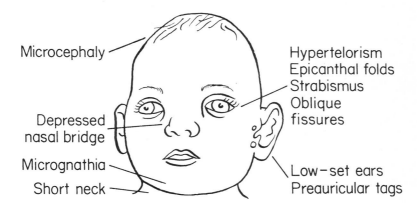

Microcephaly

Depressed
nasal bridge

Micrognathia

Short neck

Hypertelorism
Epicanthal folds
Strabismus
Oblique
fissures

Low-set ears
Preauricular tags

Round face

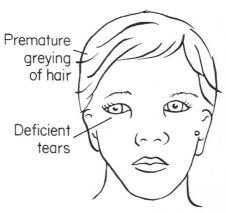

Premature
greying
of hair

Deficient
tears

Similar features
in another infant

Thin, asymmetric face
in older patient

43. 7q +

Clinical Features The syndrome of partial 7q trisomy produces rather characteristic facial malformations that should be clinically recognizable. Delayed development is usual and most have hypotonia. While head circumference is normal, there is often asymmetry of the skull with frontal bossing and/or prominence of the occiput. The scalp hair tends to be fuzzy. The palpebral fissures are horizontal but are narrow, long, and somewhat almond-shaped. Ocular hypertelorism is relatively common. The nose is rather small and with age becomes pointed. The upper lip has a tendency to overhang the lower one and macroglossia may be present. The mandible is small and cleft palate has been reported in several cases. The pinnae have a tendency to be low-set and posteriorly rotated. The neck is remarkably short. There are no characteristic limb anomalies but the nails tend to be hyperconvex.

Specific Diagnosis Diagnosis is made on chromosome karyotype.

Differential Diagnosis *Bilateral renal agenesis* (*Potter syndrome*) has a greater than chance association with this disorder.

Prenatal Diagnosis Possible, where one of the parents had a balanced translocation.

Basic Defect, Genetics, and Other Considerations Approximately 25 cases have been reported. All published examples have been due to malsegregation of a balanced parental translocation. Evidence is mounting that there are at least two syndromes: 7q31→qter and 7q32→qter. The latter is the more frequently reported disorder. Associated characteristics include severe mental retardation, hypotonia, and growth retardation. Plagiocephaly, frontal bossing, epicanthal folds, short nose with depressed bridge, and low-set poorly modeled pinnae characterize the facies and kyphoscoliosis is common. Less often noted signs include transverse palmar creases, colobomata, and various skeletal anomalies such as syndactyly and rib aplasia. Those with the larger duplication, i.e. 7q31→qter, in addition to the abovementioned signs, often have cleft palate, ocular hypertelorism, and congenital heart disease. In addition, there are a few cases in which only the segment 7q22→q31 is duplicated. The stigmata which are evident are retarded development, small palpebral fissures, ocular hypertelorism, strabismus, low-set ears, and fuzzy hair.

Prognosis and Treatment Life prognosis depends on the degree of chromosome duplication. Trisomy 7q32→qter appears to be compatible with life, while nearly all those with duplication for 7q31→qter die within the first year of life, probably due to the greater frequency of associated cerebral and cardiac malformations.

REFERENCES

Al Saadi, A. and Moghadam, A. Partial trisomy of the long arm of chromosome 7. *Clin. Genet. 9:* 250–254, 1976.

Schinzel, A. and Tönz, O. Partial trisomy 7q and probable partial monosomy of 5p. *Hum. Genet. 53: 121–124, 1979.*

Yunis, E., Ramirez, E., and Uribe, J.G. Full trisomy 7 and Potter syndrome. *Hum. Genet. 54:* 13–18, 1980.

M.R. [+ / all]

- **frontal bossing / prominent occiput**
- **narrow palpebral fissures**
- **upper lip extends over lower**
- **short neck**

7q+

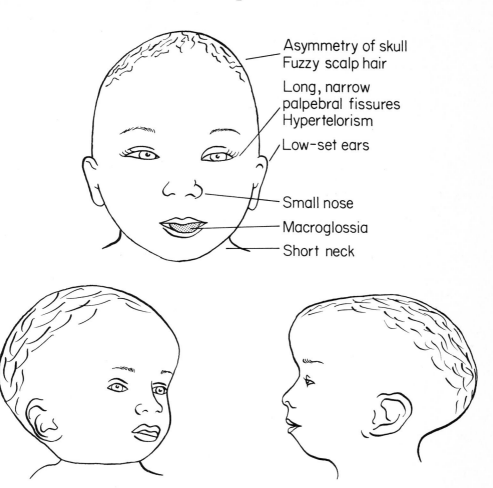

Asymmetry of skull
Fuzzy scalp hair

Long, narrow palpebral fissures
Hypertelorism

Low-set ears

Small nose

Macroglossia

Short neck

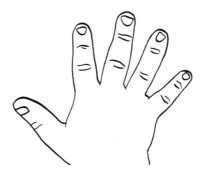

Note prominent occiput, frontal bossing, low-set ears, micrognathia

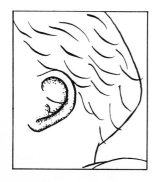

Cupping of outer helices and hyper-convex nails

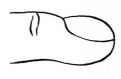

44. 8 TRISOMY

Clinical Features Trisomy 8, or more frequently trisomy 8 mosaicism syndrome, is probably the next most common autosomal chromosomal disorder following trisomies 21, 13, and 18. There does not appear to be any significant difference in phenotype between so-called pure trisomy 8 and trisomy 8 mosaicism. The most common findings are mental retardation (90%), seldom of a severe degree, contractures of the fingers and toes (70%), malformed pinnae (70%), vertebral abnormalities and/or scoliosis (55%), restricted articular functions, and progressive flexion contractures with advancing age. The forehead usually protrudes. Mild hypertelorism and strabismus are noted in over 50% of the patients. There is a broad upturned nose with anteverted nostrils and highly arched palate in about 60%. The mandible is small and retruded and the lower lip commonly everted in about 40%. Deep palmar and/or plantar furrows of a specific type have been found in about 75%. Although it has been suggested that the furrows disappear with age, we have seen examples of older individuals with very marked plantar furrows. Cryptorchidism has been noted in about 50%; hydronephrosis, hydroureter, or ureteral obstruction in 40%; and congenital heart disease in 25%.

Specific Diagnosis Most infants have normal birthweight for gestational age. The skull is often scaphocephalic. The sella may be unusually large. About one-third of the patients have had long slender trunk and slender pelvis, and about two-thirds have spinal deformity. Broad ribs, extra ribs, spina bifida occulta, and butterfly vertebrae are common. Nearly all of the patients have had contractions of the fingers or toes with generalized restricted joint function. Absent or hypoplastic patellae are frequent. Various cardiovascular defects have been seen in about 25%, usually VSD with pulmonary stenosis. The urinary tract deformities lead to hydronephrosis and/or hydroureter. Atypical agenesis of the corpus callosum may be more frequent than has been reported. Other dermatoglyphic alterations include low total finger ridge counts, bilateral arches on great toes, simian creases, and zygodactylous triradii on soles of feet.

Differential Diagnosis The phenotype is so characteristic that diagnosis can usually be arrived at clinically with great accuracy.

Prenatal Diagnosis Prenatal chromosome analysis is possible in cases where one of the parents carries a balanced translocation.

Basic Defect, Genetics, and Other Considerations The basic defect is trisomy for the number 8 chromosome. Far more common (85%) is mosaicism for trisomy 8. Several authors have found a reduction with age in the number of trisomic cells among lymphocytes, but maintenance of trisomy 8 in fibroblasts. A small but significant number of cases of partial trisomy 8 have resulted from balanced translocation from which it has been concluded that most phenotypic changes result from trisomy for the long arm. Approximately 80 cases of the disorder are known. The estimated frequency is about 1 per 25,000–50,000 children. There is a male predilection of at least 5:1. Paternal age is probably advanced. There are several examples of trisomy for 8q21→qter. In these children there are wide face, ocular hypertelorism, broad neck, unusual pinnae, cleft palate, and cardiac and renal anomalies. Trisomy for the short arm of chromosome 8 results in high forehead with frontal and parietal bossing but with temple retraction, full cheeks and round face, low nasal bridge, anteverted nostrils, wide mouth, everted lower lip, large ear lobes, and a short neck with redundant skin folds. Mental retardation is severe and absence of the corpus callosum can be demonstrated. Various congenital heart malformations have been reported.

Prognosis and Treatment The prognosis for normal life expectancy is good. The chief limitations are related to the degree of mental retardation. Especially marked is a discrepancy in language development. Orthopedic intervention may be necessary for correction of scoliosis and for treatment of contractures, which progress with age and which would otherwise be a secondary handicap problem.

REFERENCES

Annerén, G., Frodis, E., and Jorulf, H. Trisomy 8 syndrome. *Helv. Paediat. Acta 36:* 465–472, 1981.

Fineman, R.M., Ablow, R.C., Breg, W.R. et al. Complete and partial trisomy of different segments of chromosome 8: case report and review. *Clin. Genet. 16:* 390–396, 1979.

Riccardi, V.M. Trisomy 8: an international study of 70 patients. *Birth Defects 13(3C):* 171–184, 1977.

- **scaphocephaly**
- **anteverted nares**
- **thick everted lower lip**
- **deep furrows on palms and soles**

8 Trisomy

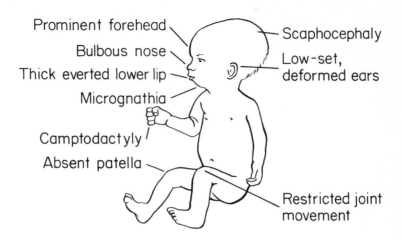

Prominent forehead — Scaphocephaly

Bulbous nose — Low-set, deformed ears

Thick everted lower lip —

Micrognathia —

Camptodactyly —

Absent patella —

Restricted joint movement

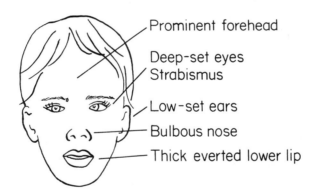

Prominent forehead

Deep-set eyes
Strabismus

Low-set ears

Bulbous nose

Thick everted lower lip

Facial features older child

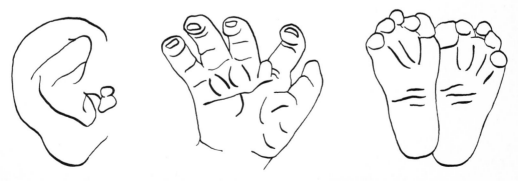

Deformed ear, contracture of digits, deep furrows on palms and soles

45. 9p−

Clinical Features A sufficient number of patients have been described so that it has become apparent that the 9p− syndrome may be clinically recognizable. All patients reported have had mental retardation and nearly all have had very mild microcephaly, trigonocephaly or prominent forehead, flat occiput, flat nasal bridge, anteverted nostrils, long philtrum; most have micrognathia or retrognathia with wide gonial angle, abnormal auricles, short neck, wide-set nipples, long fingers (usually due to long middle phalanges), and hyperconvex nails. Axial hypotonia and generalized hypertonia occur commonly in the neonatal period. Pre- and postnatal growth are usually normal. Adults are of normal height.

Specific Diagnosis In addition to the trigonocephaly and/or bulging metopic suture and flat occiput, the facies is reasonably constant in childhood but becomes less striking with age. The palpebral fissures have a mongoloid obliquity and most have epicanthal folds. The palpebral fissures are reduced in length and there is hypertelorism in approximately one-half the patients. The eyebrows are shaggy. Exotropia is less frequent. The nasal bridge is flat, the nostrils anteverted, the philtrum long, and the upper lip narrow. The mouth appears small, possibly due to short mandibular ramus with wide gonial angle. The palate is usually high-arched. The ears appear to be low-set and the ear canals narrow. The earlobes are dysmorphic. The neck is short with a low hairline. In about 50%, there is some webbing of the neck. The nipples are widely spaced. The trunk is often obese in adulthood, but the extremities are thin and fusiform. Con-genital heart defects and inguinal or umbilical hernia have been noted in about half of the patients. The less common genital abnormalities include hypospadias, small undescended testes, and small labia majora. Skeletal abnormalities have included mild scoliosis, limited flexion, clinodactyly or camptodactyly, and joint contractures. The fingernails and toenails have a tendency to be square. The fingers and/or toes have normal forms but are somewhat long, especially the second digit. Dermatoglyphic changes consist of increased numbers of whorls and excess finger creases.

Differential Diagnosis Some of these children slightly resemble those with *trisomy 21,* largely due to the mongoloid obliquity of the palpebral fissures.

Prenatal Diagnosis This is possible where one parent carries a balanced translocation.

Basic Defect, Genetics, and Other Considerations The basic defect is monosomy for the short arm of chromosome 9, the break appearing at band 9p22 in nearly all cases. In about 20% of the cases, the deletions have resulted from balanced parental translocations. The remainder are de novo deletions. There appears to be a 3:1 female predilection.

Prognosis and Treatment Mental retardation is a constant feature, no patient having an IQ greater than 50. Lifespan is of normal duration in the absence of severe internal malformations. Treatment is supportive.

REFERENCES

Fryns, J.P., Pedersen, J.C., Duyck, H. et al. Deletion of the short arm of chromosome 9. *Eur. J. Pediatr. 134:* 201–204, 1980.

Funderburk, S.J., Sparkes, R.S., and Klisak, I. The 9p− syndrome. *J. Med. Genet. 16:* 75–79, 1979.

Kuroki, Y., Yakota, S., Nakai, H. et al. A case of 9p− syndrome. *Hum. Genet. 38:* 107–111, 1977.

- **trigonocephaly**
- **flat occiput**
- **anteverted nares**
- **long philtrum**

9p−

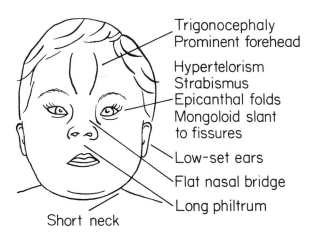

Trigonocephaly
Prominent forehead

Hypertelorism
Strabismus
Epicanthal folds
Mongoloid slant
to fissures

Low-set ears

Flat nasal bridge

Long philtrum

Short neck

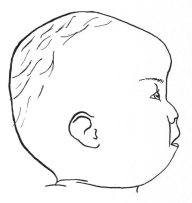

Flat occiput, trigonocephaly,
anteverted nares, long
philtrum, low-set ears
and micrognathia

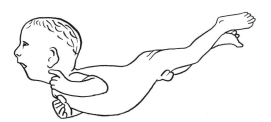

Generalized hypertonia

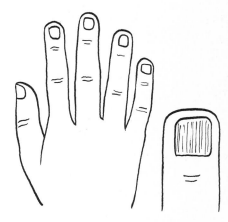

Arachnodactyly with
square, hyperconvex
finger nails

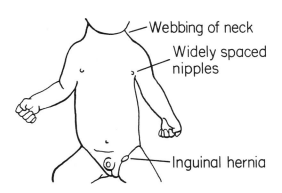

Webbing of neck

Widely spaced
nipples

Inguinal hernia

46. 9p+

Clinical Features The condition can frequently be diagnosed based on craniofacial clinical stigmata, although they are less striking than 13 or 21 trisomy. The classic features involve a characteristic facies, variable mental retardation, and hypoplasia and/or dysplasia of the terminal phalanges, especially those of the second and fifth fingers. Facial alterations include high, broad forehead with large fontanel and open metopic suture in childhood. Mild microcephaly, brachycephaly, flat occiput, moderate ocular hypertelorism, and divergent strabismus are frequent. The eyes appear relatively small and deeply set and exhibit mild antimongoloid obliquity of the palpebral fissures. The pupils may be excentric. The nose has a large globular tip with a broad nasal root. The philtrum is remarkably short. The mouth is large with the angles downturned and the lower lip everted. The grin is usually asymmetric. The pinnae are large and low-set and the auditory canals are narrow. The neck is short with a low hairline. Intelligence quotients have varied between 30 and 65. Somatic retardation is uncommon.

Specific Diagnosis The palms appear especially long relative to finger length. In addition to hypoplasia and/or dysplasia of the terminal phalanges, especially those of the second and fifth fingers, there may be mild finger contractures and hypoplastic and/or dysplastic nails with clinodactyly of the fifth fingers and mild syndactyly of the third and fourth fingers. The shoulder girdle musculature is hypoplastic in some patients. Various other skeletal anomalies include hallux valgus, cubitus valgus, genu valgum, kyphosis, and/or lumbar hyperlordosis. Sexual maturation is frequently delayed. The nipples may be darkly pigmented. Radiographically, there is delayed bone age and retarded closure of anterior fontanel, thoracolumbar scoliosis, hypoplastic terminals and middle phalanges of the fingers and toes, and proximal ossification centers of the metacarpals. Abnormal dermatoglyphics include transverse palmar crease, single flexion crease in the fifth fingers, excess of arches on fingertips and toes, absence of digital triradii *b* and *c,* hypothenar crease and a distal axial triradius *t'.*

Differential Diagnosis The phenotype is quite characteristic.

Prenatal Diagnosis This is possible where one of the parents carries a balanced translocation.

Basic Defect, Genetics, and Other Considerations The basic defect is partial trisomy of most of the short arm of chromosome 9. The disorder appears to be relatively common. There is a 2:1 female sex predilection. So-called "pure 9p trisomy" arises from breakage at the secondary constriction or by centric fusion with an acrocentric chromosome. Over half the cases of this type arise *de novo.* Other forms involve not only the short arm of chromosome 9 but the proximal half of the long arm resulting from translocation of the distal segment of 9q to a 15 or 22 chromosome. Still other cases are associated with partial monosomy or trisomy for another chromosome which has resulted from reciprocal translocation. The major phenotypic changes result from gain of the distal part of the short arm of 9. When the partial trisomy involves regions 9q2 and 9q3, the pattern of anomalies is more severe and there is marked failure to thrive, poor neurologic development, less typical craniofacial anomalies, and a large number of internal malformations. Rarely, the disorder arises from an isochromosome of 9p. These patients appear to be more severely affected.

Prognosis and Treatment The disorder does not appear to be life-threatening. There is severe speech delay which is markedly disproportionate to intelligence. Treatment is supportive.

REFERENCES

Centerwall, W.R., Miller, K.S., and Reeves, L.M. Familial partial 9p trisomy. *J. Med. Genet. 13:* 57–61, 1976.

Lewandowski, R.C., Yunis, J.J., Lehrke, R. et al. Trisomy for the distal one-half of the short arm of chromosome 9. *Am. J. Dis. Child. 130:* 663–667, 1976.

Sutherland, G.R., Carter, R.F., and Morris, L.L. Partial and complete trisomy 9: delineation of a trisomy 9 syndrome. *Hum. Genet. 32:* 133–140, 1976.

M.R. [+ / all]

- **high forehead / large fontanel**
- **deep-set eyes**
- **globular nasal tip**
- **hypoplasia of terminal phalanges**

9p+

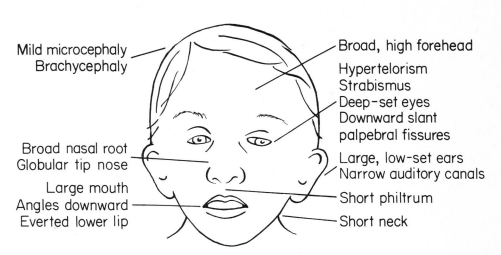

Mild microcephaly
Brachycephaly

Broad nasal root
Globular tip nose

Large mouth
Angles downward
Everted lower lip

Broad, high forehead

Hypertelorism
Strabismus
Deep-set eyes
Downward slant
palpebral fissures

Large, low-set ears
Narrow auditory canals

Short philtrum

Short neck

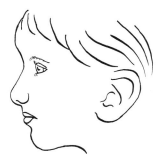

Globular tip nose,
protruding lower lip,
low-set, dysplastic ear

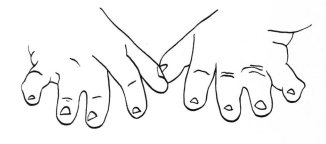

Syndactyly 3–4, clinodactyly,
hypoplasia of nails and
terminal phalanges 2 and 5

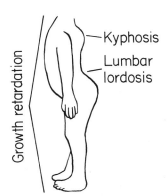

Growth retardation

Kyphosis

Lumbar
lordosis

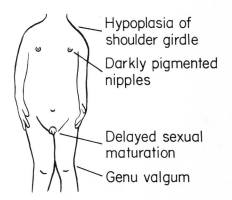

Hypoplasia of
shoulder girdle

Darkly pigmented
nipples

Delayed sexual
maturation

Genu valgum

47. 10p +

Clinical Features The most constant clinical findings include retarded growth, severe mental and psychomotor retardation, seizures, hypotonia, and joint hyperextensibility. Birth weight is low in about half the cases. Facial characteristics include dolichocephaly (less often microcephaly), high prominent forehead with low hairline, prominent cheeks, highly arched eyebrows with synophrys, wide or prominent nasal root, anteverted nostrils, long philtrum, wide rather triangular mouth, protruding upper lip, and large low-set posteriorly rotated ears. About half have cleft lip and/or cleft palate. Flexion abnormalities often involve the elbows, wrists, fingers, toes, hips, knees, or ankles, especially talipes equinovarus. The cardiac and urogenital anomalies have generally been mixed and variable. Various genital anomalies include micropenis and enlarged labia or clitoris.

Specific Diagnosis Diagnosis is made by chromosome karyotype. Radiographic changes are not marked. The sagittal sutures and fontanels are widened. The long bones are gracile and bone age is retarded. A supernumerary ulnar transverse palmar crease is relatively common in this disorder.

Differential Diagnosis Most diagnoses are arrived at by karyotype analysis of children with mental retardation and multiple malformations.

Prenatal Diagnosis Indicated after the birth of a prior affected sib and where a parent has a balanced translocation for the segment.

Basic Defect, Genetics, and Other Considerations The condition is caused by trisomy for part of the short arm of chromosome 10, in most cases 10p11→pter or 10p12→pter, but examples of 10p13→pter and 10p14→pter have been reported. Intrachromosomal duplications are rare. About 90% of the patients are unbalanced products of parental reciprocal balanced translocations involving the short arm of chromosome 10, and more often an acrocentric autosome. Meiotic segregation 2:2 has been observed in nearly all cases. It is possible that males may be more severely affected than females.

Prognosis and Treatment About 50% die early in life. Those that survive are severely retarded. Treatment is supportive.

REFERENCES

Back, E., Vogel, W., Hertel, C. et al. Trisomy 10p due to t(5;10)(p15:p11) segregating in a large sibship. *Hum Genet. 41:* 11–17, 1978.

Fryns, J.P., Deroover, J., Haegeman, J. et al. Partial duplication of the short arm of chromosome 10. *Hum. Genet. 47:* 217–220, 1979.

Stengel-Rutkowski, S., Murken, J.D., Frankenberger, R. et al. Trisomy 10p. *Eur J. Pediatr. 126:* 109–125, 1977.

- **high forehead /
  low hairline**
- **prominent cheeks**
- **triangular mouth**
- **flexion deformities**

10 p+

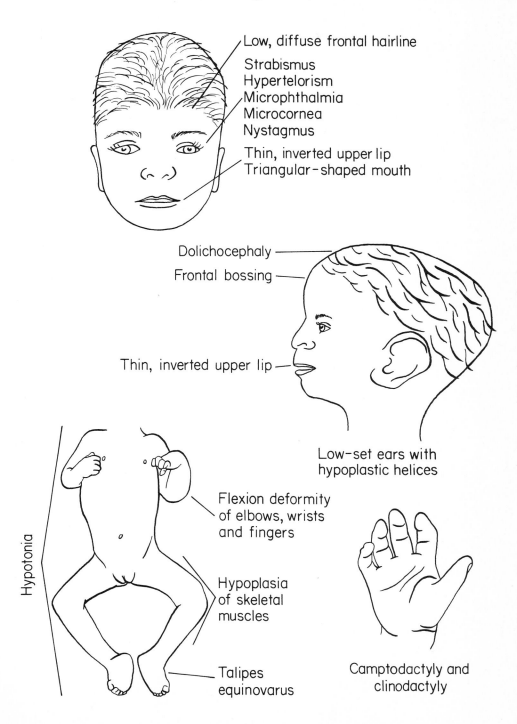

Low, diffuse frontal hairline

Strabismus
Hypertelorism
Microphthalmia
Microcornea
Nystagmus

Thin, inverted upper lip
Triangular-shaped mouth

Dolichocephaly

Frontal bossing

Thin, inverted upper lip

Low-set ears with
hypoplastic helices

Hypotonia

Flexion deformity
of elbows, wrists
and fingers

Hypoplasia
of skeletal
muscles

Talipes
equinovarus

Camptodactyly and
clinodactyly

48. 10q+

Clinical Features Trisomy for the distal portion of the long arm of chromosome 10 produces a rather distinctive clinical picture. Mental retardation is extremely marked. Height, weight, and head circumference are usually below the 3rd percentile. There is marked hypotonia. Most patients exhibit microcephaly, large forehead, a somewhat flattened face, fine arched eyebrows, especially small palpebral fissures with mild antimongoloid obliquity, microphthalmia, flat nasal bridge, small nose with anteverted nostrils, prominent cheek bones, bow-shaped mouth with prominent upper lip, small mandible, and malformed pinnae. About half the patients exhibit ptosis of eyelids, cleft palate, and long philtrum. Bilateral epicanthal folds create an illusion of ocular hypertelorism, while reduced corneal diameter (8.5–9.0 mm) may simulate the appearance of microphthalmia. Less common are prominent occiput, large ears, and narrow auditory canals. Anomalies of the hands and feet include camptodactyly, proximally implanted thumbs and/or great toes with a wide space between the hallux and second toe. Overlapping and/or fusiform fingers, rockerbottom feet, and deep plantar furrows have been noted in over a third of the patients. The plantar furrows run from between the first and second toes to the distal border of the foot. Frequently the neck is short. At least half the males exhibit cryptorchidism. Various congenital heart defects found in about half the patients include ventricular septal defect, atrial septal defect, and patent ductus arteriosus. Delayed bone age, scoliosis, and thin ribs have been noted in perhaps one-third of patients. Various kidney abnormalities include hypoplasia of kidneys, cystic alterations, hydronephrosis, hydroureter, etc.

Specific Diagnosis Diagnosis is made on chromosomal karyotype. Radiographic changes are essentially limited to kyphoscoliosis and occasionally microcephaly. Dermatoglyphic data are not diagnostic, but there is an increased incidence of transverse palmar creases, high axial triradius, and increased ulnar loops. Some patients lack a palmar *c-d* triradius.

Differential Diagnosis Blepharophimosis occurs in *blepharophimosis-ptosis syndrome, fetal alcohol syndrome,* and in *6p+ syndrome.*

Prenatal Diagnosis Indicated after the birth of a prior affected sib and where a parent has a balanced translocation for the segment.

Basic Defect, Genetics, and Other Considerations The disorder is due to trisomy for part of the long arm of chromosome 10. Over 90% of cases have resulted from a balanced translocation in one of the parents. Most examples have been trisomic for 10q25→qter. Those having a larger duplication (10q22→qter) have low birth weight (1600–1900 g), while those with trisomy for 10q25→qter apparently do not have reduced head circumference, decreased birth weight, high forehead, micrognathia, cleft palate, or congenital heart disease. Approximately 30 cases have been reported. A significant majority are male.

Prognosis and Treatment Prognosis is poor. Death has occurred prior to the age of four years in approximately half of the cases, largely due to cardiac, renal, or respiratory complications. Those that survive are severely retarded. Treatment is supportive.

REFERENCES

Berger, R., Derre, J., Murawsky, M. et al., Trisomie 10q partielle de novo. *J. Génét. Hum. 24:* 261–269, 1976.

Klep-dePater, J., Bijlsma, J.B., deFrance, H.F. et al. Partial trisomy 10q: a recognizable syndrome. *Hum. Genet. 46:* 29–40, 1979.

Prieur, M., Forabosco, A., Dutrillaux, B. et al. La trisomie 10q24→qter. *Ann. Génét. 18:* 217–222, 1975.

- microcephaly / high forehead
- arched eyebrows / eye anomalies
- prominent cheek bones
- protruding upper lip

10q+

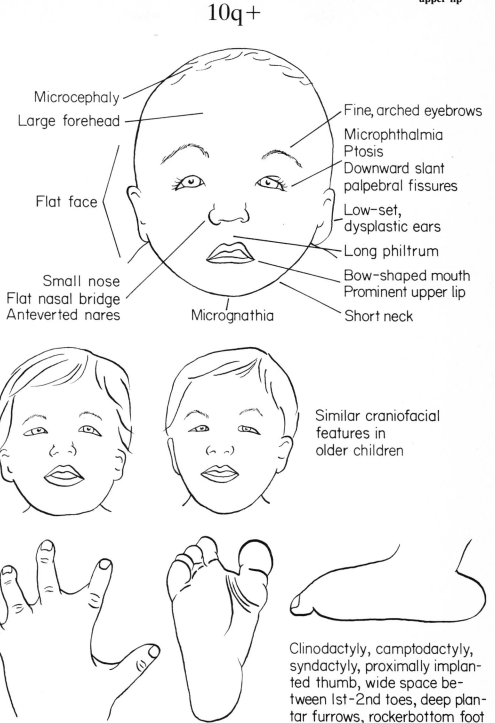

Microcephaly

Large forehead

Flat face

Small nose
Flat nasal bridge
Anteverted nares

Micrognathia

Fine, arched eyebrows

Microphthalmia
Ptosis
Downward slant
palpebral fissures

Low-set,
dysplastic ears

Long philtrum

Bow-shaped mouth
Prominent upper lip

Short neck

Similar craniofacial
features in
older children

Clinodactyly, camptodactyly,
syndactyly, proximally implanted thumb, wide space between 1st-2nd toes, deep plantar furrows, rockerbottom foot

49. 12p+

Clinical Features Pregnancy is complicated by imminent abortion or maternal toxemia in approximately 25% of cases, but birth is at term. Birth complications occurred in about 70% of the cases, making instrument delivery or Caesarean section common. The larger the chromosomal imbalance, the smaller the birth weight. Birth length is normal. Common are pospartum asphyxia, hypotonia, feeding difficulties, and a weak cry. Severe congenital malformations of the brain, heart, and intestinal tract or kidneys are more common in those with larger chromosomal imbalance; most of these infants die in the neonatal period. Cranial anomalies (macrocephaly, microcephaly, turricephaly, flat occiput) are relatively common. Characteristically the skull is broad and high and the forehead prominent. The face is rectangular and flat, the cheeks being broad and prominent. The eye axis is usually horizontal. The eyebrows are often high, broad, diffuse, and directed laterally downward. Hypertelorism, epicanthus, and almond-shaped reduced eye aperture are frequently observed. The nasal root is usually broad or flat with the nose short and nostrils anteverted. The philtrum is broad and poorly developed, the vermilion of the upper lip thin, the lower lip broad and everted. The angles of the mouth are downward slanting and there is usually micrognathia. The palate is cleft in 10% of the patients. The ears are often low set and posteriorly rotated with abnormally folded helices. The inferior crux of the anthelix is usually prominent, the superior crus underdeveloped, and the conchae deep. The neck is short and often embedded in abundant skin folds. The nipples may be low, widely spaced, or supernumerary. There may be abnormal position of the large joints and the hands and feet are often short and broad with overlapping fingers and toes and abnormally shaped distal phalanges. Clinodactyly of the fifth finger and a gap between the first and second toes are relatively common.

Specific Diagnosis Diagnosis is confirmed by chromosomal karyotype. Radiographically the changes are not striking. Dermatoglyphic studies indicate a high frequency of whorls but a relatively low total finger ridge count. Bilateral simian creases, third interdigital loops, low *a-b* ridge counts, hypoplasia of the dermal ridges, and digital axial triradii are common. An increased activity of lactic dehydrogenase-B has been found in nearly all cases.

Differential Diagnosis Facial characteristics in a mentally retarded infant may be sufficient to suggest chromosome study.

Prenatal Diagnosis This is indicated by prior birth of an affected sib.

Basic Defect, Genetics and Other Considerations The basic defect is trisomy for the short arm of chromosome 12 distal to band 12p 1.2. Approximately 25 children have been reported with this disorder. Nearly all have been born in families in which one of the parents had a balanced translocation. Various types of segregation have been reported, especially adjacent 2:2. There does not appear to be any sexual predilection. A few patients have been mosaic for the short arm of chromosome 12. There does not appear to be any significant difference in phenotype whether one is dealing with partial trisomy 12p, complete trisomy 12p, or trisomy of complete 12p and proximal parts of 12q. In cases where a parent has a balanced translocation, the estimation of risk can only be roughly estimated. A high risk is assumed when the translocated segment is small and vice-versa. These risks range from approximately 5 to 30% (see Stengel-Rutkowski et al. for specific risks).

Prognosis and Treatment Among the children who survive the neonatal period there does not appear to be diminished life expectancy. However, they have grossly impaired motor development (delayed head control, sitting, standing, walking). Hypertonia occurs in most younger patients while at least a third of the older patients exhibit variable muscular tonar spasticity. Growth in general is retarded, most patients exhibiting short stature. Severe mental retardation is a constant finding. Poor speech development is constant. Treatment is supportive.

REFERENCES

Kondo, I., Hamaguchi, H., Haneda, T. Trisomy 12p syndrome. De novo occurrence of mosaic trisomy 12p in a mentally retarded boy. *Hum. Genet. 46:* 135–140, 1979.

Parslow, M., Chambers, D., Drummond, M. et al. Two cases of trisomy 12p due to rcp t(12:21) (p11:p11) inherited through three generations. *Hum. Genet. 47:* 253–260, 1979.

Stengel-Rutkowski, S., Albert, A., Murken, J.D. et al. New chromosomal dysmorphic syndromes: trisomy 12p. *Eur. J. Pediatr. 136:* 249–262, 1981.

M.R. [+ / all]

- broad, high skull
- flat rectangular face
- eyebrows laterally downward
- thin upper lip / broad everted lower lip

12p+

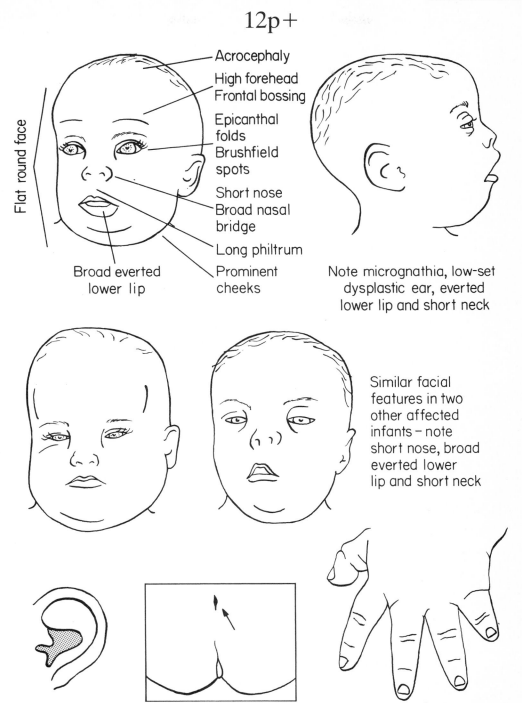

Flat round face

Acrocephaly

High forehead
Frontal bossing

Epicanthal folds
Brushfield spots

Short nose
Broad nasal bridge

Long philtrum

Prominent cheeks

Broad everted lower lip

Note micrognathia, low-set dysplastic ear, everted lower lip and short neck

Similar facial features in two other affected infants – note short nose, broad everted lower lip and short neck

Dysplastic ear with deep concha, sacral dimple (arrow), tapered digits with short 5th digit

113

50. 13q−

Clinical Features Birth weight is considerably decreased for length of gestation. Virtually constant features are psychomotor retardation, hypotonia, and microcephaly. Trigonocephaly has been seen in approximately half the patients. The facies is characterized by frontal bossing, broad prominent nasal root, protruding maxilla and incisors, and large prominent malrotated ears with deep helical sulcus. Eye anomalies consist of ptosis of the lids, epicanthal folds, microphthalmia, and colobomas. Retinoblastoma has been found in approximately 15% of the patients. The neck is short with redundant skin folds. Congenital heart anomalies have been noted in approximately 35%, but without consistent pattern. About 60% of the males have genital malformations including hypospadias, small or bifid scrotum, cryptorchism, micropenis, and perineal fistula. Anal atresia has been noted in about 20%. Skeletal anomalies are not striking. Hip dislocation and talipes equinovarus have been noted with increased frequency and hypoplastic to absent thumbs in 30%.

Specific Diagnosis Diagnosis is made by chromosome karyotype. Radiographic changes are not striking. There may be hip dislocation and, as mentioned above, the thumbs may be hypoplastic to absent. If absent, there is usually accompanying absence of the first metacarpal and synostosis of the fourth and fifth metacarpal bones.

Differential Diagnosis Absent thumbs are seen in association with absent radius, in *Fanconi pancytopenia* and in a number of other disorders that are readily distinguished from 13q− syndrome.

Prenatal Diagnosis Possible, where one of the parents has a balanced translocation.

Basic Defect, Genetics, and Other Considerations The basic defect results from partial monosomy for a segment of the long arm of a chromosome 13. At least 100 cases have been reported. Most cases involve loss of the distal two-thirds of the long arm. In some, this has resulted from deletion, in others translocation, and in others deletion and fusion producing a ring chromosome. Deletion of bands q33→qter results in severe mental retardation, microcephaly, ocular hypertelorism, frontal bossing, protruding maxilla, and large ears. Those with additional deletion of bands q31 and q32 exhibit mental retardation, microcephaly, trigonocephaly, hypoplastic or absent thumbs and metacarpals, and male genital abnormalities. Retinoblastoma is associated with deletion of band q14.

Prognosis and Treatment There is marked failure to thrive and mental retardation is nearly always severe.

REFERENCES

Cuschieri, A., Agius, P.V., and Scheres, J.M. Partial deletion of the long arm chromosome No. 13. *Hum. Genet. 36:* 341–344, 1977.

Noel, B., Quack, B., and Rethoré, M.O. Partial deletion and trisomies of chromosome 13: mapping of bands associated with particular malformations. *Clin. Genet. 9:* 593–602, 1976.

Yunis, J. and Ramsay, N. Retinoblastoma and subband deletion of chromosome 13. *Am. J. Dis. Child. 132:* 161–163, 1978.

- **microcephaly / trigonocephaly**
- **large ears**
- **ptosis eyelids / eye anomalies**
- **short neck, redundant folds**

13q−

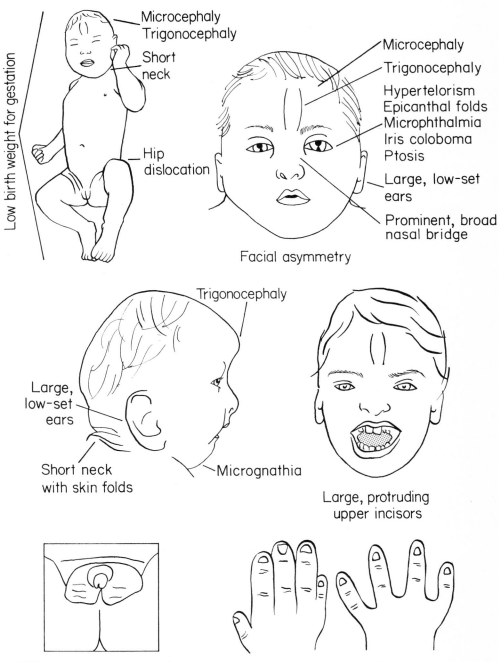

Microcephaly Trigonocephaly

Short neck

Hip dislocation

Low birth weight for gestation

Microcephaly

Trigonocephaly

Hypertelorism
Epicanthal folds
Microphthalmia
Iris coloboma
Ptosis

Large, low-set ears

Prominent, broad nasal bridge

Facial asymmetry

Trigonocephaly

Large, low-set ears

Short neck with skin folds

Micrognathia

Large, protruding upper incisors

Bifid scrotum, hypospadias and imperforate anus

Hypoplastic or absent thumbs, short 5th finger

51. 13 TRISOMY

Clinical Features The phenotype in trisomy 13 is so striking that diagnosis is usually suggested by clinical observations before cytogenetic results have been obtained. The combination of microcephaly with sloping forehead, occipitoparietal scalp defects, microphthalmia, cleft lip and/or cleft palate, broad flat nose, and postaxial polydactyly of the hands or feet readily leads to clinical diagnosis. Possibly 5% exhibit some form of holoprosencephaly.

Specific Diagnosis Mean birth weight is about 2500 g. Microcephaly is usually moderate. The forehead slopes and the sagittal sutures are usually open. Microphthalmia, coloboma of the ciliary body, cataracts, retinal detachment, retinal dysplasia, ocular hypertelorism, and malformed pinnae occur in about 80%. Capillary hemangiomas in the glabellar region and localized scalp defects in the parieto-occipital area have been noted in about 75%, cleft lip and/or cleft palate and micrognathia in 60–70%. Postaxial hexadactyly of the hands or, less often, feet is present in about 75%. The fingers are flexed and overlapping in about 60% and the nails are hyperconvex and narrow. The calcaneus is often prominent and the feet rockerbottom. Congenital heart defects (atrial septal defect, patent ductus arteriosus, ventricular septal defect, dextrocardia) and dysplastic renal anomalies are commonly noted. Genital anomalies include cryptorchidism in males and bicornuate uterus and hypoplastic ovaries in females. Dermatoglyphic changes include transverse palmar crease (60%), distal palmar axial triradius (80%), and hallucal arch fibular or loop tibial (35%). A radial loop on other than the index finger has been seen in about 50% of the cases. Polymorphonuclear neutrophils frequently have nuclear projections.

Differential Diagnosis Since some infants with trisomy 13 have holoprosencephaly, *holoprosencephaly* without trisomy 13 must be excluded. *Meckel syndrome,* because of associated polydactyly which is usually more extensive and involves all four extremities asymmetrically, may occasionally be confused with trisomy 13.

Prenatal Diagnosis Prenatal diagnosis is most likely if one of the parents is a carrier of a balanced translocation, but occasionally trisomy 13 is diagnosed following amniocentesis done on an older mother.

Basic Defect, Genetics, and Other Considerations The basic defect is trisomy of chromosome 13. About 75% are caused by primary nondisjunction. There is slight female predilection. Mean maternal age is elevated (31 years). About 20% are due to translocation. In at least 85% of these cases, the translocation, usually Robertsonian, involves chromosome 13, 14, or 15. With translocation, maternal age is not elevated and there appears to be a definite male predilection. Recurrence risk if one of the parents has a balanced 13/14 or 13/15 translocation is about 2%. About 5% of the cases are caused by mosaicism. Certain aspects of the phenotype are associated with trisomy for various bands: trisomy of the short arm and band q11 are associated with microcephaly, strabismus, and abnormal dermatoglyphics; trisomy for q12, q13, q14 with holoprosencephaly, cleft lip and/or palate, cardiac, renal, and genital anomalies; trisomy of q21 and q22 with frontal bossing, microphthalmia, narrow temporal area, wide nose, ear malformations, and elevated fetal hemoglobin; bands q31 and q32 with polydactyly and club feet; and q33 with inguinal or umbilical hernia. Trisomy 13 accounts for about 1% of spontaneous first trimester abortions. Recent estimates for nondisjunctive trisomy 13 suggest a prevalence of one case per 12,000 live births; translocation trisomy 13, 1 case per 24,000.

Prognosis and Treatment About half die within the first month, approximately 75% by the sixth month, and less than 5% survive more than three years. The oldest known person with the disorder is approximately 35 years of age. Treatment is supportive.

REFERENCES

Hodes, M.E., Cole, J., Palmer, C.G. et al. Clinical experience with trisomies 18 and 13. *J. Med. Genet. 15:* 48–60, 1978.

Noël, B., Quack, B., and Rethoré, M.O. Partial deletions and trisomies of chromosome 13; mapping of bands associated with particular malformations. *Clin. Genet. 9:* 593–602, 1976.

Schinzel, A., Hayashi, K., and Schmid, W. Further delineation of the clinical picture of trisomy for the distal segment of chromosome 13. *Hum. Genet. 32:* 1–12, 1976.

- **microcephaly / sloping forehead**
- **microphthalmia / eye anomalies**
- **cleft lip / palate**
- **postaxial polydactyly**

13 Trisomy

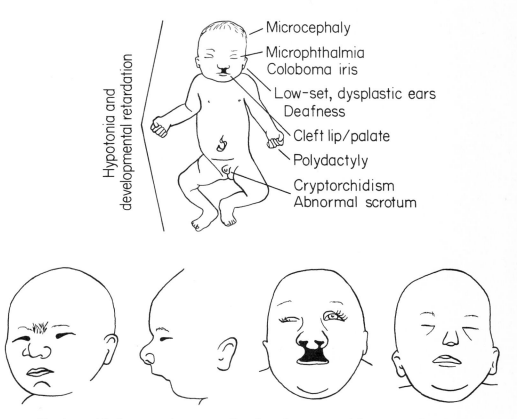

Hypotonia and developmental retardation

Microcephaly

Microphthalmia
Coloboma iris

Low-set, dysplastic ears
Deafness

Cleft lip/palate

Polydactyly

Cryptorchidism
Abnormal scrotum

Facies with hemangioma on forehead, sparse/absent eyebrows, micrognathia, sloping forehead, low-set ears, microphthalmia, anophthalmia and single nares

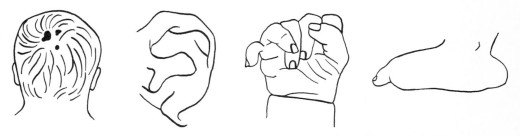

Posterior scalp lesions, dysplastic ear, postaxial polydactyly, clenched hand, narrow nails and prominent heel

117

52. 18q—

Clinical Features Mental retardation is moderate to profound and remains retarded below the 5th percentile. Birth weight at term tends to be relatively normal (ca. 3000 g). Hypotonia is almost always marked and seizures are frequent. There is a characteristic facies. The forehead is bossed. The eyes are deeply set and there is midfacial hypoplasia. The chin is prominent and the neck is short. A subcutaneous nodule is frequently present at the site of the cheek dimple. The fingers are long and tapered with fleshy tips and the thumbs are proximally placed. The second toes often overlap the third toes. Talipes equinovarus has been found in 20%. The nipples are widely spaced. Congenital heart anomalies are present in about 35%. Umbilical hernia has been noted in about one-third of the cases. The labia minora and clitoris are hypoplastic or absent in about 50% and one half the males are cryptorchid and have a small penis and scrotum.

Specific Diagnosis Microcephaly has been found in over 65% and the fontanels close late. The hair is sparse with patchy alopecia. In addition to the eyes appearing recessed, there frequently are ophthalmologic defects such as epicanthus, glaucoma, strabismus, nystagmus, and pale optic discs. The nose is short and the nasal bridge widened. The mouth is usually carp-shaped. The pinnae are somewhat unusual, the antitragus and/or antihelix being especially prominent. The ear canals are atretic with impaired hearing in about one-half of the cases. Cleft lip (10%) or cleft palate (30%) has been noted. Skin dimples may be present over the cheeks, sacrum, subacromion, and epitrochlear areas lateral to the patellae and over the knuckles. There are usually more than five fingerprint whorls present. Transverse palmar creases appear to be increased.

Differential Diagnosis While the clinical appearance is rather characteristic, the midfacial hypoplasia and atretic ear canals are not constant features and hence difficulty may be experienced in differentiating patients with 18q— syndrome from those with undiagnosed moderate to severe mental retardation.

Prenatal Diagnosis This is possible if the condition is caused by translocation. This has been found in approximately 15% of the cases.

Basic Defect, Genetics, and Other Considerations The basic defect in this rare chromosomal disorder is deletion of part of the long arm of chromosome 18, involving band q21. Translocation has been found in approximately 15% of the cases. In another 15% there has been an associated mosaicism. There is no sex predilection. Parental age is not elevated. There have been at least 65 reported cases. IgA has been diminished in over 40%.

Prognosis and Treatment The oldest known person with the disorder is approximately 20 years old. The cause of death has been variable. Treatment of the seizures is indicated as in other cases.

REFERENCES

Lurie, I. and Lazjuk, G. Partial monosomies 18. *Humangenetik 15:* 203–222, 1972.

Schinzel, A., Hayashi, K., and Schmid, W. Structural aberrations of chromosome 18. II. The 18q— syndrome. *Humangenetik 26:* 123–132, 1975.

Wertelecki, W. and Gerald, P.S. Clinical and chromosomal studies of the 18q— syndrome. *J. Pediatr. 78:* 44–52, 1971.

- **frontal bossing**
- **deeply set eyes / eye anomalies**
- **carp-shaped mouth / prominent chin**
- **long, tapered fingers**

18q−

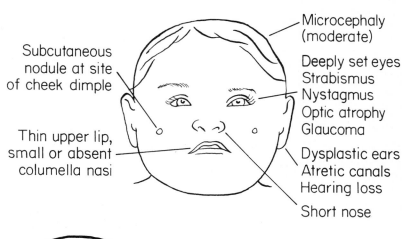

Microcephaly (moderate)

Subcutaneous nodule at site of cheek dimple

Deeply set eyes
Strabismus
Nystagmus
Optic atrophy
Glaucoma

Thin upper lip, small or absent columella nasi

Dysplastic ears
Atretic canals
Hearing loss

Short nose

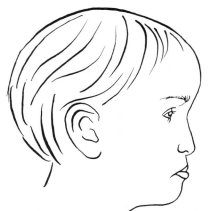

Older child with frontal bossing, midfacial retraction, thin upper lip, prominent chin and dysplastic ear

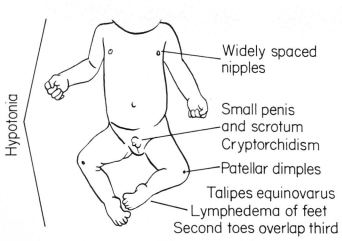

Hypotonia

Widely spaced nipples

Small penis and scrotum
Cryptorchidism

Patellar dimples

Talipes equinovarus
Lymphedema of feet
Second toes overlap third

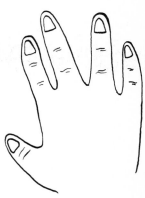

Long, tapered fingers with thumbs proximally placed

53. 18 TRISOMY

Clinical Features The most constant clinical features, noted in over 75% of the cases, include developmental retardation with failure to thrive, poor suck, feeding difficulties, hypotonia followed by hypertonia, limited hip adduction, flexion deformities and overlapping of fingers and hypoplastic nails, very short sternum, wide-spaced nipples, congenital heart disease (ventricular septal defect—90%, patent ductus arteriosus—70%, atrial septal defect—20%), short dorsiflexed halluces, rockerbottom feet, and calcaneovalgus deformity of feet. Cryptorchidism and hypoplasia of the clitoris and labia minora are noted in about 50% of the cases. Umbilical, inguinal, or diaphragmatic hernias have been noted in about 25%. There is dolichocephaly with a prominent occiput. The facies is characteristic. The nasal bridge is narrow. The palpebral fissures are short. There may be microphthalmia. The auricles are low set and often posteriorly rotated and flattened. The palate is narrow and the mandible is small. Cleft lip and/or palate have occurred in about 15%. The neck is short. The hands are often held adjacent to the head in a pleading position.

Specific Diagnosis Apart from the cardiac anomalies noted above, various findings have been noted at autopsy: hypoplastic skeletal muscles, sparse subcutaneous fat, heterotopic pancreatic tissue, thin diaphragm with eventration, Meckel's diverticulum, and various dysplastic renal anomalies. Dermatoglyphic changes are frequent: over 75% of fingerprints are simple arches; toeprints may have an even higher percentage of arches; over 35% have a transverse palmar crease and single flexion creases of the fingers are relatively frequent. There is an uncommon but definite association with aplasia of the radius. Radiographic changes are not striking. General skeletal development is gracile. The sternum has a reduced number of ossification centers. The pelvis is especially narrow and the hips dislocated.

Differential Diagnosis The phenotype is so distinctive that other syndromes are not usually confused with the condition. *Dominant distal arthrogryposis* has similar finger positions.

Prenatal Diagnosis This is most likely if one of the parents is a balanced translocation carrier. Occasionally trisomy 18 is diagnosed following amniocentesis done on an older mother.

Basic Defect, Genetics, and Other Considerations The basic defect is trisomy for chromosome 18. This occurs in approximately 1 per 7000 live births. There is about a 3:1 female predilection. About 80% of the cases are caused by nondisjunction. Mean maternal age is elevated. Trisomy 18 is caused by translocation in about 10%. Mean maternal age is lower in these cases. In perhaps 10% of the cases, mosaicism has been found. Double primary nondisjunction occurs in 5–10% of cases. Maternal age is markedly increased in this group. Small weight gain is experienced during pregnancy and fetal movements are feeble. Most examples are postmature (ca. 42 weeks), but mean birth weight is less than 2300 g. The placenta is often small with a single umbilical artery, and hydramnios has been noted in over 50%.

Prognosis and Treatment Thirty percent fail to survive more than one month. Fifty percent succumb by two months, and less than 10% live more than one year. Mean survival time is about 70 days (females—134 days, males—15 days). Treatment is supportive.

REFERENCES

Hodes, M.E., Cole, J., Palmer, C.G. et al. Clinical experience with trisomies 18 and 13. *J. Med. Genet. 15:* 48–60, 1978.

Taylor, A.I. Autosomal trisomy syndromes: a detailed study of 27 cases of Edward's syndrome and 27 cases of Patau's syndrome. *J. Med. Genet. 5:* 227–252, 1968.

Weber, W.W. Survival and the sex ratio in trisomy 17–18. *Am. J. Hum. Genet. 19:* 369–377, 1967.

- dolichocephaly / prominent occiput
- short palpebral fissures / eye anomalies
- overlapping fingers
- rocker bottom feet

18 Trisomy

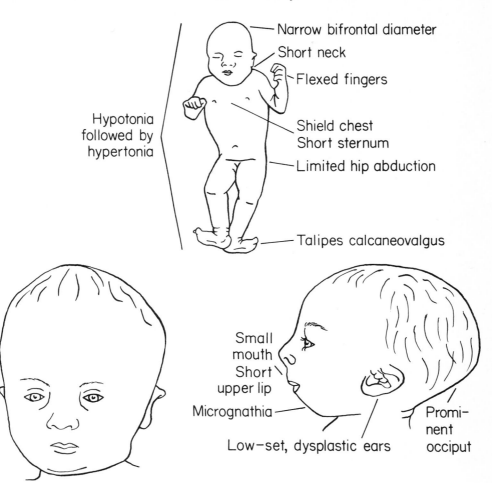

Narrow bifrontal diameter

Short neck

Flexed fingers

Hypotonia followed by hypertonia

Shield chest
Short sternum

Limited hip abduction

Talipes calcaneovalgus

Small mouth
Short upper lip

Micrognathia

Low-set, dysplastic ears

Prominent occiput

Microphthalmia, epicanthal folds, short palpebral fissures, corneal opacities are common eye findings

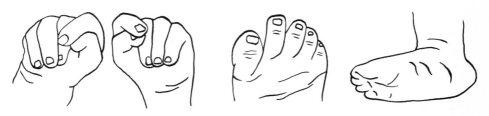

Clenched hand, overlapping index fingers, short hallux dorsiflexed and prominent heel

54. 21 TRISOMY
(Down syndrome, mongolism)

Clinical Features The phenotype is so characteristic (save in the newborn) that karyotype study is needed only to ascertain whether one is dealing with nondisjunction or translocation. Most evident aspects are the facies, hypotonia, absent moro reflex, cardiac anomalies, and dermatoglyphic alterations. The skull is brachycephalic with flattening of the occiput. Development of the midface is poor with relative prognathism and ocular hypotelorism and hypoplasia of the nasal bones. The palpebral fissures slant upward while the outer canthus is slightly higher than the inner. Epicanthal folds, speckled iris (Brushfield spots), blepharitis, convergent strabismus, and nystagmus are common. Ear anomalies include angular overlapping helix, prominent antihelix, and small or absent earlobes. The mouth is often open with the tongue often thrust beyond the lips. The lips and tongue are often fissured. The cry and voice are low and raucous.

Specific Diagnosis The hands are characteristically short and broad, the fifth finger usually being abbreviated and clinodactylous. Hypotonia is especially marked in infancy and joints are usually hyperextensible. The moro reflex is absent in over 80%. The penis and scrotum are usually small, about 25% have cryptorchidism, and pubic hair is straight. Congenital cardiac anomalies, present in about 40%, in decreasing order of frequency are: ventricular septal defect, A/V communis, atrial septal defect, and patent ductus arteriosus. A host of anomalies may be present at low frequency, such as diastasis recti, duodenal atresia, umbilical hernia, and syringoma. Radiographically, a metopic suture is found in about 50%. Absence of frontal and sphenoid sinuses and hypoplasia of the maxillary sinuses are common. There is reduced iliac and acetabular angles in the young infant and hypoplastic middle phalanx of the fifth finger. Dermatoglyphic anomalies include distal axial triradius in the palm in over 80%, bilateral transverse palmar creases in about 30%, single flexion creases in the fifth finger in 20%, a marked increase in ulnar loops, a hallucal arch tibial in approximately 70%, or small loop distal in about 30%.

Differential Diagnosis Phenotype usually is quite distinctive but at birth may be over- or underdiagnosed. Some patients with *9p− syndrome* share many of the stigmata.

Prenatal Diagnosis Indicated for mothers over 35 years of age, for those who have already had a child with trisomy 21, or who are known carriers of a balanced translocation.

Basic Defect, Genetics, and Other Considerations The basic defect is trisomy for chromosome 21 which occurs about once in every 650 births regardless of race. Technically the phenotype depends on trisomy for the distal segment q22. There is a mild male predilection. About 92% are due to nondisjunction (maternal meiosis I—70%, paternal meiosis I and II—each 15%). In nondisjuction, there is often elevated maternal age. The risk at 35 years is about 1 per 350, at 40 years about 1 in 100, and at 45 years about 1 in 30. About 5% arise from translocation, which is age-independent. Over half are to a 13–15-group chromosome, most often (60%) chromosome 14, less often (20% each) to 13 or 15. In half the cases these arise de novo. About 40% involve translocation to a G-group chromosome (85% to a 21, 15% to a 22). These nearly all arise de novo. Three percent are mosaics. Regarding recurrence risks: nondisjunction—about 1%; for 13–15-group, if mother carries balanced translocation—about 15%, if father, about 5%, for t(21q,22q), 10% risk for mother, 2% risk for father, but for t(21q,21q), 100% for either 21 trisomy or spontaneous abortion.

Prognosis and Treatment Most patients with Down syndrome three years of age or less have IQs of 50–59, but slip with increasing age to 25 to 49. Sociability is high. Height, less often weight, is reduced (mean male adult—155 cm, mean female adult 145 cm). Because of susceptibility to respiratory infection, early mortality used to be great. With the introduction of antibiotics and cardiac surgery, the mean survival age is almost 20 years. There appears to be premature aging. There is a twenty-fold increased association with acute leukemia.

REFERENCES

Breg, W.R. Down syndrome: a review of recent progress in research. *Pathobiol. Annual 7:* 257–303, 1977.

Hook, E.B. and Lindsjö, A. Down syndrome in livebirths by single year maternal age interval in a Swedish study. Comparison with results from a New York State study. *Am. J. Hum. Genet. 30:* 19–27, 1978.

Johnson, R.C. and Abelson, R.B. Intellectual, behavioral and physical characteristics associated with trisomy, translocation and mosaic types of Down's syndrome. *Am. J. Ment. Defic. 73:* 852–855, 1969.

M.R. [+ / all]

- **brachycephaly / flat occiput**
- **upward slanting palpebral fissures / epicanthal folds**
- **open mouth / protruding tongue**
- **brachydactyly / clinodactyly / simian crease**

21 Trisomy
[Down syndrome, mongolism]

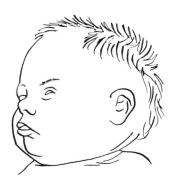 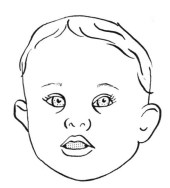 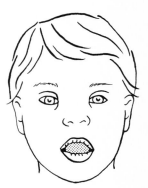

Short neck with skin folds, brachycephaly, flat face, protruding tongue, epicanthal folds, straight hair and small, low-set ears

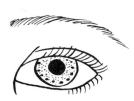 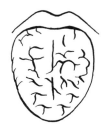 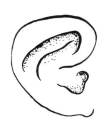 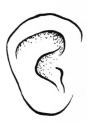

Epicanthal fold, Brushfield spots in iris, fissured tongue, angular overlapping helix, prominent antihelix and small ear lobes

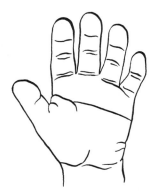 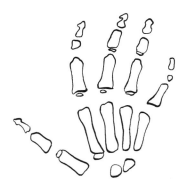 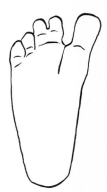

Brachydactyly, clinodactyly, simian crease, small middle phalanx 2nd and 5th digits, syndactyly toes 2-3, wide space and furrow between toes 1-2

55. CAT-EYE SYNDROME

Clinical Features The term "cat-eye syndrome" refers to the clinical association of ocular coloboma and anal atresia. While the syndrome is usually ascribed to the presence of an extra small satellited chromosome fragment, there are reports in which no chromosomal abnormality has been apparent in the presence of the typical phenotype. There does not appear to be any marked difference between those patients having the marker and those that do not have the marker present. Mental retardation of variable degree has been present in 55 to 80%. Approximately 40% exhibit microcephaly. Low-set, malformed pinnae are extremely common. About 25% have cleft lip and/or cleft palate. Various eye anomalies have included microphthalmia (25%), epicanthus (30%), hypertelorism (40%), and iris coloboma (60% in those with the marker, and 100% in those without the marker). Cardiovascular anomalies have been found in about 55%. Genital malformations and kidney malformations each have been noted in about 20%. These have included agenesis or hypoplasia of a single kidney and/or ureter, bladder neck obstruction or bladder hypoplasia with reflux, and hydronephrosis. Anal atresia or stenosis has been found in 60–70% of patients. The anal atresia is usually associated with a rectoperineal, rectourethral, or rectovaginal fistula. The palpebral fissures are often downward slanting. Preauricular tags, sinuses, or fistulas are extremely common. Congenital heart defects most commonly found are ASD and VSD.

Specific Diagnosis Diagnosis is established on clinical grounds and by chromosome karyotype. Simian creases have been found in 20–40% of patients.

Differential Diagnosis As indicated below, there is similarity to *partial trisomy 13*. There is also some overlap with the *VATER association*. Banding techniques have not, so far, proved to be efficient in identifying the abnormal chromosomal marker. Perhaps the continued search for a gene-dosage effect might be of some value.

Prenatal Diagnosis Theoretically possible when a small marker chromosome is found in fetal amniotic cells.

Basic Defect, Genetics, and Other Considerations It is not known what the marker represents. Such small extra satellited fragments may also be found in normal people. Several authors have suggested that it represents a deleted chromosome 13, and there are many similarities between the two conditions. Comparison between patients with cat-eye syndrome and those with trisomy for the proximal region of the long arm of chromosome 13 is reasonably strong. This problem has been especially well discussed by Guanti et al. It is possible that those without the marker originally had the marker and it has been lost from the cells. If it does involve chromosome 13 it is probably in the 13q13 region. There is some resemblance to trisomy 22, but to complicate matters even more, some cases reported as trisomy 22 really represent a chromosome derived from a t(11;22) translocation largely containing distal 11q material.

Prognosis and Treatment Life span may be shortened due to cardiac and/or renal malformations. More than half of the patients are mentally retarded. Therapy should be symptomatic. Surgery is necessary for correction of the anal atresia and associated fistula, cleft palate, and often for the bladder reflux.

REFERENCES

Bofinger, M.K. and Soukup, S.W. Cat-eye syndrome: partial trisomy 22 due to translocation in the mother. *Am. J. Dis. Child. 131:* 893–897, 1977.
Guanti, G. The aetiology of the cat-eye syndrome reconsidered. *J. Med. Genet. 18:* 108–118, 1981.
Kunze, J., Tolksdorf, M., and Wiedemann, H.R. Cateye-Syndrom. *Humangenetik 26:* 271–289, 1975.

- **microcephaly**
- **ocular coloboma / eye anomalies**
- **anal atresia / stenosis**
- **low-set ears / ear tags**

Cat-Eye Syndrome

EYE ANOMALIES

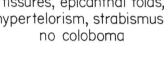

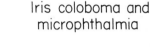

Down-slanting palpebral fissures, epicanthal folds, hypertelorism, strabismus, no coloboma

Iris coloboma and microphthalmia

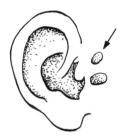
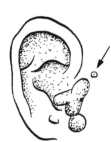
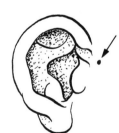
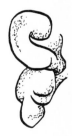

Bilateral iris colobomas

Down–slanting palpebral fissures, partial and total iris colobomas

EAR ANOMALIES

Preauricular tags, pits and sinuses (arrows) and malformed pinnae

ANAL/RECTAL ANOMALIES

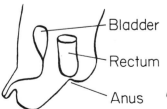
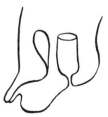
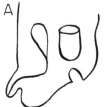

- Bladder
- Rectum
- Anus

Membrane stenosis

Stenosis

Atresia (A), with rectourethral fistula (B)

56. TRIPLOIDY

Clinical Features Pure triploidy is found in 12% of all spontaneous abortions and 20% of chromosomally abnormal abortuses prior to the 12th week of gestation. Those who survive are mosaic, that is, have a normal as well as a triploid cell line. Bleeding during the first trimester, hydramnios, preeclampsia, and postpartum hemorrhage are common complications of the pregnancy. Clinical features of liveborn infants with pure triploidy include low birth weight (males—1900 g, females—1500 g) and prematurity. The posterior fontanel is enlarged in 50% and the occipital and parietal bones are reduced in size. Microphthalmus and/or coloboma of the iris and choroid are noted in 30%. The pinnae are malformed. Cutaneous 3–4 syndactyly of the fingers occurs in 50% and 1–2 and 3–4 syndactyly of the toes in 30%. Talipes equinovarus and enlarged thigh muscles are frequent. Hypospadias, micropenis, cryptorchidism, and hypoplastic scrotum are common in males, but females have normal genitalia. Those with 46,XX/69,XXY constitution frequently have ambiguous genitalia. A number have exhibited hydrocephalus (50%), spina bifida (25%), holoprosencephaly, cleft palate (25%), and hypertelorism. Omphalocele, umbilical hernia, and diastasis recti are increased. Among mosaics, most of the same features are present. The longer living mosaics are usually mentally retarded and about 50% have asymmetric body or head.

Specific Diagnosis Clinical features of the patient, embryo, or placenta should lead to the chromosomal studies. The placenta is large with hydatidiform degeneration of chorionic villi. The conceptus ranges from being relatively normal to there being no visible embryo present. Among the abortuses, about 57% are 69,XXY; 40% are 69,XXX; and only 3% are XYY. Those that have 69,XYY karyotype manifest the least embryonic development. Culture of skin biopsy of the embryo or patient is necessary to reveal the true karyotype because triploid cells are selectively eliminated from lymphocytes but not from fibroblasts. Thus, many mosaics have likely been missed. Furthermore, the triploid cell line may disappear from prolonged cell culture. In 69,XXX infants, the ovaries are hypoplastic with few follicles. Most male triploids have hypoplastic Leydig cells. Dilated cerebral ventricles, agenesis of the corpus callosum, ASD, VSD, and various renal anomalies (cystic, hypoplastic, hydronephrotic kidneys) and adrenal hypoplasia are not rare in this syndrome. About 50% have transverse palmar creases and digital whorls are increased.

Differential Diagnosis Because of body asymmetry, *Russell-Silver syndrome* must be excluded. Asymmetric growth has been seen in individuals mosaic for various trisomies, such as *trisomies 13, 14, 18, and 22.*

Prenatal Diagnosis In those with neural tube defect or omphalocele, the α-fetoprotein is elevated.

Basic Defect, Genetics, and Other Considerations It has been estimated that 65% are due to dispermy, 25% arise from fertilization of a haploid ovum by a diploid sperm due to an error in the first meiotic division in the male. The remaining 10% arise from a diploid egg due to error in the first meiotic division in the female. Commonly, there is more than one active X chromosome which appears to be independent of the origin of the extra haploid set. The frequency may be as high as 1 in 2500 live births.

Prognosis and Treatment Pure triploidy is lethal. At least 90% of liveborn pure triploids succumb within the first 24 hours of life. It is possible that 69,XXX triploids have a greater chance of being stillborn, while 69,XXY triploids have a slightly grater chance for surviving a day or two. While mosaic individuals may die neonatally, most live a normal life span.

REFERENCES

Graham, J.M., Jr., Hoehn, H., Lin, M.S. et al. Diploid-triploid mixoploidy. Clinical and cytogenetic aspects. *Pediatrics 68:* 23–28, 1981.

Jacobs, P.A., Angell, R.R., Buchanan, I.M. et al. The origin of human triploids. *Ann. Hum. Genet. 42:* 49–57, 1978.

Wertelecki, W., Graham, J.M., and Sergovitch, F.R. The clinical syndrome of triploidy. *Obstet. Gynecol. 47:* 69–73, 1976.

- **large posterior fontanel**
- **microphthalmia / eye anomalies**
- **dysplastic ears**
- **malformed external genitalia in males**

Triploidy

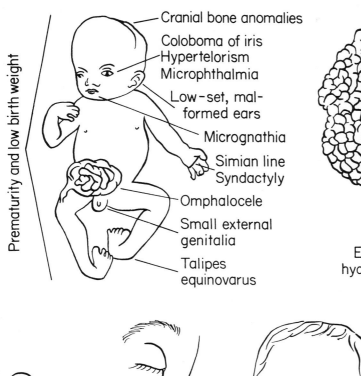

Prematurity and low birth weight

Cranial bone anomalies

Coloboma of iris
Hypertelorism
Microphthalmia

Low-set, malformed ears

Micrognathia

Simian line
Syndactyly

Omphalocele

Small external genitalia

Talipes equinovarus

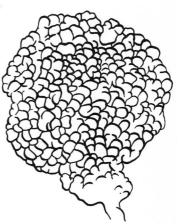

Enlarged and/or hydatid form placenta

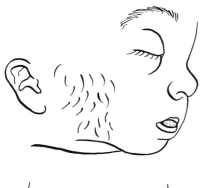
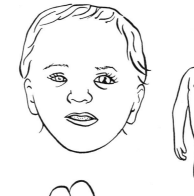
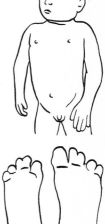

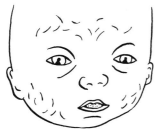

Lanugo, iris colobomas, macroglossia, micrognathia and low-set ears

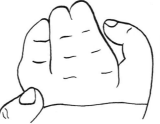

Facial/body asymmetry, syndactyly fingers 3–4, toes 2–3, clinodactyly and simian line

57. TURNER SYNDROME

Clinical Features Turner syndrome is characterized by sexual infantilism, primary amenorrhea, sterility, webbed neck, and cubitus valgus in postpubertal females. Adult height is usually less than 144 cm (57 inches). Epicanthal folds, ptosis of upper eyelids, prominent ears, and micrognathia are common features. Low hairline at the nape is seen in 75%. Breast development is poor and the chest is shield-shaped (60%) with seemingly wide-spaced, hypoplastic nipples. External genitalia are infantile and pubic hair is sparse. Birth weight is below the third percentile in about 50%. During embryonic life, neck blebs or cystic hygroma are common. In infants, excess skin on the nape and peripheral lymphedema have been noted in about 40%. With age, the excess skin metamorphoses into pterygium colli (about 50%) and, with improvement of deep lymphatic circulation, the peripheral edema gradually disappears. Toenails are hypoplastic, hyperconvex, and deep-set in 75%; increased numbers of cutaneous nevi occur in 60%. Coarctation of the aorta and idiopathic hypertension occur in about 25%, various renal anomalies, especially horseshoe kidney, in over 40%, and telangiectasia of the small bowel in 5%. Hearing loss has been documented in about 50%.

Specific Diagnosis The dysgenetic gonad found in Turner syndrome consists of long streaks of white wavy connective tissue stroma without follicles. Follicles are present, however, in the fetal and infantile ovaries, but in diminished numbers. Thyroid antibodies are elevated in 45,X Turner syndrome, but less frequently than in the X-isoX mosaic. Various skeletal anomalies include cubitus valgus (about 75%), short fourth metacarpals (about 50%), deformity of medial-tibial condyle (about 65%), osteoporosis (about 50%), hypoplasia of cervical vertebrae (about 80%), and small carpal angle.

Differential Diagnosis Turner syndrome must be differentiated from *Noonan syndrome,* an autosomal dominantly inherited disorder characterized by webbed neck, short stature, and lymphangiectatic edema of the extremities; and also from the *multiple pterygium syndrome.*

Prenatal Diagnosis If abnormal cervical blebs are noted on ultrasonography and/or there is elevated α-fetoprotein levels in amniotic fluid, a karyotype is recommended. About 20% of spontaneous abortuses have Turner syndrome.

Basic Defect, Genetics, and Other Considerations Turner syndrome occurs about 1 per 5000 live female births and constitutes approximately 25% of abortuses lost during the first trimester of pregnancy. Turner syndrome is due to partial or complete monosomy X. This most often results from meiotic nondisjunction in gametogenesis in the mother or father or in a postzygotic mitotic error. In about 50% of cases there is only one X chromosome. Another 15% have an iso-X chromosome resulting from replication of the long arm of an X-chromosome and over 65% of this group are mosaics. The clinical spectrum of mosaicism is wide. About 20% menstruate and fertility is markedly reduced. In contrast to patients with 45,X Turner syndrome, who are prone to aortic coarctation, those with X/XX karyotypes are more likely to have pulmonary stenosis with or without atrial septal defects. Deletion of the short arm of an X chromosome (XXp-) results in the Turner phenotype. They are as short as individuals with 45,X Turner syndrome, but are less likely to have associated malformations. Ring chromosome X (XXr) differs phenotypically according to the size of the ring, reflecting the amount of deletion of both short and long arms. The smaller the ring, the greater the deletion and the closer the resemblance to classic 45,X Turner phenotype. XXp- and XXr cases together comprise no more than 10% of Turner syndrome. About 5% are mosaic 45X/46XY. Some virilization may occur at puberty. The Y-bearing cell line predisposes the patient to gonadal neoplasia.

Prognosis and Treatment Prognosis is good for normal life span in the absence of hypertension, cardiovascular anomaly, or gonadal tumor. Psychological problems may result from short stature and sexual infantilism. Cyclic estrogen substitution therapy should be given from the age of about 10 years until the age of menopause. Surgical intervention may be necessary for correction of the coarctation of the aorta or webbing of the neck. Laparotomy and removal of remaining gonadal structures should be done in the case of 45X/46XY karyotype.

REFERENCES

Ferguson-Smith, M.A. Karyotype-phenotype correlations in gonadal dysgenesis and their bearing on the pathogenesis of malformations. *J. Med. Genet. 2:* 142–155, 1965.

Palmer, C.G. and Reichmann, A. Chromosomal and clinical findings in 110 females with Turner syndrome. *Hum. Genet. 35:* 35–43, 1976.

Simpson, J.L. Gonadal dysgenesis and abnormalities of the human sex chromosome: current status of phenotypic-karyotypic correlations. *Birth Defects 11(4):* 23–59, 1975.

- **excess skin neck**
- **lymphedema hands / feet**
- **shield chest / widely spaced nipples**
- **hyperconvex, deep-set nails**

Turner Syndrome

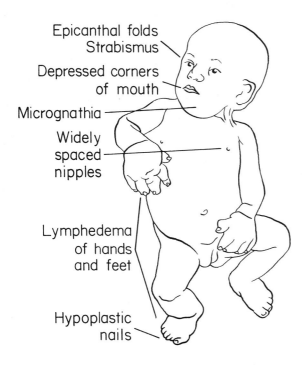

Epicanthal folds
Strabismus
Depressed corners of mouth
Micrognathia
Widely spaced nipples
Lymphedema of hands and feet
Hypoplastic nails

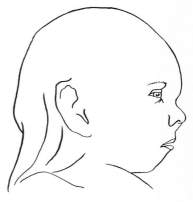

Redundant skin of posterior neck and prominent ear

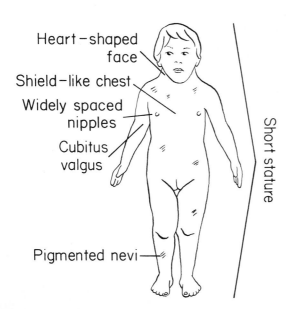

Heart−shaped face
Shield−like chest
Widely spaced nipples
Cubitus valgus
Short stature
Pigmented nevi

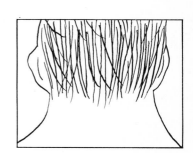

Low posterior hairline and pterygium colli

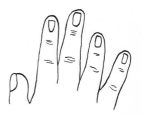

Short 4th metacarpal, narrow, deep-set, hyperconvex nails

58. X-LINKED MENTAL RETARDATION

Clinical Features X-linked mental retardation appears to be second only to Down syndrome in its prevalence. It represents a heterogeneity and has been classified into four groups: (a) Renpenning syndrome, (b) macro-orchidism and fragile X (Martin-Bell), (c) Howard-Peebles syndrome, and (d) Allen-Herndon-Dudley syndrome. *Renpenning syndrome* is characterized by relatively severe mental retardation without other CNS involvement, small head, short stature, normal facies, normal ears, and normal or small testes. In the *macro-orchidism/fragile X syndrome,* mental retardation is moderately severe. Birth weight may be increased, stature is normal, and head circumference is normal or somewhat enlarged. The forehead and mandible are especially prominent and there is some degree of midface retraction. The ears tend to be very large and outstanding with simple helices. The eyes are usually blue. The nose is usually broad-based. Mild scoliosis is not uncommon. The macro-orchidism, unilateral or bilateral, is rarely noted prior to puberty. However, this is not an invariable finding. Speech delay is common and often there is characteristic rhythmic intonation (litany speech). Patients usually exhibit alternating anxiety and hilarity. Seizures occur only in those with the lowest intelligence. The *Howard-Peebles syndrome* phenotype is like that of the macro-orchidism/fragile X syndrome, but without either one of these cardinal features. The *Allen-Herndon-Dudley syndrome* also exhibits mental retardation, hypotonia, weakness, muscle atrophy, and speech retarded beyond the degree of mental retardation.

Specific Diagnosis In the fragile X syndrome, chromosomes grown for a prolonged period (up to 96 hours) in a folic acid-deficient medium (such as TC199) at elevated pH supplemented with only 5% serum exhibit a fragile site at Xq27–28 in 5–75% of the cells of the hemizygote (median 20%). Methotrexate and/or fluorodeoxyuridine is added for the last 24 hours of culture, and colchicine is not used. Air drying of the preparation helps increase the number of fragile sites manifested. The female carrier exhibits the fra(X)(q28) in 0.5 to 6.5% (median 3%) of cells. There is good evidence to indicate that the fragility decreases with age. Hence diagnosis of the heterozygote over 25 years of age may be extremely difficult. Testicular volume is usually measured by the formula $\pi/6 \times$ length $\times$ width^2. Testicular volume is significantly increased (25 to 65 ml); normal values for postpubescent males range from 9 to 25 ml (mean 19 ml).

Differential Diagnosis In the absence of a family history one must exclude other forms of *nonspecific mental retardation.* R-banded chromosomes can be used to rule out a fragile site near 6qter. It should be borne in mind that macro-orchidism is not an invariable finding in the macro-orchidism and fragile X syndrome. Conversely, one may find *macro-orchidism in otherwise normal males.*

Prenatal Diagnosis With recently published techniques for culturing fibroblasts, prenatal diagnosis seems possible.

Basic Defect, Genetics, and Other Considerations As the name implies, the disorder is due to one of several genes—whether allelic is not known—located on the X chromosome. The prevalence of X-linked mental retardation is roughly 1.8 per 1000 males and may account for as many as 25% of males in institutions for the mentally retarded. Macro-orchidism/marker X syndrome may constitute 50% of the cases. Studies on mildly retarded females have demonstrated that about 4% exhibited the fragile X. However, it should be stressed that many obligate heterozygotes are of normal intelligence. Where there is a family history and/or the presence of the marker X, genetic counseling presents no problem, but in the absence of both, a figure of 10% recurrence risk is usually employed for nonspecific mental retardation in the case of an isolated male proband.

Prognosis and Treatment Lifespan does not seem to be markedly affected in any of the disorders. However, in the Allen-Herndon-Dudley syndrome there is often contracture of the hamstring muscles and muscular atrophy making mobility difficult. Currently there is no therapy for these disorders.

REFERENCES

Hecht, F., Jacky, P.B., and Sutherland, G.R. Fragile X chromosome: current methods. *Am. J. Med. Genet. 11:* 489–496, 1982.

Turner, G. and Opitz, J.M. X-linked mental retardation. *Am. J. Med. Genet. 7:* 407–415, 1980.

Turner, G., Daniel, A., and Frost, M. X-linked mental retardation, macro-orchidism and the Xq27 fragile site. *J. Pediatr. 96:* 837–841, 1980.

[Fragile X type]
- **prominent forehead**
- **large, simple ears**
- **prognathism**
- **large testes after puberty**

X-Linked Mental Retardation

MACRO-ORCHIDISM/FRAGILE X SYNDROME

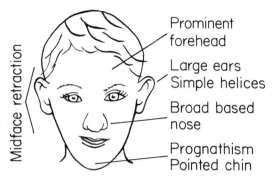

Midface retraction

Prominent forehead

Large ears
Simple helices

Broad based nose

Prognathism
Pointed chin

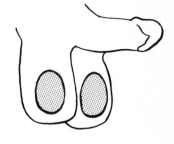

Macro-orchidism,
usually after puberty

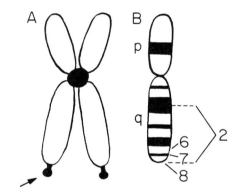

A) fragile X-chromosome (arrow)
B) fragile site at Xq28

RENPENNING SYNDROME

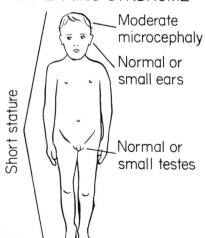

Short stature

Moderate microcephaly

Normal or small ears

Normal or small testes

ALLEN-HERNDON-DUDLEY SYNDROME

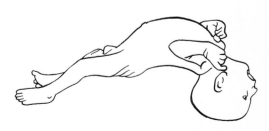

Hypotonia, muscular atrophy and later unintelligible speech

59. XXXXY and XXXXX SYNDROMES

Clinical Features Nearly all reported patients with XXXXY and XXXXX syndromes are mentally retarded, intelligence quotients ranging from 20 to 60. In contrast to XXY Klinefelter syndrome, in which the child is essentially normal up to the time of puberty, those with XXXXY chromosome complement exhibit poor development of the external genitalia. The penis is always minute, the testes extremely small and undescended, the scrotum usually hypoplastic. Birth weight is somewhat low and height is often below the third percentile. Nearly all exhibit muscular hypotonia. Microcephaly is a mild but common feature. Ocular hypertelorism is present in approximately 90%, epicanthus in 80%, strabismus in 50%, mild obliquity of palpebral fissures in 35%, and myopia in 25%. Redundant skin of the nape with subsequent pterygium colli has also been noted. The neck is short in about 80%. Perhaps 5% exhibit cleft palate. In infancy the face is often rounded, but this disappears with age and midface growth is retarded, producing relative mandibular prognathism, especially following puberty, in about 60%. In contrast to XXY syndrome, gynecomastia is not a feature of the XXXXY syndrome. The ability to pronate the forearm is reduced in about 50%. Congenital heart disorders, most frequently PDA or VSD, have been noted in about 15%. The phenotype of XXXXX syndrome closely resembles that of the XXXXY male. The breasts remain infantile, the external genitalia are normal. There are scant pubic hair and infantile uterus but gonadal dysfunction has not been definitely established.

Specific Diagnosis Diagnosis is done by chromosome karyotype analysis. Buccal smears may be examined for Barr bodies. Roentgenographic changes present in most of the cases of XXXXY syndrome include thickened calvaria, radioulnar synostosis, epiphyseal dysplasia, cubitus valgus, retarded bone age, coxa valga, genua valga, elongation of distal ulna and proximal radius, dislocation of radial head, hypoplasia of middle phalanx of fifth digit, squared vertebral bodies, pseudoepiphyses of metacarpals and metatarsals, scoliosis, overlapping toes, and pes planus. Taurodontism is a frequent finding. Simian creases are common. Finger ridge count tends to be low. Microscopically, sections of the testes reveal a marked reduction in spermatogonia. The skeletal changes in the XXXXX syndrome are similar to those in XXXXY. The ovaries in the XXXXX syndrome in some patients are microscopically normal.

Differential Diagnosis Because of the redundant skin at the nape, one might wish to exclude *Noonan syndrome.*

Prenatal Diagnosis While this is possible, it is not probable that diagnosis would be made in this way.

Basic Defect, Genetics, and Other Considerations Postzygotic nondisjunction in an XXY zygote appears to be the cause for the XXXXY state, all the supernumerary X chromosomes coming from the mother. There have been over 100 cases of XXXXY syndrome and about 20 cases of XXXXX syndrome published. All the extra X chromosomes in pentasomy X syndrome are also of maternal origin from double meiotic nondisjunction. There appears to be imperfect inactivation of the supernumerary X chromosomes.

Prognosis and Treatment Mental retardation and sterility are virtually constant findings. There does not appear to be a reduced life span. Treatment is supportive.

REFERENCES

Funderburk, S.J., Valente, M., and Klisak, I. Pentasomy X: report of patient and studies of X-inactivation. *Am. J. Med. Genet. 8:* 27–30, 1981.

Terheggen H.G., Pfeiffer, R.A., Haug, H. et al. Das XXXXY Syndrom. *Z. Kinderheilkd. 115:* 209–234, 1973.

Tumba, A. Le phénotype XXXXY. Étude analytique et synthétique. À propos de 3 cas personnels et de 67 autres cas de la literature. *J. Génét. Hum. 20:* 9–48, 1972.

- excess skin neck
- microcephaly /
  eye anomalies
- round face
- **XXXXY small penis /
  scrotum**
- **XXXXX normal external
  genitalia**

XXXXY and
XXXXX Syndromes

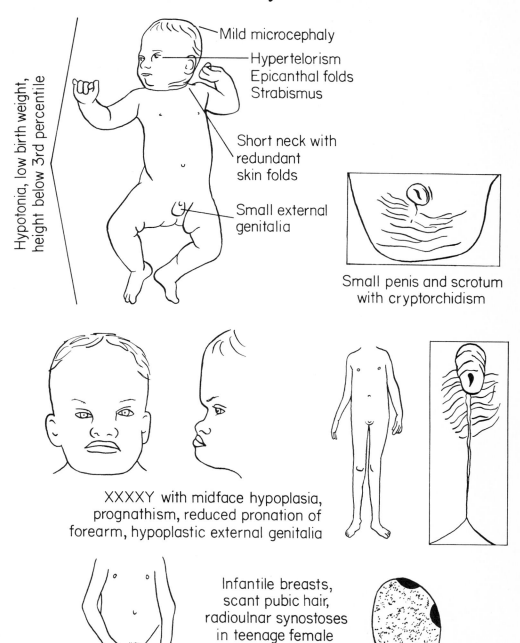

Mild microcephaly

Hypertelorism
Epicanthal folds
Strabismus

Short neck with
redundant
skin folds

Small external
genitalia

Hypotonia, low birth weight,
height below 3rd percentile

Small penis and scrotum
with cryptorchidism

XXXXY with midface hypoplasia,
prognathism, reduced pronation of
forearm, hypoplastic external genitalia

Infantile breasts,
scant pubic hair,
radioulnar synostoses
in teenage female
with XXXXX having
4 sex chromatin bodies

133

C. Genetic Syndromes
b. Connective Tissue

60. CONGENITAL CONTRACTURAL ARACHNODACTYLY

Clinical Features A history of breech delivery appears to be more frequent than normal. At birth, the infants have marked flexion contractures (almost 90°) of the large joints (especially the knees). Muscle mass is disproportionately slender. In infancy there is usually mild kyphosis. With time, scoliosis develops. Early growth and development are normal but motor development is usually impaired because of the contractures. Elbows cannot be completely extended and there is limitation of supination and pronation. The fingers are long and narrow with flexion contractures of the proximal interphalangeal joints. The thumb may be adducted into the palm. The feet are dorsiflexed and excessively long and narrow.

Specific Diagnosis Diagnosis is entirely clinical. Radiographic studies demonstrate gracile bones. The diaphyseal cortices are thin and the trabeculae are sparse. The long bones may be bowed. The proximal phalanges of the fingers and toes are elongated. Scoliosis is progressive. The skull is usually dolichocephalic with frontal bossing. The eyes are deepset. The nose is small with anteverted nostrils and the philtrum is long. The oral opening appears small with microretrognathia. The ears are abnormally shaped, crumpled, and/or outstanding. The antihelix has a prominent crux which partially obliterates the concha allowing for flattening of the helix and giving a crumpled appearance.

Differential Diagnosis One must exclude all other conditions in which there is flexion contracture of the fingers. Among them are various *arthrogrypotic syndromes. Osteogenesis imperfecta* should be excluded because of its manifestation of osteopenia. Patients with *Marfan syndrome, Marfanoid hypermobility syndrome, or homocystinuria,* while exhibiting arachnodactyly, do not manifest flexion contractures. Conversely, patients with congenital contractural arachnodactyly generally have neither cardiovascular abnormalities nor dislocated lenses.

Prenatal Diagnosis This is not currently possible.

Basic Defect, Genetics, and Other Considerations The basis defect is unknown. The disorder has autosomal dominant inheritance with variable expressivity. The condition is relatively rare.

Prognosis and Treatment With time, the kyphoscoliosis may become more severe. The generalized osteopenia may result in fractures, but the flexion contractures improve with age. Treatment consists of early physical therapy and various orthopedic measures both mechanical and surgical to correct the kyphoscoliosis.

REFERENCES

Beals, R.K. and Hecht, F. Congenital contractural arachnodactyly: heritable disorder of connective tissue. *J. Bone Joint Surg. 53A:* 987–993, 1971.

Lipson, E.H., Viseskul, C., and Herrmann, J. The clinical spectrum of congenital contractural arachnodactyly: a case of congenital heart disease. *Z. Kinderheilkd. 118:* 1–8, 1974.

Sanger, R.G. and Wieman, W.B. The C.C.A. syndrome (congenital contractural arachnodactyly): a new differential syndrome for Marfan's syndrome and homocystinuria. *Oral Surg. 40:* 354–361, 1975.

- **flexion contractures**
- **arachnodactyly**
- **kyphoscoliosis**
- **crumpled ears**

Congenital Contractural Arachnodactyly

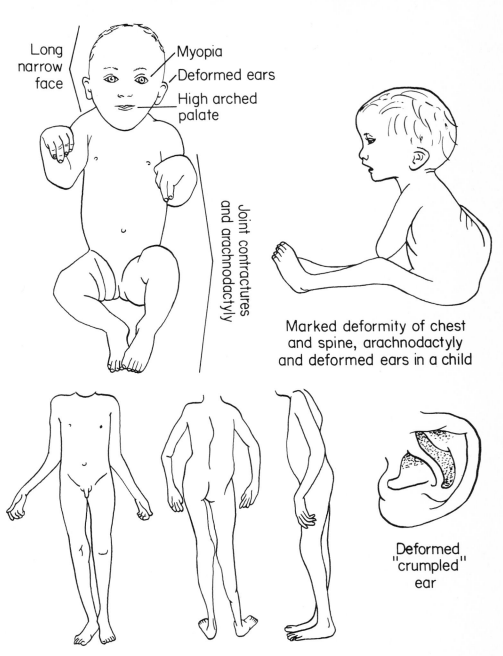

Long narrow face

Myopia

Deformed ears

High arched palate

Joint contractures and arachnodactyly

Marked deformity of chest and spine, arachnodactyly and deformed ears in a child

Deformed "crumpled" ear

Sparse cutaneous fat, joint contractures and kyphoscoliosis in older child

61. CUTIS LAXA SYNDROMES

Clinical Features Cutis laxa is a group of conditions characterized by skin which hangs in loose folds. Blepharochalasis and ectropion of the eyelids together with sagging facial skin (jowls), a long philtrum, and accentuation of the nasolabial and other facial folds produces an aged appearance. The skin of the entire body appears too large for the individual, often hanging in folds. The skin is not hyperplastic and there is no fragility or difficulty in healing. The most common is the severe or lethal form (Type II). In Type II cutis laxa, emphysema is a constant finding. It is apparently congenital and associated with tachypnea, prolonged expiration, or apparent asthma. Associated are right ventricular enlargement, bundle branch block, and cor pulmonale. Pulmonary stenosis, proximal aortic dilatation, and extremely tortuous blood vessels have been reported. Inguinal, diaphragmatic, and umbilical hernia are also frequently noted, as well as diverticulae of the small intestines and bladder, redundant ureter, and prolapse of the gastric, vaginal, and rectal mucosae. Frequent urination is common. The voice is usually hoarse, harsh, deep, and resonant in quality, resulting from laxity of the vocal chords. The patient with the relatively benign form (Type I) exhibits *only* loose skin and it is not uncommon for an affected pubertal child to look older than his unaffected parents. Type III cutis laxa is associated with retarded development. In addition to pre- and postnatal growth retardation there are large fontanels with delayed closure, ocular hypertelorism, congenital hip dislocation, and lax joints. Height is usually below the 10th percentile and intelligence is normal to mildly retarded. Less frequently noted are epicanthal folds, bilateral macular colobomas with fine retinal pigmentation, and low-set ears. Type IV cutis laxa (also known as EDS type IX) is characterized by mild skin hyperextensibility, characteristic facies, occipital horns, ligamentous laxity, scoliosis, pectus excavatum, inguinal hernia, bladder diverticulae, and hydronephrosis.

Specific Diagnosis With elastic fiber stains, one can demonstrate generalized fragmentation and granular degeneration of elastic fibers which result in their marked diminution. The defect is not known in any except the X-linked recessive forms (Type IV) where lysyl oxidase deficiency has been demonstrated in dermal fibroblasts with intermediate activity in female heterozygotes. Serum copper is low.

Differential Diagnosis So-called *acquired cutis laxa* may follow cutaneous inflammation. A congenital acquired form follows chronic penicillamine therapy during pregnancy (*fetal penicillamine syndrome*). *Geroderma osteodysplastica,* an X-linked disorder, is characterized by general retardation, predisposition to skeletal fractures, and platyspondyly. The *wrinkly skin syndrome,* a recessively inherited disorder, is characterized by excessive wrinkling of the skin of the chest, abdomen, and dorsa of the hands and feet. Loose skin, especially in the neck and axillas, may be seen in *pseudoxanthoma elasticum.*

Prenatal Diagnosis Theoretically this should be possible in Type IV cutis laxa, but attempts to date have not been successful. Fetal skin fibroblasts may provide a means of diagnosis, as well as possible histologic changes seen in a fetal skin biopsy obtained by fetoscopy.

Basic Defect, Genetics, and Other Considerations The basic defect is known only for Type IV. Lysyl oxidase acts on residues in collagen to produce reactive aldehydes which effect intermediate cross-links and thus abnormal collagen fibrillogenesis. Type IV thus represents a defect in collagen and not in elastin as exists in Types I, II, and III. The skin changes are mildest in the autosomal dominant Type I form. Type II clearly has autosomal recessive inheritance. It is hard to know whether patients with retarded development, severe mental retardation, athetosis, and cloudy corneas have the same disorder as Type III, which possibly has autosomal recessive inheritance. Type IV has X-linked recessive transmission.

Prognosis and Treatment Type II is lethal, most children dying from emphysema prior to the age of two to three years. Patients with Type III may be retarded. Plastic surgical procedures seem to be of limited value.

REFERENCES

Agha, A., Sakati, N.O., Higginbottom, M.C. et al. Two forms of cutis laxa presenting in the newborn period. *Acta Paediatr. Scand. 67:* 775–780, 1978.

Beighton, P. The dominant and recessive forms of cutis laxa. *J. Med. Genet. 9:* 216–221, 1972.

Byers, P.H., Siegel, R.C., Holbrook, K.A. et al. X-linked cutis laxa. Defective cross-link formation in collagen due to decreased lysyl oxidase activity. *N. Engl. J. Med. 303:* 61–65, 1980.

M.R. [+ / few
in some types]

- sagging skin
- prematurely aged
  appearance
- blepharochalasis
- long philtrum /
  short columella

Cutis Laxa Syndromes

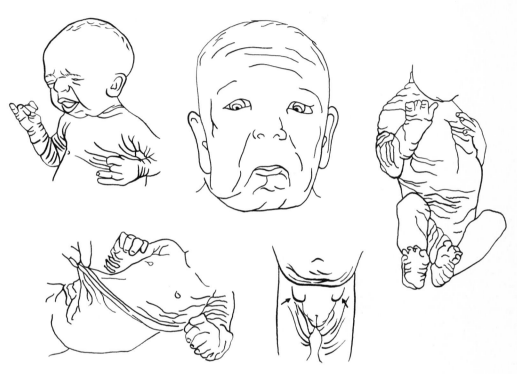

Generalized laxity of skin in infants giving
prematurly aged appearance – inguinal hernias (arrows)

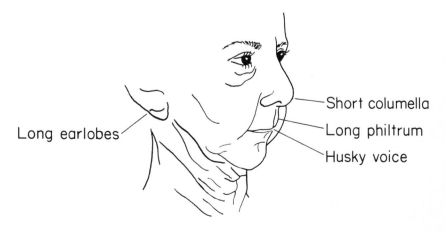

Long earlobes

Short columella

Long philtrum

Husky voice

Teenage girl with marked wrinkling of face and neck

62. EHLERS-DANLOS SYNDROMES

Clinical Features Ehlers-Danlos syndromes (EDS) represent a large genetic heterogeneity. Classic or severe (*Type I*) disease manifests hyperelastic skin, skin hemorrhages, loose-jointedness, cutaneous pseudotumors over the heels and major joints, skin fragility, and subcutaneous spherules of bony prominences of forearms and shins. Prematurity due to early rupture of fetal membranes is common. Hypotonia, blue sclerae, epicanthal folds, and loose-jointedness may be noted at birth. Usually there are scars on the forehead and chin. The ears are often outstanding. The skin is stretchable (especially over joints) and has a velvety feel. Skin wounds gape and heal with a pigmented papyraceous scar. Secondary skin creases in the palm are common and there is often a redundancy of the skin of the hands and feet. Varicose veins and acrocyanosis are frequent. The hand clasp is weak. Recurrent joint dislocations are not rare and kyphoscoliosis and/or hernia are seen in 15–20%. *Type II* is mild, manifesting only moderate skin elasticity and fragility, mild joint hyperextensibility, and moderate bruising. *Type III* or benign hypermobile form usually exhibits marked skin and joint hypermobility but only minimal skin fragility and bruising. *Type IV* or ecchymotic form is characterized by skin translucency exhibiting prominent venous vascular markings, severe bruising of the entire lower leg and elastosis perforans, spontaneous perforations of the intestine or massive gastrointestinal hemorrhage, occasionally arterial rupture, aortic dissection, or peripheral pulmonary artery stenoses. Hyperextensibility is minimal. *Type V* is manifested by marked cutaneous hypermobility, but loose-jointedness is limited to the digits. Skin fragility and bruises are minimal. *Type VI* exhibits fragility of the cornea and sclera and retinal detachment. There is marked joint and skin hypermobility and minimal skin fragility and bruising. *Type VII* is characterized by short stature, multiple joint dislocation, moderate skin hypermobility, fragility, and bruising. *Type VIII* shows minimal skin hypermobility, moderate joint hypermobility limited to digits, marked skin fragility, minimal bruising, and early advanced periodontitis. Lesions on the shins resemble those of necrobiosis diabeticorum. *Type IX* is the same as *cutis laxa*, type IV. *Type X* is characterized by skin and joint hypermobility with a platelet aggregation abnormality. There are undoubtedly many more types.

Specific Diagnosis Diagnosis for the various types is based on clinical manifestations, inheritance patterns, and biochemical abnormalities in Types V–IX (except VIII). Type IV, which is highly heterogeneous (at least four subtypes), requires ultrastructural differentiation. Microscopically, in classic EDS, skin biopsy shows an increase in the number of elastic fibers.

Differential Diagnosis Joint hypermobility is seen in a number of disorders (*Marfan syndrome, Marfanoid hypermobility syndrome,* etc.), but they can be excluded on clinical grounds.

Prenatal Diagnosis In the case of those forms associated with known enzyme defects, it is possible to diagnose the disorders prenatally.

Basic Defect, Genetics, and Other Considerations The basis defect is not known in Types I, II, and III, but a defect in cross-linkage has been suggested. Type IV is due to a deficiency in type III collagen. The cause for Type V is lysyl oxidase deficiency. In Type VI there is lysyl hydroxylase deficiency and in Type VII there is procollagen peptidase deficiency. The cause in Type VIII is unknown. Type IX is associated with defective fibronectin. Inheritance is autosomal dominant in Types I, II, III, IVb, and VIII, autosomal recessive in Types IVa, VI, VII, and IX; and X-linked recessive in Type V. Their approximate frequency is Type I 30%, Type II 45%, Type III 10%, Type IV 5%, Type V 10%. The other forms are extremely rare.

Prognosis and Treatment Death in youth or early adulthood may occur in Type IV (ecchymotic form). Friable tissues and operative difficulties due to abnormal bleeding may occur in both Types I and IV. Avoidance of trauma and contact sports is important in the more severe forms, while special wound closure is necessary for those who make poor scar tissue. Repeated joint dislocations may lead to arthritic changes.

REFERENCES

Beighton, P., Price, A., Lord, J. et al. Variants of the Ehlers-Danlos syndrome: clinical, biochemical, hematological and chromosomal features of 100 patients. *Ann. Rheum. Dis.* 28: 228–245, 1969.

Byers, P.H., Holbrook, K.A., McGillivray, B. et al. Clinical and ultrastructural heterogeneity of type IV Ehlers-Danlos syndrome. *Hum. Genet.* 47: 141–150, 1979.

Stewart, R.E., Hollister, D.W., and Rimoin, D.L. A new variant of Ehlers-Danlos syndrome: an autosomal dominant disorder of fragile skin, abnormal scarring and generalized periodontitis. *Birth Defects* 13(3B): 85–93, 1977.

Ehlers-Danlos Syndromes

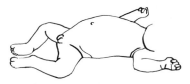

Hypotonia at birth

Epicanthal folds and blue
sclerae in childhood

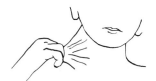 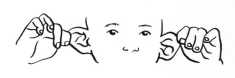

Hyperextensibility of skin   Tongue to nose   Stretchable ears

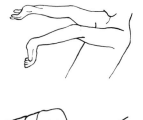 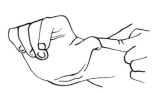 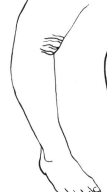 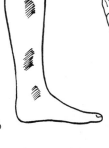 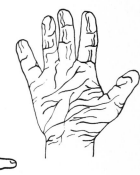

Joint hypermobility, fine scar tissue about knee,
genu recurvatum, pes planus, easy
bruisability and increased palmar creases

63. FIBRODYSPLASIA OSSIFICANS PROGRESSIVA

Clinical Features Fibrodysplasia ossificans progressiva (FOP) is characterized by progressive accumulation of heterotopic bone in connective tissue, skeletal muscle, tendons, and ligaments and by several typical malformations of the foot and hand. Ossification first occurs in the head, neck, spine, or shoulders, or somewhat less often in the lower extremities. Occasionally multiple sites of onset are noted. Onset is noted prior to the age of four years in about 65% (range: 3 months—puberty). With time there is extension to involve most frequently the shoulders, chest, hip, elbow, abdomen, knee, jaw, heels, ankle, head, wrist, foot, and hand, in that order. Unilateral involvement is relatively infrequent. The lesions are painful even to palpation in the early stages, and the overlying skin is erythematous. Within a few weeks, the soft tissue swelling subsides, leaving a bony remnant. Associated fever is experienced by less than 20%. Hearing loss is experienced by 30%. Easy bruisability is noted in about 30%. Joint mobility is accordingly reduced. Nearly all patients have bilateral shortening and valgus deformity of the great toe and about half have short thumbs and clinodactyly of the little fingers.

Specific Diagnosis Biopsy of the bony lesion is not indicated since the hand and, especially, the foot anomalies are quite diagnostic and the biopsy site may serve as a nidus for ectopic ossification. Radiographic studies show complex bony structures in the soft tissues. The proximal phalanx of the first toe is usually broader and squarer than normal and frequently fused with the terminal first phalanx. The first metatarsal is often abnormal, ranging from distortion of the distal tip to a cylindrical foreshortened bone lacking distal metaphyseal or epiphyseal outlines. At least half the patients exhibit fusion anomalies of the middle and terminal phalanges of the second through fifth toes. Hand changes are less severe, the most common being short first metacarpal and small middle phalanx of the fifth digit with associated clinodactyly. The short, broad first metacarpal may be fused with the proximal phalanx of the thumb. Only rarely is there fusion of the middle and terminal phalanges of other digits of the fingers. There is no correlation between the degree of hand and foot malformation and the ossification disorder. The vertebral bodies are often bridged through the spinal processes from the cervical to the lumbar levels. Midthoracic scoliosis is rather frequent.

Differential Diagnosis *Congenital hallux valgus* can be inherited as an autosomal dominant disorder but it is not known whether these cases represent incomplete expression of FOP. Biopsy of the bony lesions may be erroneously diagnosed as *osteosarcoma*.

Prenatal Diagnosis Possibly FOP could be diagnosed by fetoscopic visualization of abbreviation of the large toe and its valgus positioning.

Basic Defect, Genetics, and Other Considerations The basic defect in FOP is not known. It clearly has autosomal dominant inheritance, but the majority of reported cases have been sporadic. Perhaps this is due to the general failure of the individuals, because of their infirmities, to marry and have children. A paternal age effect has been demonstrated. It has been suggested that the abnormal cells which differentiate into heterotopic chondroosseous tissue and the anomalies of the hands and feet arise in alterations which occur about the 43rd to 44th day of fetal development.

Prognosis and Treatment Normal physical activity becomes progressively reduced. In time, such tasks as getting out of bed, sitting in a chair, walking, climbing stairs, dressing, bathing, and using a toilet become increasingly difficult or impossible without aid. Drug therapy with disodium etidionate (diphosphonate) appears to have little or no effect on the course of the disease. Surgery does not increase the range of motion of an impaired joint.

REFERENCES

Rogers, J.G. and Geho, W.B. Fibrodysplasia ossificans progressiva, a survey of forty-two cases. *J. Bone Joint Surg. 61A:* 909–914, 1979.

Schroeder, H.W., Jr. and Zasloff, M. The hand and foot malformations in fibrodysplasia ossificans progressiva. *Johns Hopk. Med. J. 147:* 73–78, 1980.

Smith, R. Myositis ossificans progressiva: a review of current problems. *Sem. Arth. Rheum. 4:* 369–380, 1975.

- **microdactyly of thumbs and big toe**
- **hallux valgus**
- **calcified masses over body**
- **strabismus / facial asymmetry**

Fibrodysplasia Ossificans Progressiva

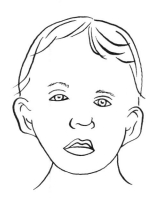
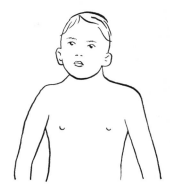

Note strabismus, torticollis and facial asymmetry

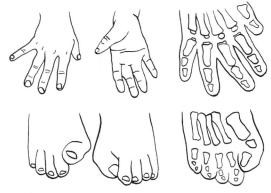
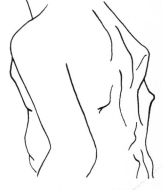

Microdactyly of thumbs, small halluces in valgus position

Multiple calcified masses over back

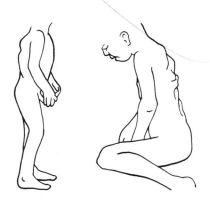
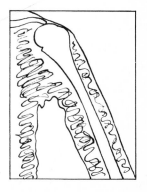

Rigid stance and posture

Extensive soft tissue calcification

64. MARFAN SYNDROME

Clinical Features The main features of Marfan syndrome include disproportionate skeletal growth with dolichostenomelia and arachnodactyly, ectopia lentis, and fusiform and dissecting aneurysms of the aorta. The facies is not really characteristic, for while dolichocephaly is common, the face is not always long, and mandibular prognathism is not always present. More striking are body proportions. The elongated fingers and toes are especially striking. Hammer toes are not uncommon. Pectus excavatum and carinatum, late developing kyphoscoliosis, pes planus, and hyperextensibility of joints with habitual dislocation (hips, patella, clavicle) are common. Hernia (inguinal, femoral) is frequent. There is often deficiency of subcutaneous fat. Eye changes (more common in males) are characteristic. Dislocation of the lens is preceded by iridodonesis. The suspensory ligaments of the lenses break, producing bilateral dislocation in at least 70%. The lenses become displaced superonasally and superotemporally in about 75%. Myopia is common. Aortic regurgitation and floppy mitral valve with mitral regurgitation are found in at least 65%. There is diffuse generally progressive dilatation of the ascending aorta with or without dissecting aneurysm. Aneurysms of the thoracic and abdominal aorta or pulmonary artery are less common. There is an increased frequency of aortic coarctation.

Specific Diagnosis Diagnosis is clinical. The lower segment of the body (pubis to sole) is longer than the upper segment (vertex to pubis). The US/LS ratio in whites averages 0.85 (normal = 0.93). Other indices such as the metacarpal index, relative slenderness index, Walker-Murdoch wrist sign, and Steinberg thumb sign may be helpful. The metacarpal index (the sum of the length of the four metacarpals divided by the sum of the widths of the metacarpals at the exact midpoints) should not exceed 8.5. However, we have found the thumb sign to be positive in many thin females. Ultrasonography of the aortic root in children appears to be indicated for early detection of aneurysms.

Differential Diagnosis A Marfanoid habitus may be observed in a number of conditions: *homocystinuria, congenital contractural arachnodactyly, Marfanoid hypermobility syndrome, eunuchoidism, Klinefelter syndrome, sickle cell anemia, multiple mucosal neuroma syndrome*, and occasionally in the *nevoid basal cell carcinoma syndrome*. Ectopia lentis may occur in *Weil-Marchesani syndrome, Ehlers-Danlos syndromes, homocystinuria*. Aortic dilatation is also seen in *Erdheim's cystic medial necrosis* and in *tertiary syphilis*. Joint hypermobility occurs in a number of disorders, including *osteogenesis imperfecta*, the *Ehlers-Danlos syndromes, homocystinuria*, the *Stickler syndrome*, and the *Marfanoid hypermobility syndrome*.

Prenatal Diagnosis Sonography in the second trimester has been done in pregnancies at risk and, in one, significantly longer limbs were demonstrated.

Basic Defect, Genetics, and Other Considerations The disorder is thought to result from a deficiency in chemically stable collagen cross-links. Collagen production is disturbed at the cellular level, and there appears to be an increase in the ratio of soluble to insoluble collagen. The disorder is inherited as an autosomal dominant trait with a high degree of penetrance and very variable expressivity. Roughly 85% of the cases are familial. The prevalence of Marfan syndrome is at least 1.5 per 100,000 in the general population.

Prognosis and Treatment Prognosis for normal life largely depends on whether there is sudden death resulting from dissecting aneurysm or heart difficulties resulting from aortic regurgitation or mitral regurgitation. Rarely there is hypertension resulting from narrowing of one or both renal arteries. Surgical measures for treatment and prevention of aneurysms and heart valve replacement may be necessary, as well as orthopedic intervention for correction of scoliosis.

REFERENCES

Koenigsberg, M., Factor, S., Cho, S., Herskowitz, A., Nitowsky, H., and Morecki, R. Fetal Marfan syndrome: prenatal ultrasound diagnosis with pathological confirmation of skeletal and aortic lesions. *Prenatal Diag. 1:* 241–247, 1981.

Phornphutkul, C., Rosenthal, A., and Nadas, A.

Cardiac Manifestations of Marfan syndrome in infancy and childhood. *Circulation 47:* 587–596, 1973.

Pyeritz, R.E. and McKusick, V.A. The Marfan syndrome: diagnosis and management. *N. Engl. J. Med. 300:* 772–777, 1979.

- **dolichostenomelia**
- **arachnodactyly**
- **hyperextensible joints**
- **pectus excavatum / carinatum**

Marfan Syndrome

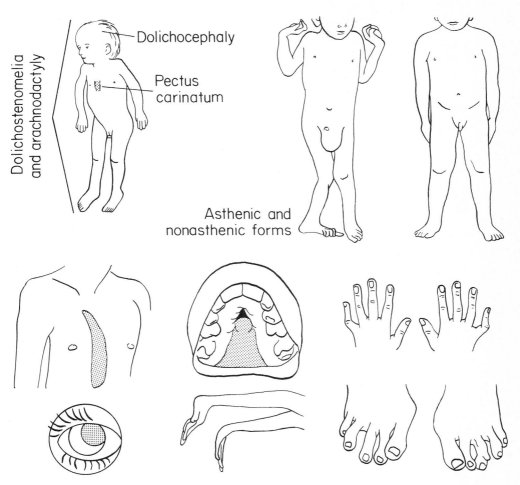

Dolichostenomelia and arachnodactyly

Dolichocephaly

Pectus carinatum

Asthenic and nonasthenic forms

Pectus excavatum, high arched palate, arachnodactyly and camptodactyly 5th fingers, ectopia lentis — upward displacement of lens, joint hypermobility

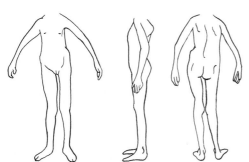

Dolichostenomelia, winging of scapulae, kyphoscoliosis and pes planus

65. OSTEOGENESIS IMPERFECTA SYNDROMES

Clinical Features Osteogenesis imperfecta is a genetic heterogeneity and hence its clinical features depend on the specific type under discussion. Its involvement may be diffuse for not only the skeletal system but the eye, ear, skin, teeth, and blood vessels may be affected. Because of the heterogeneity, the clinical picture can range from infants with a congenital lethal disorder to adult individuals with only a slightly increased tendency toward bone fractures, but with dentinogenesis imperfecta.

Specific Diagnosis Diagnosis is largely clinical, although exceptions will be noted. While the classification of Sillence et al. has some problems, it nevertheless should serve as a working basis for discussion. *Type I:* only about 10% appear to have congenital fractures; most have their first fractures before five years of age. Although bone fracture is frequent, bowing and curvature of long bones and spine are usually mild. Kyphosis with loss of skeletal height occurs with age due to osteopenia of the spine. Otosclerosis with mixed hearing loss is noted with almost 100% frequency by age 50. All affected have blue sclerae. While some families have opalescent dentin, others have normal-appearing teeth. Radiographic changes show characteristic osteopenia, Wormian bones in the skull, and if clinical tooth changes are present the characteristic short tooth roots and obliterated pulp canals and chambers with constriction at the neck of the teeth. *Type II* is characterized by extreme bone fragility, huge numbers of intrauterine fractures especially evident in the ribs and accordion-like alterations in long bones. Radiographic alterations in addition to beaded ribs and crumpling of long bones include poor ossification of the skull vault and base. *Type III* represents the classic concept of osteogenesis imperfecta, the affected individual having severe short stature with progressive deformity of long bones and spine. While the sclerae may be somewhat blue at birth, with age they assume a normal opacity. *Type IV* is the mildest type of osteogenesis imperfecta. Fractures, if they occur at all, are seen during the first few years of life. Some have congenital bowing. During adulthood, there is a tendency toward progressive kyphoscoliosis. Some families appear to have dentinogenesis imperfecta, while others have normal teeth. Subtypes of Types I and IV have now been recognized.

Differential Diagnosis Similar dental color changes are seen in *hereditary opalescent dentin* and in the primary teeth in *dentin dysplasia Type II*. Wormian bones are seen in a number of conditions: *cleidocranial dysplasia, pyknodysostosis, progeria, mandibuloacral dysplasia, acroosteolysis* and a number of other disorders. However, there are sufficient clinical differences to make the diagnosis clearly distinct. Blue sclerae may be seen in *normal infants,* may be inherited as an *isolated autosomal dominant* trait, or in various other disorders such as the *Ehlers-Danlos syndromes.* Prenatal bowing of limbs occurs in *campomelic dysplasia,* in *hypophosphatasia,* and *idiopathically. Osteogenesis imperfecta* in combination with *microcephaly* and *cataracts* exists as an autosomal recessive syndrome.

Prenatal Diagnosis Type II has been diagnosed prenatally at 17.5 weeks using sonography. By 21 weeks, analysis of procollagen synthesis in amniotic fluid cells was abnormal and radiographs showed fractures and short limbs.

Basic Defect, Genetics, and Other Considerations The disorder is pathogenetically heterogeneous. No consistent biochemical findings have been noted. There appears to be a decreased synthesis of Type I collagen, at least in Type II osteogenesis imperfecta, and failure of synthesis of α-2-polypeptide of type I collagen in fibroblasts from Type III osteogenesis imperfecta. Whether these are consistent findings has not been established. Type I osteogenesis imperfecta is transmitted as an autosomal dominant disorder. Type II is autosomal recessive, Type III appears to have autosomal recessive and dominant forms and Type IV is autosomal dominant. The frequency of the various types has not been precisely established, but Type I is approximately 3.5 per 100,000 live births and Type II, 1.6 per 100,000 live births in Australia.

Prognosis and Treatment Various agents such as sodium fluoride, calcitonin and vitamin C have been tried, but there is no evidence to indicate that they are effective. Intramedullary rodding is ordinarily employed as well as spinal fusion. Prognosis depends essentially upon the type of osteogenesis imperfecta one is dealing with. Types I and IV are compatible with normal lifespan. Type II is lethal. Type III individuals often die in the fourth or fifth decade from cardiac valvular anomalies.

REFERENCES

Shapiro, J. E., Phillips, J. A., Byers, P. H. et al. Prenatal diagnosis of lethal perinatal osteogenesis imperfecta (OI Type II). *J. Pediatr. 100:* 127–133, 1982.

Sillence, D.O. Osteogenesis imperfecta: an expanding panorama of variants. *Clin. Orthop. Res. 159:* 11–25, 1981.

Sillence, D.O., Senn, A., and Danks, D.M. Clinical heterogeneity in osteogenesis imperfecta. *J. Med. Genet. 16:* 101–116, 1979.

- **fractures /
  bowing of bones**
- **blue sclerae**
- **kyphoscoliosis**
- **hearing loss**

Osteogenesis Imperfecta Syndromes

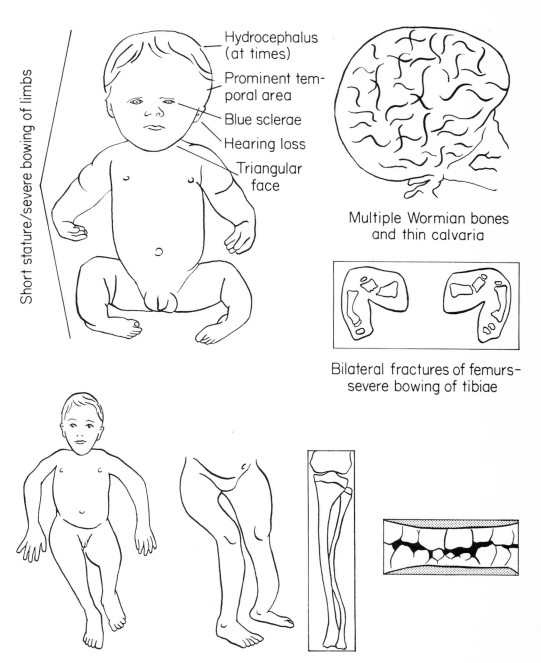

Short stature/severe bowing of limbs

Hydrocephalus (at times)

Prominent temporal area

Blue sclerae

Hearing loss

Triangular face

Multiple Wormian bones and thin calvaria

Bilateral fractures of femurs-severe bowing of tibiae

Short stature, bone deformities, saber-like shape of tibiae, slenderness and bowing of long bones and poor dentition

66. PSEUDOXANTHOMA ELASTICUM SYNDROMES

Clinical Features Pseudoxanthoma elasticum (PXE) is a genetic heterogeneity consisting of alterations of skin, recurrent severe gastrointestinal hemorrhages, weak peripheral pulses, failing vision, and angioid streaks of the retina. The skin becomes thickened and inelastic with the markings accentuated by raised yellowish flat papules, especially about the mouth, neck, axillas, elbows, groin, and periumbilical area. The changes are usually recognized after the second decade but may be present much earlier. The mucosa of the lips, especially the lower, may exhibit yellowish intramucosal nodules in about 10%. Buccal mucosa, soft palate, tonsillar pillars, and vaginal, gastric, or rectal mucosas may be similarly involved. Visual disturbances have been noted in approximately 30% of older patients, often following organization of retinal hemorrhage. Hypertension has been noted in about 20%. Angina pectoris is seen in at least 50% and abdominal angina due to stenosis of the celiac artery is common. Weakness of peripheral pulses and intermittent claudication is noted in about 20% by the third decade. Hemorrhage, especially gastrointestinal, occurs in about 15% and may be recurrent and difficult to manage. Bleeding may also occur in the retina, kidney, uterus, or bladder. Some patients have peptic ulcer.

Specific Diagnosis The involved skin or mucous membrane presents a characteristic microscopic appearance. In the middle and lower corium, the elastic tissue appears as fragmented granular masses. The deposit of calcium salt can be demonstrated by von Kossa staining. Collagen fibers are reduced while reticulum fibers are increased in number. Fundoscopic examination shows white, red-brown, or gray (angioid) streaks in over 85% in the second decade or later due to disruption of Bruch's membrane. Retinal pigment epithelial disturbances, atypical drusen, and neovascularization may also be noted. The fundus following injection of fluorescent dye clearly exhibits the angioid streaks. Abdominal arteriography shows tortuosity and narrowing of arterioles and arteries and angiomatous formation. Radiographic examination reveals calcification of peripheral arteries, especially those of the lower extremities, in about 15%. Calcification of the falx cerebri and subcutaneous tissues has also been noted.

Differential Diagnosis Angioid streaks may be seen in *Paget's disease of bone, sickle cell disease, trauma, osteoectasia with macrocranium (hyperphosphatasia), tumoral calcinosis,* and *hyperphosphatemia.* Clinical skin changes in *senile elastosis* somewhat resemble those in PXE. A combination of *Paget's disease and PXE* has been described by several authors.

Prenatal Diagnosis This has not been accomplished.

Basic Defect, Genetics, and Other Considerations The primary alteration is calcification of elastic fibers. Medium-sized arteries are severely affected by degenerative arteriosclerosis. The internal elastic lamina calcifies and the medial layer thickens, resulting in arterial disease: hypertension, angina, transient cerebral ischemic attacks, and intermittent claudication. There are two recessive and two dominant forms. The combined prevalence of the four types has been estimated at 1 per 40,000. In dominant form I, common findings are flexural lesions, angina, claudication and hypertension, and severe choroiditis with angioid streaks in perhaps 35%. In dominant form II, the most common aspects are macular rash, increased extensibility of the skin, myopia, blue sclerae, and joint hypermobility and angioid streaks in approximately 50%. In recessive form I, classic findings are the orange-peel skin changes, severe choroiditis, and angioid streaks in approximately half the patients. In the recessive form II, the only finding is general cutaneous changes. No primary biochemical defect is known, though elastin metabolism is deranged in most cases.

Prognosis and Treatment Psychiatric disorders have been noted in about 5%. The arteries of the gastrointestinal mucosa are particularly susceptible to spontaneous rupture and hemorrhage is a frequent cause of morbidity and mortality. There is no specific therapy for PXE available at present. Prognosis for visual acuity depends on the degree of atrophic changes and neovascularization of choroidal vessels. Visual acuity gradually worsens. One must attempt to avoid factors predisposing to ocular trauma and vascular disease.

REFERENCES

Altman, L.K., Fialkow, P.J., Parker, F., and Sagebiel, R.W. Pseudoxanthoma elasticum. An underdiagnosed genetically heterogeneous disorder with protean manifestations. *Arch. Intern. Med. 134:* 1048–1054, 1974.

Pope, F.M. Autosomal dominant pseudoxanthoma elasticum. *J. Med. Genet. 11:* 152–157, 1974.

Pope, F.M. Two types of autosomal recessive pseudoxanthoma elasticum. *Arch. Dermatol. 110:* 209–212, 1974.

- **yellow, pebbled skin in body creases**
- **angioid streaks / decreased vision**
- **peripheral vascular disease**
- **upper G.I. hemorrhage**

Pseudoxanthoma Elasticum Syndromes

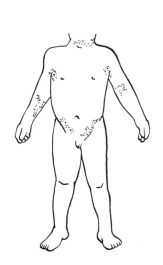
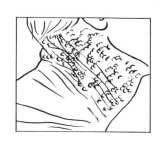
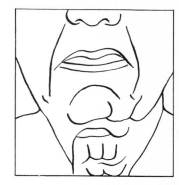
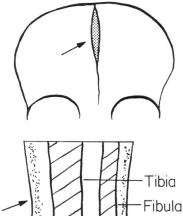
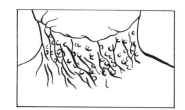
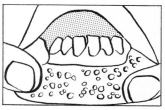

Yellow, pebbled skin in flexural areas, wrinkling and redundant skin folds, mucosal involvement of lip

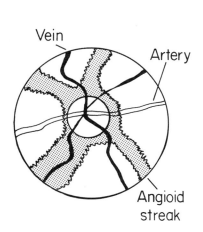

Vein

Artery

Angioid streak

Angioid streaking of fundus

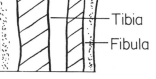
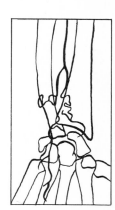

Tibia

Fibula

Calcification of falx cerebri, cutis portion of skin (arrows)— obstruction of radial and ulnar arteries in an adult

67. STICKLER SYNDROME
(hereditary progressive arthroophthalmopathy)

Clinical Features This syndrome whose manifestations are extremely variable consists of progressive multiple dysplasia of the epiphyses and of other skeletal changes, round asymmetric facies, long philtrum, epicanthal folds, joint hypermobility, myopia, retinal detachment, cleft palate, micrognathia, and sensorineural hearing loss. About 85% of the patients exhibit midfacial flattening. The nasal bridge is depressed or saddle-shaped in about 65%. Cleft palate or submucous cleft palate has been present in about 15% of the cases. Bony enlargement of the ankles, knees, and wrists may occur in the first few years of life. The joints at times are painful with use and become stiff at rest. Rarely they are reddened and warm. The patient may experience difficulty in walking if the capital femoral epiphyses are involved. Premature and progressive arthritis is noted with increased frequency. Thoracic kyphosis or scoliosis are noted in about 25% with joint hypermobility in about 40%. Other less common skeletal anomalies include pectus carinatum, genu valgum, and pes planus. Congenital progressive myopia as great as 20 diopters with vitreous degeneration has been noted in about 75–80%. Before the tenth year of life, broad zones of retinal detachment are experienced in about 20%. By 30 years, 75% have detachment. Vitreous and chorioretinal degeneration occur in 80–90%. Cataract (40%) and glaucoma (15%) complicate the clinical picture. About 80% will show sensorineural hearing loss if tested but are usually asymptomatic until middle age.

Specific Diagnosis Diagnosis is purely clinical, there being no test for Stickler syndrome. Radiographically, about one-third of patients exhibit multiple epiphyseal ossification disturbances and diminution in the width of the shafts of tubular bones. The overly thin diaphyses contrast with the normally broad metaphyses. The pelvic bones may be hypoplastic and the femoral neck poorly modeled and plump. There may be some coxa valga. Vertebral bodies tend to be flattened and irregular with a tendency to anterior wedging. The distal tibial epiphysis is usually wedge-shaped. Thoracic kyphosis, as noted above, is common.

Differential Diagnosis It is not known whether this disorder differs from the *Marshall syndrome;* most likely they are the same entity. It is interesting that the original patients described by Wagner with *hyaloideovitreous degeneration* exhibiting autosomal dominant inheritance apparently do not have retinal detachment or cleft palate or bony anomalies, and hence represent another syndrome.

Prenatal Diagnosis There is no technique currently available for prenatal diagnosis of this disorder.

Basic Defect, Genetics, and Other Considerations The basic defect is unknown. The syndrome has autosomal dominant inheritance but remarkably variable expressivity. Historically, the syndrome has been independently described by a number of specialists, usually emphasizing their specific area of interest, so that it has appeared periodically in the literature under various names.

Prognosis and Treatment There is a normal life span. For most patients the chief difficulty lies not in bony involvement but in severe myopia and the constant threat of retinal detachment and glaucoma. Periodic eye examinations should be scheduled with proper treatment given for retinal detachment and other ocular findings. Mental retardation has been reported in a few patients.

REFERENCES

Knobloch, W.H. and Layer, J.M. Clefting syndromes associated with retinal detachment. *Am. J. Ophthalmol. 73:* 517–530, 1972.

Liberfarb, R.M., Hirose, T., and Holmes, L.B. The Wagner-Stickler syndrome: a study of 22 families. *J. Pediatr. 99:* 394–399, 1981.

Maumenee, I.H.: Vitreoretinal degeneration as a sign of generalized connective tissue diseases. *Am. J. Ophthalmol. 88:* 432–449, 1979.

M.R. [+ / few]

- **enlarged joints**
- **myopia /
  retinal detachment**
- **cleft palate**
- **flat midface**

Stickler Syndrome
[hereditary progressive
arthroophthalmopathy]

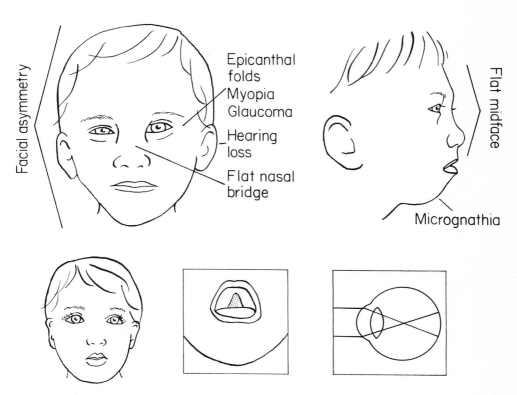

Facial asymmetry

Epicanthal
folds
Myopia
Glaucoma

Hearing
loss

Flat nasal
bridge

Flat midface

Micrognathia

Rounded facies with asymmetry, cleft palate,
myopia prone to retinal detachment

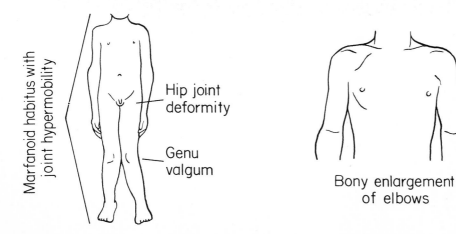

Marfanoid habitus with
joint hypermobility

Hip joint
deformity

Genu
valgum

Bony enlargement
of elbows

151

C. Genetic Syndromes
c. Endocrine / Metabolic

68. ADRENOGENITAL SYNDROMES

Clinical Features The adrenogenital syndromes represent a heterogeneity. Over 90% of patients have 21-hydroxylase deficiency. Less frequently the disorder is due to 11-β-hydroxylase deficiency or 3-β-dehydrogenase deficiency. There are other forms, but they are extremely rare. Since 21-hydroxylase deficiency is most common, it will be described in detail. Newborn females exhibit variable degrees of masculinzation ranging from mild clitoral enlargement to complete fusion of labioscrotal folds, simulating a scrotum without testes. Some females have a male phallus and a developed prostate, but ovaries and uterus are also present. Rarely, complete external virilization of newborn females may lead to erroneous gender assignment. Untreated females do not exhibit pubertal changes. The genitalia and/or nipples may exhibit excessive pigmentation. Newborn males appear clinically normal but may develop premature penile enlargement and early development of secondary sexual characteristics. Bone maturation is accelerated in both sexes with premature fusion of the epiphyses resulting in short stature. Salt loss, manifested by vomiting, hyponatremia, hypercalcemia, dehydration, and renal salt excretion is exhibited by about 65% of patients with 21-hydroxylase deficiency. The incidence would even be higher were plasma renin activity used as an index. In 11-β-hydroxylase deficiency, one notes similar virilization of female genitalia but no loss of salt. Hypertension is frequent. In the 3-β-dehydrogenase type, the patients lose large amounts of salt and males are incompletely virilized with hypospadias with or without cryptorchidism.

Specific Diagnosis In 21-hydroxylase deficiency, all patients have elevated urinary and plasma levels of 17-ketosteriods and pregnanetriol. There is marked elevation of plasma 17-α-hydroxyprogesterone. Neonatal screening for 21-hydroxylase deficiency may be done by measuring plasma 17-α-hydroxyprogesterone in an assay done on a drop of blood dried on filter paper.

Differential Diagnosis Salt loss with its attending manifestations may be mistaken for *pyloric stenosis,* especially in newborn males who lack the genital stigmata. The effect of hyperkalemia on the myocardium may lead to erroneous diagnosis of *congenital heart disease.* An ECG should exhibit elevated T-waves typical of hyperkalemia. Mild female cases may present first in adult life and stimulate *Stein-Leventhal syndrome.* Rarely, adrenogenital syndrome (11-β-hydroxylase type) may be associated with adrenal cortical adenoma or especially carcinoma.

Prenatal Diagnosis Successful antenatal detection has been reported for all forms of adrenogenital syndrome. In the case of 21-hydroxylase deficiency, its linkage with the HLA complex makes prenatal diagnosis possible.

Basic Defect, Genetics, and Other Considerations In the adrenogenital syndromes there is a block at one of the stages in the biosynthesis of cortisol by the adrenal. The 21-hydroxylase deficiency occurring in about 1 in 40,000 in the United States involves failure to convert progesterone and 17-α-hydroxyprogesterone to deoxycorticosterone and 11-deoxycortisol, which require 21-hydroxylations. Since cortisol is involved in a negative feedback mechanism, there is excessive production of ACTH by the pituitary. Metabolic conversions in extra-adrenal sites of ACTH stimulate androgen precursors leading to elevated androgen levels which cause virilization. Those with and without salt loss are fairly specific. In 11-hydroxylase deficiency, the block results in a buildup of compound S (desoxycortisol) and desoxycorticosterone, the latter resulting in hypertension. In 3-β-dehydrogenase deficiency, the block affects the glucocorticoid, mineralocorticoid, and sex steroid pathways. All forms of the adrenogenital syndromes exhibit autosomal recessive inheritance.

Prognosis and Treatment Intrauterine therapy may be effected to minimize virilization in female embryos. With appropriate therapy there is no reduced life span or height. Administration of cortisol prevents progressive virilization. Female fertility is reduced if treatment is inadequate. If there is salt loss, treatment with hydration, a mineralocorticoid, and additional salt intake are required. Plastic surgical repair of the ambiguous appearance of the genitalia is ordinarily done within the first few years to allow appropriate sex rearing. Definitive plastic repair of the urogenital sinus is deferred until adolescence.

REFERENCES

Nichols, J. and Gibson, G.G. Antenatal diagnosis of the adrenogenital syndrome. *Lancet 2:* 1068–1069, 1969.

Pang, S., Hotchkiss, J., Drash, A.L. et al. Microfilter paper method for 17-alpha-hydroxy progesterone radioimmunoassay: its application for rapid screening for congenital adrenal hyperplasia. *J. Clin. Endocrinol. Metab. 45:* 1003–1008, 1977.

Simopoulos, A.P., Marshall, J.R., Delea, C.S., et al. Studies on the deficiency of 21-hydroxylation in patients with congenital adrenal hyperplasia. *J. Clin. Endocrinol. Metab. 32:* 438–443, 1971.

Adrenogenital Syndromes

21−HYDROXYLASE DEFICIENCY

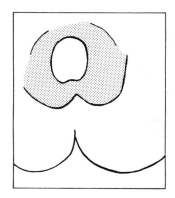 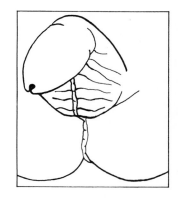

External genitalia of female infants
showing moderate and complete virilization

3 BETA− DEHYDROGENASE DEFICIENCY

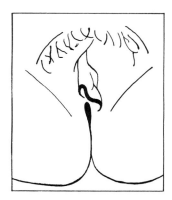 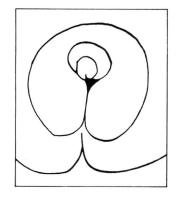

Female infant with
clitoral hypertrophy
and pubic hair

Male infant with
bifid scrotum, hypospadias
and small penis

69. ASCHER SYNDROME

Clinical Features Ascher syndrome consists of blepharochalasis, double lip, and nontoxic thyroid enlargement. In the presence of all three anomalies, the diagnosis is easy. The sagging eyelids and abnormal lip seen during smiling or talking are quite striking. The lids are usually involved first. The upper lid manifests relaxation of the supratarsal fold. This allows the edge of the lid to hang slack over the palpebral fissure. The lid skin is markedly thin and atrophic. Several patients have indicated that the atrophy and drooping of the lid have followed repeated angioneurotic edema-like episodes. At some time between the eighth and fifteenth years of life the swelling of the lids and enlargement of the lips may occur simultaneously. There may be some association with sexual maturation. The lip, almost always the upper, is the site of a horizontally running duplication located between the inner and outer parts of the lip. The fold cannot be seen when the lips are closed. The enlargement of the lip also exists from childhood. Rarely the lower lip is enlarged. Thyroid gland enlargement is variable and is not associated with toxic symptoms. It appears several years after eyelid involvement, but usually during the second decade and its presence is the least consistent of the triad.

Specific Diagnosis Gross examination of the relaxed skin of the eyelid has shown prolapsed orbital fat or more frequently hyperplastic lacrimal gland tissue. The excessive labial tissue usually reveals loose areolar tissue and hyperplastic mucous glands, numerous blood-filled capillaries, and perivascular infiltration with plasma cells and lymphocytes.

Differential Diagnosis *Double lip* may occur as an isolated anomaly. The *Melkersson-Rosenthal syndrome* (cheilitis glandularis, facial paralysis, and fissured tongue) and *vascular neoplasms* (hemangioma, lymphangioma) should be considered. *Blepharochalasis*, either unilateral or bilateral, may be an isolated finding or seen in the *cutis laxa* syndromes. It has been estimated that Ascher syndrome constitutes about 10% of cases of blepharochalasis.

Prenatal Diagnosis This is not possible.

Basic Defect, Genetics, and Other Considerations The cause of the disorder is unknown. Various theories have included hormonal dysfunction and vasomotor instability. While autosomal dominant transmission has been suggested, we are skeptical that the disorder has single gene inheritance. At least 50 cases have been reported.

Prognosis and Treatment Minor surgery by an ophthalmologist and dentist or oral surgeon will correct the eye and labial anomalies. There is no therapy other than surgical correction. There is no evidence to indicate that there are functional abnormalities of the thyroid in this disorder.

REFERENCES

Barnett, M.L., Bosshardt, L.L., and Morgan, A.F. Double lip and double lip with blepharochalasis (Ascher's syndrome). *Oral Surg. 34:* 727–733, 1972.

Findlay, G.H. Idiopathic enlargements of the lips: cheilitis granulomatosa, Ascher's syndrome, and double lip. *Br. J. Dermatol. 66:* 129–138, 1954.

Papanayotou, P.H. and Hatziotis, J.C. Ascher's syndrome. *Oral Surg. 35:* 467–471, 1973.

Ascher Syndrome

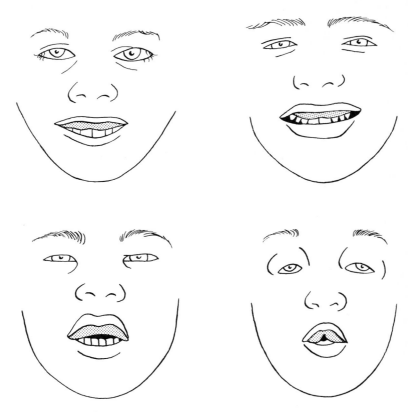

Degrees of horizontal duplication
of upper lip and blepharochalasis

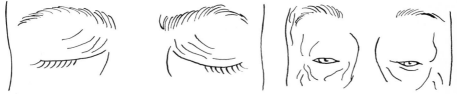

With age upper eyelids become more wrinkled,
thin and atrophic with drooping

70. BARDET-BIEDL SYNDROME

Clinical Features There has been much attendant confusion due to close overlap of several syndromes. Since the Bardet-Biedle syndrome appears to be most common, it shall be described in detail. Classic features include mental retardation, pigmentary retinopathy, polydactyly, obesity, and hypogenitalism. Birth weight is usually elevated, about 70% falling above the 50th percentile and 40% above the 90th percentile for gestational age. About one-third are obese by the age of one year. The obesity is almost invariably of the truncal type and is present in over 90%. Patients tend to be short. Pigmentary retinopathy is present in over 80% and nystagmus in about 20%. The hypogenitalism, probably due to primary gonadal failure, has been noted in about 85% of men and in 50% of women. Approximately 70% have postaxial hexadactyly of one or more extremities. About 5% exhibit an associated mild syndactyly or brachydactyly. Psychological or neurological disorders have been observed in approximately 85% of males and 70% of females. Most commonly there are mental retardation, a labile personality, and an infantile affect. In about 10% there is a mild spasticity of the extremities or extrapyramidal abnormality. Approximately 10–15% exhibit renal problems: glomerulonephritis, pyelonephritis, dilatation of the calices. Sensorineural hearing loss has been noted in approximately 10%. There is no characteristic facies, but mild macrocephaly is commonly noted.

Specific Diagnosis Diagnosis is essentially clinical, based on the above features. Urinary gonadotropin levels are decreased.

Differential Diagnosis The *Laurence-Moon syndrome* patients have pigmentary retinopathy and spastic paraplegia, but not polydactyly or obesity and hence have a different disorder. *Alstrom syndrome* is characterized by retinitis pigmentosa, obesity, diabetes mellitus, sensorineural hearing loss, and normal intelligence. To further compound the confusion, an Alstrom-like family has been reported with mental retardation. *Biemond II syndrome* consists of mental retardation, obesity, polydactyly, and iris colobomas. Many so-called "atypical" cases of Bardet-Biedl syndrome are examples of Alstrom syndrome in which urinary gonadotropin levels are elevated. *Prader-Willi syndrome* shares obesity and mental retardation, but there are neither polydactyly nor pigmentary retinopathy. The *Carpenter syndrome* should be readily distinguished.

Prenatal Diagnosis May be possible by fetoscopy or sonography if extra digits are present.

Basic Defect, Genetics, and Other Considerations The Bardet-Biedl syndrome, Laurence-Moon syndrome, Beimond syndrome, and Alstrom syndrome are all inherited as autosomal recessive disorders. In the case of Bardet-Biedl syndrome, consanguinity is high, hence the gene must be extremely rare. Alstrom syndrome probably has greater frequency than the number of published cases indicates. The Laurence-Moon cases may be unique and the Biemond syndrome has only a few published examples.

Prognosis and Treatment About 35% of patients with Bardet-Biedl syndrome die from renal failure. Therapy is largely supportive.

REFERENCES

Bauman, M.L. and Hogan, G.R. Laurence-Moon-Biedl syndrome. *Am. J. Dis. Child. 126:* 119–126, 1973.

Edwards, J.A., Sethi, P.K., Scoma, A.J., Bannerman, R.M., and Frohman, L.A. A new familial syndrome characterized by pigmentary retinopathy, hypogonadism, mental retardation, nerve deafness and glucose intolerance. *Am. J. Med. 60:* 23–32, 1976.

Schachat, A.P. and Maumenee, I.H. Bardet-Biedl and related disorders. *Arch. Ophthalmol. 100:* 285–288, 1982.

- **obesity**
- **polydactyly**
- **retinopathy**
- **hypogenitalism**

Bardet-Biedl Syndrome

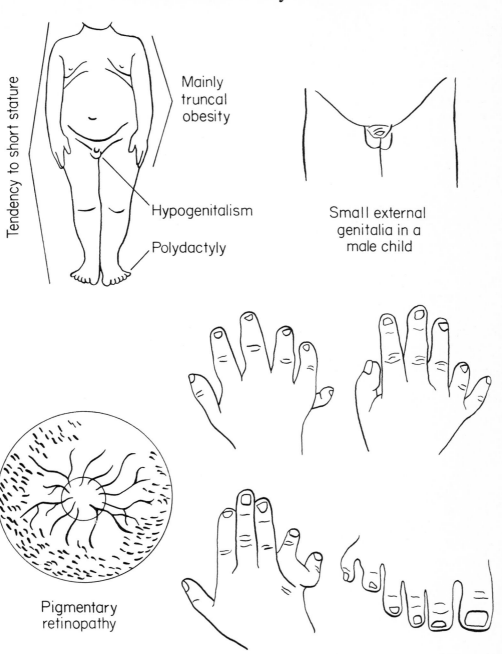

Tendency to short stature

Mainly truncal obesity

Hypogenitalism

Polydactyly

Small external genitalia in a male child

Pigmentary retinopathy

Postaxial hexadactyly with mild syndactyly and brachydactyly

71. FABRY DISEASE

Clinical Features Fabry syndrome is characterized by systemic accumulation of the glycosphingolipid, trihexosyl ceramide, particularly in the cardiovascular-renal system, skin, eyes, and oral mucosa. The cutaneous and mucosal telangiectatic lesions usually appear during childhood and increase in size and number with age. They appear as clusters of individual macular or papular punctate superficial dark red angiectases which do not blanch on pressure. There is a predilection for the iliosacral area, scrotum, posterior thorax, buttocks, thighs, umbilicus, and lips. Hypohidrosis is a frequent finding. Ocular changes include aneurysmal dilatation and tortuosity of conjunctival and retinal vessels. Diffuse haziness or whorled streaks may be seen in the corneal epithelium under slit-lamp microscopy in all hemizygous males and in some heterozygous females. The cardiovascular-renal system becomes progressively involved with age. Proteinuria, isosthenuria, and gradual deterioration of renal function with development of azotemia occur in the second to fourth decades. Cardiovascular findings in late maturity may include hypertension, left ventricular hypertrophy, myocardial ischemia or infarction, and cerebrovascular death.

Specific Diagnosis Growth retardation and delayed puberty are commonly noted. During childhood or adolescence, frequently there is periodic excruciating incapacitating acroparesthesia, which may become frequent and severe with age. The painful crises may last for several days and are associated with low-grade fever and elevation of the erythrocyte sedimentation rate. There may be mild microcytic hypochronic anemia. Nausea, vomiting, diarrhea, and abdominal or flank pain are common gastrointestinal symptoms. Less frequent are massive lymphedema of the legs and dyspnea. Casts, red cells, and lipid inclusions with characteristic birefringent maltese crosses appear in the urinary sediment relatively early in the disease. There is deficient activity of specific ceramide trihexosidase or nonspecific

α-galactosidase in plasma, leukocytes, cultured fibroblasts, hair follicles, urine, and tears of the hemizygote and in 60–70% of heterozygotes. The identification rate of heterozygotes is improved to 90% if an α/β-galactosidase activity ratio is employed.

Differential Diagnosis The skin lesions are so characteristic that the need for differential diagnosis is extremely limited. They may also be seen in *fucosidosis*. The lesions of *hereditary hemorrhagic telangiectasia* are larger, less numerous, and do not involve the lower trunk and thighs. The *Fordyce type of angiokeratoma* is usually limited to the scrotum. The painful extremities and elevated sedimentation rate may lead to the erroneous diagnosis of *rheumatic fever*.

Prenatal Diagnosis This is possible as there is deficient α-galactosidase in cultured cells obtained by amniocentesis.

Basic Defect, Genetics, and Other Considerations The basic defect is deficient activity of the α-galactosidase, ceramide trihexosidase which normally catabolizes the accumulated glycosphingolipid. The latter is deposited in endothelial cells of the glomeruli and in smooth muscle cells of blood vessels. The disorder exhibits X-linked recessive inheritance with variable expression in heterozygotes. The genetic loci for Xg^a and Fabry syndrome have been shown to be linked. A rough estimate for the frequency of the disorder is 1 in 50,000 U.S.A. whites.

Prognosis and Treatment Most hemizygotes die either from uremia or cerebrovascular accident by the fourth decade. Currently there is no effective general treatment, i.e. enzyme replacement. The acroparesthesia and painful crises are helped greatly by use of diphenylhydantoin or carbamazepine. The cardiovasculorenal, neurologic, pulmonary, and musculoskeletal problems are treated symptomatically.

REFERENCES

Desnick, R.J. et al. Fabry's disease: enzymatic diagnosis of hemizygotes and heterozygotes: alpha-galactosidase activities in plasma, serum, urine, and leukocytes. *J. Lab. Clin. Med. 81:* 157–171, 1973.
Pyeritz, R.E., Bender, W.L., and Lipford, E.H. III. Anderson-Fabry disease. *Johns Hopk. Med. J. 150:* 181–187, 1982.

Sheth, K.J., Good, T.A., and Murphy, J.V. Heterozygote detection in Fabry disease utilizing multiple enzyme activities. *Am. J. Med. Genet. 10:* 141–146, 1981.

- **cutaneous and mucosal angiectases**
- **vascular eye changes**
- **hypohidrosis**
- **acroparesthesias**

Fabry Disease

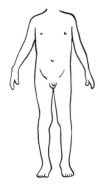

In childhood—
periodic fever
with burning
pain in skin
and extremities
plus diminished
sweating

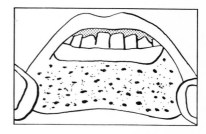

Angiokeratoma about
labial mucosa

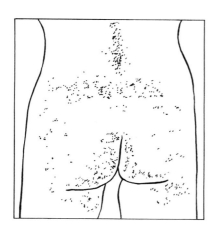

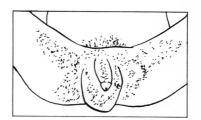

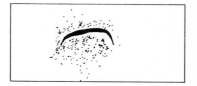

Angiokeratoma about buttocks, back, penis,
scrotum, inner thighs and periumbilical area

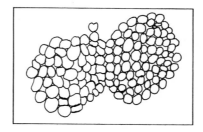

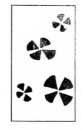

Fundus with tortuous veins, renal epithelial cells filled with lipid
steroids (mulberry cells), "Maltese cross" material in urinary sediment

72. FUCOSIDOSIS SYNDROMES

Clinical Features There appear to be three, possibly four, forms of fucosidosis. In all known types, initial psychomotor development appears normal. In the most severe (Type I) and in a less severe (Type II) form, psychomotor development stops at 10 and 18 months, respectively. Progressive neurologic deterioration then occurs with increasing spasticity, tremor, and gradual loss of environmental contact eventuating in a state of total unresponsiveness. Type III, a milder form, is initially manifest at a later time, probably close to 3 years. In all subtypes, muscular weakness and hypotonia are observed. In Type I and Type II there is progression to decorticate and/or decerebrate rigidity. Type III is characterized by a less rapid rate of psychomotor and neurologic deterioration and by skin lesions (angiokeratomata) especially in the pubic area. The skin is thick. Gingival angiokeratomata have also been reported. Sweating is deficient. In Type II and in some cases of Type III there is coarse facies characterized by prominent forehead, ocular hypertelorism, broad and flat nose, heavy eyebrows, thick lips and tongue. Growth retardation is evident. The thorax is broad and there is usually lumbar hyperlordosis. All types exhibit severe hepatosplenomegaly and recurrent upper respiratory tract infections. There may be a fourth type which resembles Type III but exhibits dry thin skin and no angiokeratomata.

Specific Diagnosis There is low serum and leukocyte activity of α-L-fucosidase. In all types of fucosidosis, radiographic studies show changes of mild dysostosis multiplex: diploic thickening, premature cranial suture closing, cervical platyspondyly, thoracolumbar kyphosis, anterior beaking of lumbar spine, and absent or rudimentary coccyx.

Differential Diagnosis Angiokeratoma corporis diffusum is also seen in *Fabry disease*. The radiographic changes are essentially those of dysostosis multiplex and must be differentiated from the mild forms of *mucopolysaccharidosis, mucolipidosis,* and *mannosidosis.* Fucosidosis, Types I and II, must be differentiated from various storage diseases such as *Tay-Sachs disease, Sandhoff disease,* etc.

Prenatal Diagnosis Should be possible by demonstrating the lysosomal deficiency from cultured fetal fibroblasts obtained by amniocentesis.

Basic Defect, Genetics, and Other Considerations The basic defect is deficiency of the lysosomal hydrolase α-L-fucosidase, with consequent abnormal intracellular accumulation of fucose-containing compounds (glycolipids, lipoproteins, oligosaccharides, polysaccharides) in lysosomes of cells in almost all organ systems. At least 35 cases have been reported. Fucosidosis has autosomal recessive inheritance but there is a marked male predilection. The disorder may have higher frequency in individuals of Italian descent. It is not known whether the different forms represent different allelic mutations, but there is suggestion that they do not.

Prognosis and Treatment The progress of the disease in Types I and II is rapid. No patient has survived beyond six years of age. Patients with Type III and Type IV may survive into the third decade. It is likely that there is further heterogeneity. Treatment is supportive.

REFERENCES

Borrone, C., Gatti, R., Trias, X. et al. Fucosidosis: clinical, biochemical, immunologic and genetic studies in two new cases. *J. Pediatr.* 84: 727–730, 1974.

Lee, F.A., Donnell, G.N., and Gwinn, J.L. Radiographic features of fucosidosis. *Pediatr. Radiol. 5:* 204–209, 1977.

Schoonderwaldt, H.C., Lamers, K.J.B., Kleijnen, F.M. et al. Two patients with an unusual form of Type II fucosidosis. *Clin. Genet. 18:* 348–354, 1980.

M.R. [+ / all]

- angiokeratomata
- thick skin
- hepatosplenomegaly
- muscle weakness / neurologic deterioration

Fucosidosis Syndromes

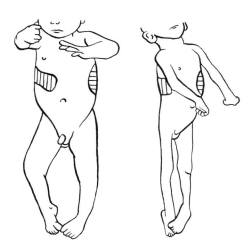

Types I and II with hepatosplenomegaly, muscular weakness and spasticity progressing to decerebrate rigidity

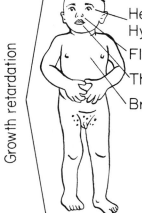

Growth retardation

Prominent forehead
Heavy eyebrows
Hypertelorism
Flat nose
Thick lips
Broad chest

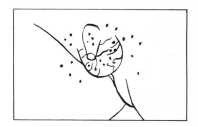

Type III with coarse facies, psychomotor deterioration, deficient sweating and angiokeratomata about pubic area

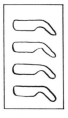 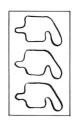 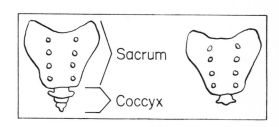

Sacrum

Coccyx

Cervical platyspondyly, anterior beaking lumbar spine, normal coccyx and hypoplasia of coccyx in fucosidosis

73. GAUCHER DISEASE

Clinical Features There are three subtypes of Gaucher disease: (a) acute neuropathic or infantile form, (b) the most common (perhaps 90%) subacute neuropathic or juvenile form, (c) non-neuropathic chronic or adult form. Onset of the classic infantile form presents at two to four months of life as failure to thrive. Affected infants have opisthotonus, spasticity, and severe psychomotor retardation. The subacute neuropathic type is characterized by onset of hepatosplenomegaly during infancy or early childhood. These patients exhibit gradually increasing dementia with seizures and/or extrapyramidal and cerebellar signs. The so-called adult type, which is somewhat of a misnomer, may present within the first year of life. In this form hepatosplenomegaly may be enormous. Bone and joint pain, pathologic fractures, thrombocytopenia with associated easy bruising and epistaxis, and aseptic necrosis, especially of the capital femoral epiphysis, are characteristic features. Often there is failure of tubulation, producing the so-called Erlenmeyer-flask alteration of the femur. There may be areas of dissolution in long bones and vertebrae. Increased pigmentation of the face and extremities may occur and pingueculae (yellow patches of the sclerae) are seen in about 30% of adults.

Specific Diagnosis So-called Gaucher cells can be found in bone marrow. These are large histiocytic cells, 20–100 μm in diameter, with an eccentric nucleus and wrinkled cytoplasm. They are PAS positive. Elevated glucocerebrosides may be found in the liver, spleen, or plasma, and there is a deficiency of β-glucosidase in tissues or in circulating white blood cells. There is an increase in tartrate-resistant serum acid phosphatase activity which is also histochemically demonstrable in the cytoplasm of Gaucher cells in all three forms.

Differential Diagnosis The infantile subtype must be differentiated from other neurodegenerative disorders both with hepatosplenomegaly (*Niemann-Pick, mannosidosis, mucopolysaccharidoses I-H and VIII, sialodosis, G$_M$2 gangliosidosis*) and without hepatosplenomegaly (*Tay-Sachs disease, Krabbe disease, metachromatic leukodystrophy*) as well as various *congenital infections* by the presence of the characteristic Gaucher cells in bone marrow. However, these cells are not specific and may be seen in some leukemias and in idiopathic thrombocytopenic purpura. The juvenile and non-neuropathic subtypes are differentiated from other disorders exhibiting splenomegaly by the presence of the characteristic bone marrow cells. Similar macrophages which are not PAS-positive occur in chronic myelogenous leukemia.

Prenatal Diagnosis Possible, by demonstration of deficient β-glucosidase activity in aminocytes cultured from amniotic fluid.

Basic Defect, Genetics, and Other Considerations The basic defect is deficient activity of acid β-glucosidase, a glucocerebroside-cleaving enzyme whose absence causes accumulation of glucocerebroside in histiocytes and in lysosomes of reticuloendothelial cells. All forms of Gaucher disease are inherited as autosomal recessive disorders. The infantile form is seen in various ethnic groups. The majority of cases of the subacute neuropathic type have occurred in an inbred isolate of Sweden above the Arctic Circle. Approximately 80% of patients with the adult form of Gaucher disease are of Ashkenazi Jewish ancestry. The carrier rate is approximately that of Tay-Sachs disease (about 1 in 30 Ashkenazi Jewish individuals).

Prognosis and Treatment In the infantile patient, aspiration pneumonia and debilitation usually lead to death by one year of age. Death in the juvenile subacute neuropathic form usually occurs by the second decade. In the adult form, fractures of the femoral neck and vertebral bodies and aseptic necrosis of the femoral head are common. With extensive involvement of the hips, total hip replacement may be carried out with good results. Painful infarcts are best managed by bedrest, fluids, and analgesics. Splenectomy should be undertaken only to control hemorrhagic symptoms or when it is so massive that it causes mechanical obstruction.

REFERENCES

Lee, R.E., Peters, S.P., and Glew, R.H. Gaucher's disease: clinical, morphologic and pathogenetic considerations. *Pathol. Annual 12:* 309–339, 1977.

Peters, S.P., Lee, R.E., and Glew, R.H. Gaucher's disease, a review. *Medicine 56:* 425–442, 1977.

Sack, G.H., Jr. Clinical diversity in Gaucher's disease. *Johns Hopk. Med. J. 146:* 166–170, 1980.

- opisthotonus /
  spasticity
- progressive psycho-
  motor retardation
- hepatosplenomegaly /
  thrombocytopenia

Gaucher Disease

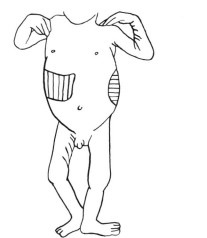
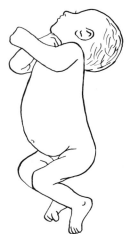
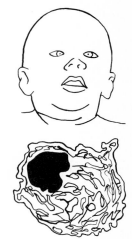

Protuberant abdomen with hepatosplenomegaly,
opisthotonus, spasticity, masklike face with
strabismus and Gaucher cell from bone marrow

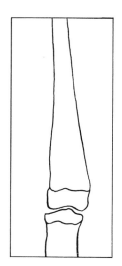
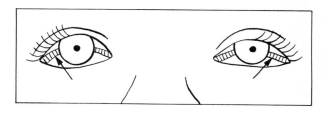
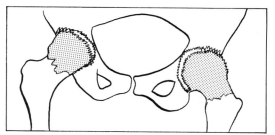

Erlenmeyer – flask deformity of femur, bilateral
pingueculae (arrows) – osteolytic changes in head
and neck of femurs in the adult form

74. G_M1 GANGLIOSIDOSIS

Clinical Features There are two classic types. In Type I, during the neonatal period, there is marked mental and motor retardation. The characteristic facies includes a prominent forehead with hirsutism, ocular hypertelorism, transverse skin fold below eyes, flattened nose, gingival enlargement, large mouth with macroglossia, hepatomegaly, less often splenomegaly, and generalized edema. In approximately 50%, there are cherry red macular changes noted. Clonic-tonic convulsions soon become evident. Type II has its onset somewhat later than Type I, the mental and motor aspects usually being normal during the first year of life. From then on, there is progressive weakness, locomotor ataxia, dementia, and seizures. The facial changes are extremely mild or absent and cherry red spots in the macula are not present. The viscera are not enlarged. In addition, there are several rare types reviewed by Sandhoff and Christomanou.

Specific Diagnosis Radiographically, in Type I there is initially diaphyseal cloaking followed by dysostosis multiplex. In Type II, bone changes are absent or only mildly abnormal. In both types foam cells are found in the bone marrow and circulating lymphocytes appear vacuolated. Renal biopsy shows vacuolization of glomerular epithelial cytoplasm. G_M1-ganglioside is increased in viscera and especially brain. There is marked deficiency of ganglioside G_M1-β-galactosidase activity in cultured skin fibroblasts, leukocytes, urine, brain, and liver. Additional accumulation of a keratan-like material and of oligosaccharides and glycopeptides has been demonstrated.

Differential Diagnosis Cherry red spot can be seen in *Sandhoff disease* and in *Tay-Sachs disease*. The coarse facial features can also be seen in the various *mucopolysaccharidoses* and *mucolipidoses*.

Prenatal Diagnosis This can be done by laboratory analysis of the levels of β-galactosidase in cultured fetal fibroblasts obtained at amniocentesis.

Basic Defect, Genetics, and Other Considerations The basic defect is deficiency of lysosomal β-galactosidase in brain and other organs. This enzyme is involved as the name implies in cleaving galactose from a number of substances—gangliosides, glycoproteins, and galactose-containing mucopolysaccharides. If cleavage does not take place, further degradation cannot occur. The accumulation of G_M1-ganglioside, especially in neurons, leads to progressive damage of the nervous system while failure to degrade the acid MPS, oligosaccharides and glycopeptides leads to hepatosplenomegaly and dysostosis multiplex. Both forms exhibit autosomal recessive inheritance. There have been approximately 75 cases of Type I reported, and 25 cases of Type II.

Prognosis and Treatment In Type I there is gradual deterioration in the child with progressive growth failure, seizures, and recurrent bronchopneumonia. Therapy is only supportive. Death usually occurs by two years, although in a few cases, children have reached the age of four. Patients with Type II usually die between four and fifteen years, although a few individuals have survived into their twenties.

REFERENCES

O'Brien, J.S. Ganglioside storage diseases. *Adv. Hum. Genet. 3:* 39–98, 1977.

Sandhoff, K. and Christomanou, H. Biochemistry and genetics of gangliosidoses. *Hum. Genet. 50:* 107–143, 1979.

Wolfe, L.S., Callahan, J., and Fawcett, J.S. G_M1-gangliosidosis without chondrodystrophy or visceromegaly. *Neurology 20:* 23–44, 1970.

M.R. [+ / all]

G_M1 Gangliosidosis

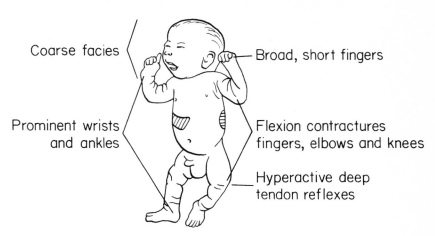

Coarse facies

Broad, short fingers

Prominent wrists and ankles

Flexion contractures fingers, elbows and knees

Hyperactive deep tendon reflexes

Hepatosplenomegaly after 6 months

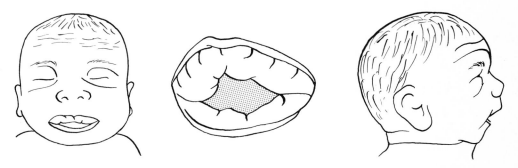

Prominent brow, hirsutism on forehead, transverse skin fold below eyes, flat nose, large mouth with macroglossia and gingival hypertrophy

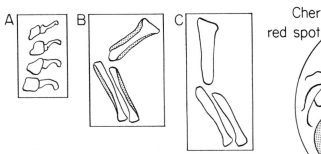

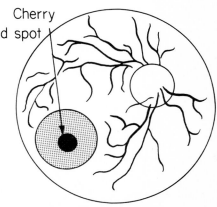

Cherry red spot

A) hypoplasia of anteriorsuperior lumbar vertebrae, B) periosteal cloaking C) later widening of bones

75. HOMOCYSTINURIA

Clinical Features Homocystinuria is characterized by ectopia lentis, myopia, thromboembolic episodes involving medium sized arteries and veins, malar flushing and livedo reticularis, osteoporosis, and various skeletal anomalies. Nonprogressive mental retardation occurs in about 80%. A Marfanoid appearance, joint laxity (especially flat feet), genu valgum, pes cavus, kyphoscoliosis, pectus carinatum, dolichostenomelia, and arachnodactyly have been reported in about 35% of the patients. Restricted joint mobility of the fingers, and contractures have also been noted. Generalized progressive osteoporosis first noticed around puberty is present in at least a third of affected adults, which may lead to vertebral body collapse and/or fracture. Malar flushing is seen in about 50%, which becomes more intense upon exertion. Ectopia lentis is present in about 90%, displacement in over half the cases being nasal, inferonasal, and inferior. The myopia, progressive in nature, usually is manifested before lens dislocation is discernible. Thrombosis of medium sized arteries, especially the coronary and renal arteries, is common.

Specific Diagnosis Initial screening is done by the cyanide-nitroprusside test which is positive in both cystinuria and homocystinuria. This should be followed by high-voltage electrophoresis or chromatographic amino acid analysis of urine for homocystine (normal 5–49 μM), methionine (normally undetectable), and cysteine (normal 44–96 μM). If the former two are elevated while the last is deficient, one may assume that one is dealing with cystathionine β-synthase deficiency. If homocystine levels are normal or reduced, there is a defect in remethylation. Radiographic changes consist of generalized osteoporosis, codfish vertebrae, and calcified metaphyseal spicules in the distal radius and ulna. This last sign, combined with a large capitate and small lunate bones, is almost pathognomonic for homocystinuria. The upper segment/lower segment ratio is less than normal.

Differential Diagnosis Affected individuals have sometimes been reported as having the *Marfan syndrome*. Body habitus may also resemble that seen in *congenital contractural arachnodactyly,* but in the latter ectopia lentis and mental retardation are not present.

Prenatal Diagnosis This has been accomplished utilizing normal amniotic cells for control.

Basic Defect, Genetics, and Other Considerations Homocystinuria is a group of disorders of methionine metabolism which eventuate in accumulation of homocystine in plasma and urine. It is a heterogeneity resulting from several autosomal recessively inherited or, at times, nongenetic causes (diet deficient in methionine, formula supplemented with DL-methionine, defective intestinal resorption of vitamin B_{12}, ingestion of excessive amounts of protein, liver disease). The major form is due to deficiency of cystathionine β-synthase, an autosomal recessive disorder. Two major pathways of methionine metabolism, transmethylation and transsulfuration, share the same initial steps, the paths diverging at the level of homocystine. Homocystine may be remethylated to form methionine or may condense with serine to form cystathionine. The most common form due to cystathionine β-synthase deficiency prevents the formation of cystathionine, thus resulting in increased homocystine and methionine in the plasma and urine. The other forms involve defective homocysteine remethylation and do not result in concomitant methionine accumulation. These include primary deficiency of the vitamin B_{12} cofactor; 5,10-methylene tetrahydrofolate reductase; and two inherited defects in the formation of the methylcobalamine cofactor of 5-methyl tetrahydrofolate homocysteine methyl transferase. Since there is no accumulation of methionine in these transmethylation defects, one can easily differentiate transmethylation from transsulfuration defects. It is assumed that the clinical manifestations result from slowly progressive toxic effects of homocysteine and its metabolites. Prevalence appears to be higher in those of Irish extraction.

Prognosis and Treatment Approximately half the patients benefit greatly from ingestion of pyridoxine, which may ameliorate or completely correct the biochemical abnormalities. Response to pyridoxine is usually evident within 10 days. Those who do not respond to pyridoxine may benefit from a methionine-restricted diet supplemented with L-cystine, or from various antiplatelet agents such as aspirin or dipyridimole which may decrease the likelihood of thromboembolic complications.

REFERENCES

Carey, M.C., Donovon, D.E., Fitzgerald, O. et al. Homocystinuria: a clinical and pathological study of nine subjects in six families: *Am. J. Med. 45:* 7–25, 1968.

Fowler, B., Kraus, J., Packman, S. et al. Homocystinuria: evidence for three distinct classes of cystathio-nine beta-synthetase mutants in cultured fibroblasts. *J. Clin. Invest. 61:* 645–653, 1978.

Poole, J.R., Mudd, S.H., Conerly, E.B. et al. Homocystinuria due to cystathionine synthase deficiency. *J. Clin. Invest. 55:* 1033–1048, 1975.

- **dolichostenomelia**
- **myopia / ectopia lentis**
- **malar flushing**
- **livedo reticularis**

Homocystinuria

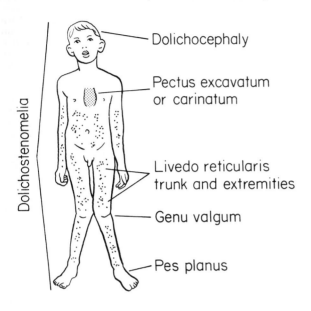

Dolichostenomelia

- Dolichocephaly
- Pectus excavatum or carinatum
- Livedo reticularis trunk and extremities
- Genu valgum
- Pes planus

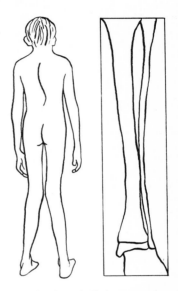

Scoliosis, dolichostenomelia with slender fibula and tibia

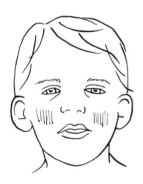

Malar flush

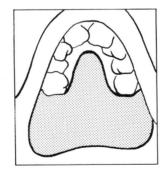

Narrow, high arched palate

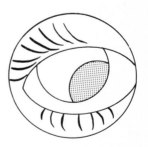

Ectopia lentis with lens displaced downward

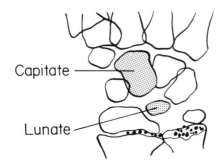

Capitate

Lunate

Large capitate, small lunate and calcified spicules in the distal ulna and radius

76. HYPERPHOSPHATASIA

Clinical Features This disorder has been described under a large number of designations (juvenile Paget's disease, hyperostosis corticalis juvenilis deformans, familial osteoectasia with macrocranium, etc.). It is characterized by fever and pain and swelling of the extremities during the first year of life. During the second and third year, enlargement of the calvaria up to 65 cm or more associated with headache is noted. There may be sporadic cranial nerve involvement. Visual acuity may be diminished because of optic atrophy. There are numerous fractures and bending and widening of the bones of the extremities. However, healing of fractures is normal. Anterior bowing of the legs is common. Growth is not seriously diminished. Muscle weakness retards running, walking, or jumping. There is often inability to extend at the elbow. Frontal bossing, pectus carinatum, barrel-shaped chest, and kyphoscoliosis are frequent. Hypertension has been reported in several cases. Progressive mixed hearing loss (60 to 80 dB) has been evident from the fourth to the fourteenth year of life. The ear canals are narrowed. The sclerae are blue.

Specific Diagnosis Radiographic changes in the calvaria resemble those seen in Paget's disease. Long bones exhibit bending, over cylindricalization, and general diaphyseal cortical widening. Coxa vara is frequent. Cysts have been described in the metaphyses of the long bones. The bone structure is coarse. Short bones are involved to a lesser degree, mostly on the endosteal side. Only rarely are facial bones involved. Microscopically there is intensive metaplastic fibrous bone formation as well as increased osteoblastic and osteoclastic activity very similar to that seen in Paget's disease, but without typical mosaic or regression lines. The spine and ribs may be osteoporotic. Ophthalmologic examination may reveal angioid streaks and/or macular hemorrhage. Both serum acid and alkaline phosphatase levels are elevated, but calcium and phosphorus levels are normal. Alkaline phosphatase may range from 100 to 500 King-Armstrong units. Urinary hydroxyproline and proline-containing peptides are increased and mild microcytic hypochromic anemia has been noted in several cases.

Differential Diagnosis One must rule out *polyostotic fibrous dysplasia, Van Buchem disease, Paget's disease, craniodiaphyseal dysplasia,* and *osteogenesis imperfecta.*

Prenatal Diagnosis To the best of our knowledge, this condition has not been diagnosed prenatally.

Basic Defect, Genetics, and Other Considerations The basic defect is unknown but it leads to broadening of the diaphyses of the long bones and the rapid turnover of lamellar bone and bone collagen. Fibrous bone does not become compact bone. This results in weak bone and growth retardation. The inheritance is autosomal recessive.

Prognosis and Treatment Treatment is largely symptomatic, although sodium fluoride has been given at a dose of 1 mg/kg/day with mildly encouraging results. Calcitonin has been stated to have considerable beneficial effect.

REFERENCES

Caffey, J. Familial hyperphosphatasemia with ateliosis and hypermetabolism of growing membranous bone: review of the clinical, radiographic and chemical features. *Bull. Hosp. Joint Dis. 33:* 81–110, 1972.

Eyring, E.J. and Eisenberg, G. Congenital hyperphosphatasia: a clinical, pathological, and biochemical study of two cases. *J. Bone Joint Surg. 50A:* 1099–1117, 1968.

Whalen, J.P., Horwith, M., Krook, L. et al. Calcitonin treatment in hereditary bone dysplasia with hyperphosphatasemia: a radiographic and histologic study of bone. *Am. J. Roentgenol. 129:* 29–35, 1977.

- **enlargement of the calvaria / frontal bossing**
- **fractures**
- **bowing of legs**
- **pectus carinatum / kyphoscoliosis**

Hyperphosphatasia

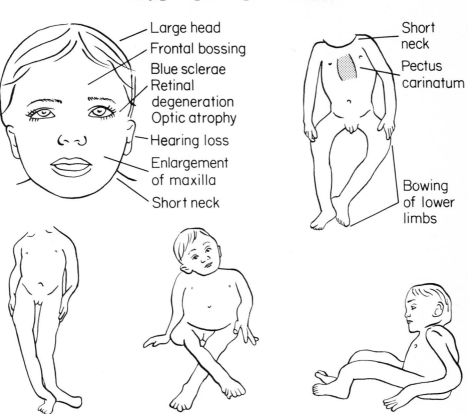

Large head
Frontal bossing
Blue sclerae
Retinal degeneration
Optic atrophy
Hearing loss
Enlargement of maxilla
Short neck

Short neck
Pectus carinatum
Bowing of lower limbs

Bowing of long bones, large head, short neck, increased chest diameter and kyphoscoliosis

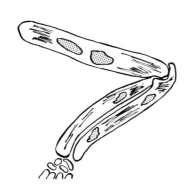

Large cylindrical bones bowing and pseudocysts

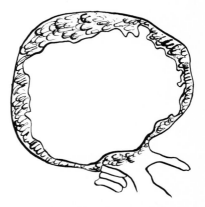

Widened diploe with cotton-like dense islands

77. HYPOPHOSPHATASIA

Clinical Features There appear to be at least three forms of hypophosphatasia, divided according to age of onset and severity: (a) *infantile*, the most severe, is characterized by onset in utero. The child is often stillborn. The skull may have the quality of a paper bag. The limbs are short and bowed and the wrists, knees, and ankles enlarged and deformed. The ribs are soft and beaded. Irritability, twitching, seizures, vomiting and high-pitched cry are common. Pyrexia and a bleeding tendency occur in those that survive a few days. The (b) *childhood form* is milder, exhibits gradual development of signs after 6 months of age which include craniosynostosis with sutural ridging and bulging of anterior fontanel, growth retardation, rachitic skeletal changes (narrow chest with rosary, enlarged wrists, knees, and ankles, bowed legs), increased susceptibility to infection, and premature loss of primary anterior teeth. The (c) *adult* or mildest *form* exhibits osteoporosis, an occasional fracture or pseudofracture, at times with a history of childhood vitamin D-resistant rickets or premature loss of deciduous anterior teeth.

Specific Diagnosis Radiographically, in the infantile form there may be severe widespread undermineralization, the calvaria being essentially noncalcified. In the childhood form, there are delayed closure of the fontanel and widened cranial sutures, a "beaten silver" appearance to the calvaria, and generalized ragged metaphyseal mineralization. Less common signs are mid-shaft diaphyseal spurs, abnormally shaped distal phalanges, mild S-shaped tibiae. Hypercalcemia and calcification of the kidney may be noted. Microscopic examination of exfoliated teeth reveals essentially intact root structure, but only spotty deposits of cementum on the roots of the incisor teeth, which explains their exfoliation due to minimal trauma. The canine and molar teeth are less severely involved and are rarely lost. The pulp chambers are enlarged. The histologic picture of bone is the same as that of rickets. Hypercalcemia may be present in severely affected infants. Serum alkaline phosphatase activity is low and urinary and plasma phosphoethanolamine and inorganic pyrophosphate levels are elevated in most homozygotes. Furthermore, not all heterozygotes have altered chemistries.

Differential Diagnosis Clinically, the infantile form simulates *osteogenesis imperfecta, campomelic dysplasia*, and the *"short-limbed dwarf"* syndromes. Radiographically, the childhood form cannot be distinguished from *rickets*. On ultrasonography, the apparently absent head may simulate *anencephaly*. The adult form should be differentiated from *osteomalacia* and *Paget's disease*. Delayed closure of the anterior fontanel may be seen in a host of disorders: *hypothyroidism, Down syndrome, cleidocranial dysplasia, fetal hydantoin syndrome, osteogenesis imperfecta, Beckwith-Wiedemann syndrome*, etc. Premature loss of teeth may result from *trauma, premature periodontal disease*, etc. Various disorders associated with premature fusion of cranial sutures must be excluded. Urinary phosphoethanolamine can be elevated in *celiac disease, scurvy, hypothyroidism*, and *hypomagnesemia*.

Prenatal Diagnosis May be carried out by identifying greatly reduced alkaline phosphatase activity in fetal cells obtained from amniocentesis. In severe cases, ultrasonography at 16 weeks may aid in the diagnosis by showing poor visualization of the fetal head.

Basic Defect, Genetics, and Other Considerations The basic defect is not known. There is inadequate to total lack of calcification of bone matrix in cartilage. It is likely that the defect rests in defective regulation of various alkaline phosphatase isozymic forms. Hypophosphatasia exhibits autosomal recessive transmission. It is probable that there are several allelic forms rather than variable expression of a single gene, since recurrent cases are usually of the same form. Not all heterozygotes exhibit intermediate values of alkaline phosphatase and phosphoethanolamine levels. Over 200 cases have been reported. The frequency is about 1 per 100,000 live births for the lethal form.

Prognosis and Treatment In the infantile form, about half the children are stillborn or die in infancy. Craniosynostosis occuring in the childhood form may need surgical correction. The bone lesions heal and the permanent teeth are not affected. There is some evidence that high oral phosphate (1–3 g neutral sodium phosphate) given in four to five divided doses is beneficial.

REFERENCES

Beumer, J., Trowbridge, H.E., Silverman, S., Jr. et al. Childhood hypophosphatasia and the premature loss of teeth. *Oral Surg. 35:* 631–640, 1973.

Kozlowski, K., Sutcliffe, J., Barylak, A., et al. Hypophosphatasia. Review of 24 cases. *Pediat. Radiol. 5:* 103–117, 1976.

Macpherson, R.I., Kroeker, M., and Houston, C.S. Hypophosphatasia. *J. Canad. Assoc. Radiol. 23:* 16–26, 1972.

- poor formation of skull
- short bowed limbs
- enlarged joints
- high-pitched cry

Hypophosphatasia

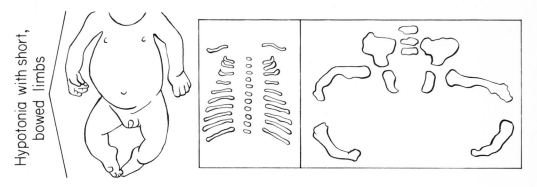

Hypotonia with short, bowed limbs

Infantile form – small thoracic cage, enlarged, deformed joints, hypoplastic ribs and vertebrae, severe bowing of lower limbs

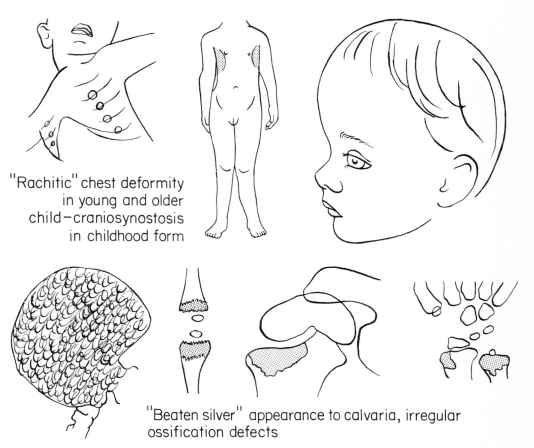

"Rachitic" chest deformity in young and older child – craniosynostosis in childhood form

"Beaten silver" appearance to calvaria, irregular ossification defects

78. LESCH-NYHAN SYNDROME

Clinical Features Classic features include mental retardation, spastic cerebral palsy, choreoathetosis and bizarre, self-mutilating, aggressive behavior. Infants appear normal at birth and commonly develop normally for the first six to eight months of life. Often the first recognizable signs are orange uric acid crystals which may resemble sand in the diaper. Some develop nephrolithiasis or hematuria in the early months of life. Gouty tophi may be noted about the posterior part of the pinna. Cerebral manifestations are insidious. Increased irritability may be noted by the third month. An infant that has been sitting and supporting his head will lose the ability. Involuntary movements of choreic and athetoid type will be noted. Spasticity is usually prominent. Deep tendon reflexes are increased and clonus and Babinsky responses are often present. Self-mutilation may result in massive destruction of the lower and less often upper lip. The fingers are badly chewed and the ears and nose are occasionally injured. However there is no loss of pain sensation and patients are often more comfortable when restrained. The degree of mental retardation varies but is usually severe. However, most patients learn to talk and appear more intelligent than test results would indicate.

Specific Diagnosis Cultured skin fibroblasts may be used to identify the hemizygote who has marked reduction in HGPRTase. Serum uric acid levels, normally 2.5 to 6.0 mg/dl, are raised to 8.5 to 15.0 mg/dl. Occasionally a megaloblastic anemia has been observed. Heterozygotes can easily be detected by electrophoresis of a single hair-root lysate. Despite severe CNS signs, both gross and microscopic findings in the brain are relatively unremarkable.

Differential Diagnosis Clinical findings are striking and essentially distinctive. However, self-mutilation may occur in *congenital indifference to pain* and occasionally in the *deLange syndrome.*

Prenatal Diagnosis Prenatal diagnosis can be done by the finding of reduced enzyme activity in cultured amniotic fluid cells.

Basic Defect, Genetics, and Other Considerations The basic defect is virtual absence of hypoxanthine guanine phosphoribosyltransferase. This results in excess uric acid production. There also appears to be a dysfunction of brain neurotransmitters. The disorder exhibits X-linked recessive transmission. Its frequency has been estimated to be approximately 1 per 100,000 births. The carrier state may be diagnosed. "Partial" deficiency has been described in adult males who exhibit gouty arthritis, early renal complications, less often epilepsy, spasticity, and incoordination.

Prognosis and Treatment The excessive uric acid production is managed with allopurinol, a xanthine oxidase inhibitor which blocks the final step in uric acid formation. However this produces no decrease in self-mutilative behavior or improvement in mental function. Hand restraints and selective tooth extractions of deciduous teeth prevent extensive self-inflicted injury. The permanent dentition is usually spared, since lip-biting behavior decreases with age. Urate stone prevention is facilitated by increased fluid intake to increase the renal output of uric acid. Death usually occurs in the second or third decade from infection or renal failure.

REFERENCES

Bakay, B., Tucker-Pian, C., and Seegmiller, J.E. Detection of Lesch-Nyhan syndrome carriers: analysis of hair roots for HPRT by agarose-gel electrophoresis and autoradiography. *Clin. Genet. 17:* 369–374, 1980.

Emmerson, B.T. and Thompson, L. The spectrum of hypoxanthine guanine phosphoribosyltransferase deficiency. *Q. J. Med. 42:* 423–440, 1973.

Kelly, W.N. Biochemistry of the X-linked uric aciduria enzyme defect and its genetic variants. *Arch. Internal. Med. 130:* 199–206, 1972.

- tophi about ears
- choreoathetosis
- spasticity
- self-mutilation

Lesch-Nyhan Syndrome

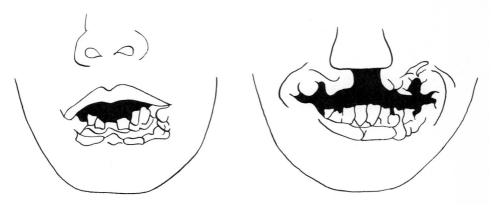

Varying degrees of self-mutilation of lips

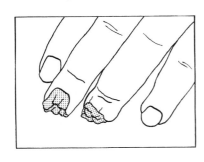

Self-mutilation of fingers

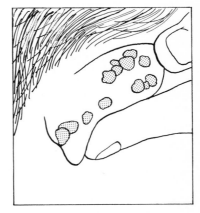

Tophi on pinna

79. LIPOATROPHIC DIABETES
(Berardinelli-Seip syndrome)

Clinical Features Lipoatrophic diabetes is manifest by generalized disappearance of body fat, insulin-resistant diabetes, and hepatomegaly. Skeletal growth is often accentuated during the first ten years of life. However, it then tapers off and there is average or even short stature after puberty. The phenotype is further altered by the enlarged joints of the hands and feet. Loss of the subcutaneous adipose tissue in the face, especially that of the buccal fat pad, causes the cheeks to have a gaunt appearance. This, combined with large ears and hirsutism, produces a distinctive appearance. Hepatosplenomegaly may be pronounced in infancy. There may be cardiac murmurs and cardiomegaly and the kidneys are often enlarged. A few have had hydronephrosis and hydroureter. Mental retardation of variable degree has been noted in about half the patients. The muscles are prominent, due in part to lack of subcutaneous fat, but may be absolute. This may be evident from birth. Increased skeletal maturation has been commonly noted during the first four years of life. The penis or clitoris is often enlarged and cystic ovaries are a common feature. Hirsutism of the face, neck, arms, and legs is often marked at birth and increases with age. Scalp hair often becomes excessively curly and thick, the hair growing nearly to the eyebrows. Acanthosis nigricans is a prominent feature in nearly all patients. Especially common in the axillas and on the wrists and ankles, it tends to decrease with increasing age and may disappear after puberty.

Specific Diagnosis Liver biopsies in the older children or young adults have shown fatty infiltration of the liver with moderate early fibrosis and increased glycogen deposits. The fatty infiltration is secondary to hypertriglyceridemia and lack of functional fat storage deposits. There is absence of mesenteric and perinephric fat. Lipoatrophic diabetes is clearly distinct from diabetes mellitus. The diabetes, which is insulin-resistant, appears after the onset of the lipodystrophy, usually between six and 20 years of age. Ketosis is rarely present. Infants do not have glycosuria except when challenged with large amounts of glucose. Hyperlipemia is a constant feature, usually preceding the onset of hyperglycemia. The serum of these patients is intermittently turbid or milky, with increased triglycerides and contains very low-density lipoprotein. A lack of insulin receptors has been demonstrated.

Differential Diagnosis Many features of lipoatrophic diabetes are noted in *leprechaunism:* liver enlargement, lipodystrophy, enlarged clitoris or penis, neurologic damage, hirsutism, and disturbances of glucose metabolism. It is conceivable that leprechaunism represents a lethal form of lipoatrophic diabetes. The *diencephalic syndrome* caused by a tumor in the region of the anterior hypothalamus is manifested by profound emaciation with accelerating early growth, increased motor activity, and euphoria. The affected infants are normal at birth but become symptomatic with age. Progressive emaciation leads to a loss of subcutaneous fat but without the muscularity of lipodystrophic patients. The hands and feet may also be large. Hepatomegaly, genital enlargement, and hyperlipemia have not been reported. Differentiation from *autosomal dominant lipodystrophy* should be easy since the lipodystrophy extends only to the waist with large buttocks in that form.

Prenatal Diagnosis This has not been described.

Basic Defect, Genetics, and Other Considerations The basic defect has not been established, but it may be in part related to absence of insulin receptors. Insulin binding to cultured fibroblasts has been normal in some patients; in others it has been decreased. Lipoatrophic diabetes is clearly autosomal recessive. Parental consanguinity has been noted in about 25% of the affected families.

Prognosis and Treatment There is no effective therapy. Most of these patients die during their teenage years from diabetes.

REFERENCES

Oseid, S., Beck-Nielsen, H., Pedersen, O. et al. Decreased binding of insulin to its receptor in patients with congenital generalized lipodystrophy. *N. Engl. J. Med. 296:* 245–248, 1977.

Reed, W.B., Dexter, R., Corley, C. et al. Congenital lipodystrophic diabetes with acanthosis nigricans: the Seip-Lawrence syndrome. *Arch. Dermatol. 91:* 326–334, 1965.

Seip, M. Generalized lipodystrophy. *Ergeb. Inn. Med. Kinderheilk. 31:* 59–95, 1971.

- loss of subcutaneous fat tissue / gaunt appearance
- large ears and genital enlargement
- hirsutism
- hepatomegaly

Lipoatrophic Diabetes
[Berardinelli-Seip syndrome]

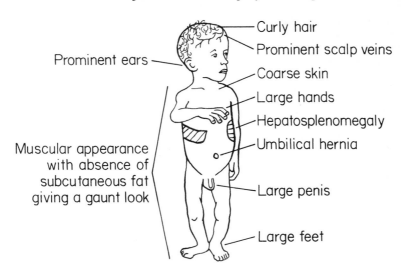

Prominent ears

Curly hair
Prominent scalp veins
Coarse skin
Large hands
Hepatosplenomegaly
Umbilical hernia
Large penis
Large feet

Muscular appearance with absence of subcutaneous fat giving a gaunt look

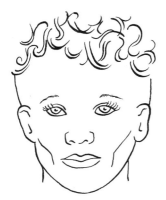

Absent buccal
fat pad

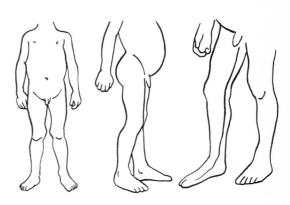

Muscular build, protruding abdomen
large penis and phlebomegaly

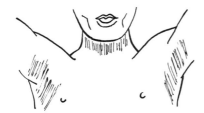

Acanthosis nigricans
of neck and axillae

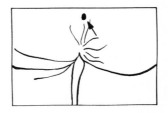

Coccygeal dimple (arrow)

80. MANNOSIDOSIS

Clinical Features Mannosidosis is heterogeneous. Children with the more common form are essentially normal for the first year of life, but exhibit a propensity toward recurrent respiratory infections. The coarse facies is noted after the first few years of life and becomes progressive. The nasal bridge tends to be low, the forehead is high, and the mandible is prominent. The neck is somewhat short. There is delayed early motor development which becomes manifest as clumsiness. Growth is retarded and speech is delayed. Stabilized intelligence quotients are usually in the 50–75 range. Tendon reflexes are brisk. Wheel-like or spoke-shaped opacities have been noted in the lenses in several patients. Severe high-frequency mixed hearing loss is a common if not constant feature along with large auricles. There is a general mild hypotonia. The abdomen is protuberant but hepatosplenomegaly is mild and possibly transient. Lumbar gibbus has been noted in several patients. Umbilical and inguinal hernia are common. Those with the less severe form of mannosidosis exhibit mild mental retardation, delayed speech, somewhat coarse facies, and reduced mobility of large joints.

Specific Diagnosis The condition is diagnosed by finding reduced α-mannosidase in leukocytes, cultured fibroblasts, or in serum at or below pH 4.0. Thin-layer chromatography of urinary glycoproteins demonstrates a characteristic pattern. Radiographically, there is thickened calvaria, the long bones are osteoporotic, and the ulna and radius are broad with curved diaphyses and a thin cortex. The clavicles and ribs are widened. The upper lumbar vertebrae are somewhat trapezoidal in form. The iliac bases are overconstricted, the femoral necks and metacarpals widened, the epiphyses are sloped and trabeculae coarse throughout the skeleton. The mastoids and sinuses may not be pneumatized. Peripheral lymphocytes are vacuolated in 20–90% of the cells counted. Coarse dark granules are present in neutrophils.

Differential Diagnosis Urinary acid mucopolysaccharide excretion is normal in mannosidosis but glycoprotein excretion is elevated, thus separating this disorder from the various *mucopolysaccharidoses*. The phenotype of *aspartylglycosaminuria* is similar but biochemically distinct. Several patients diagnosed as having *mucolipidosis* have been demonstrated to have mannosidosis.

Prenatal Diagnosis Possible by showing reduced α-mannosidase in cultured amniotic fluid cells.

Basis Defect, Genetics, and Other Considerations Absence of acidic (pH 4.0–4.5) isoenzymes of α-mannosidase results in the accumulation of mannose-rich glycosylated compounds (oligosaccharides) in lysosomes in liver, spleen, and brain and in leukocytes. There is excretion of similar substances in the urine. The mild form is due to partial deficiency of the acidic component(s) of α-mannosidase. Heterozygotes have reduced levels of α-mannosidase. At least 50 cases have been reported of this autosomal recessive disorder. There is some concentration in the Scandinavian population.

Prognosis and Treatment Prognosis apparently depends on the specific genetic form one is dealing with, since several of these individuals have died in early childhood. While zinc or cobalt may stimulate residual enzyme activity, there is no evidence that zinc therapy results in clinical improvement.

REFERENCES

Aylsworth, A.S., Taylor, H.A., Stuart, C.M. et al. Mannosidosis: phenotype of a severely affected child and characterization of α-mannosidase activity in cultured fibroblasts from the patient and his parents. *J. Pediatr. 88:* 814–818, 1976.

Desnick, R.J., Sharp, H.L., Grabowski, G.A. et al. Mannosidosis: clinical, morphological, biochemical, and immunologic studies. *Pediatr. Res. 10:* 985–996, 1976.

Montgomery, T.R., Thomas G.H., and Valle, D. Mannosidosis in an adult. *Johns Hopk. Med. J. 151:* 113–117, 1982.

- coarse facies / prominent mandible
- high forehead
- large ears / deafness
- lens opacities

Mannosidosis

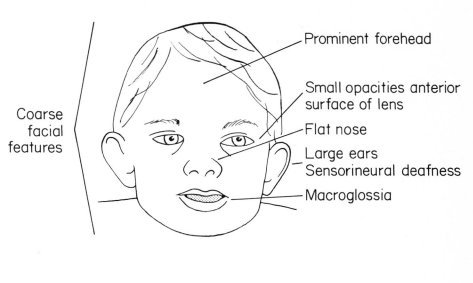

Coarse facial features

Prominent forehead

Small opacities anterior surface of lens

Flat nose

Large ears
Sensorineural deafness

Macroglossia

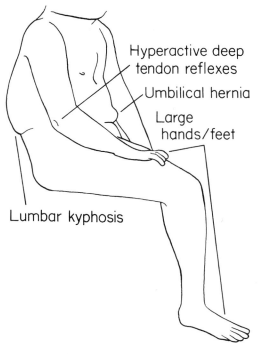

Hyperactive deep tendon reflexes

Umbilical hernia

Large hands/feet

Lumbar kyphosis

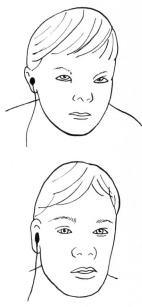

Older children –
similar facial features,
note hearing aid

81. MENKES SYNDROME

Clinical Features The patient appears normal at birth. Prematurity occurs in over half the patients. Near the end of the first month of life, drowsiness, increased difficulties with feeding, and a tendency to hypothermia become evident. There appears to be deficient visual development. By three months, clonic seizures become manifest and there is a gradual inexorable CNS degeneration and pyramidal signs (spasticity, hyperreflexia, quadriparesis) leading to death. There is marked failure to thrive with severe retardation in both growth and mental development. An increased susceptibility to infection has been noted. The scalp and eyebrow hair is characteristically unruly. However, some patients have been described with normal hair. The hair lacks lustre and is often depigmented. It easily breaks off, leaving short stubbles that exhibit a wiry texture. The nose has a tendency to be short and broad, the mandible small, and the cheeks full. There may be failure or delay of tooth eruption. Bladder diverticulae have been described in several patients. They probably result from abnormal bladder innervation.

Specific Diagnosis The hair exhibits a variety of microscopic patterns such as pili torti (twisted hair), monilethrix (beaded hair), trichorrhexis nodosa (beaded hair manifesting paintbrush fractures at the nodes). Electroencephalographic studies reveal multiple spike discharges. Radiographic findings include mild microcephaly, metaphyseal spurring, and diaphyseal cloaking of long bones, that is, thickening of the periosteum. There may be flaring of rib-ends and Wormian bones in the parietal area of the calvaria. Abnormal cerebral vasculature on angiograms (marked vessel tortuosity, "loop-the-loop" anterior cerebral arteries) has been described. Peripheral systemic arteries show similar tortuosity. Grossly the brain is small and atrophic with the cerebral gyri narrowed and the sulci widened. Microscopic study of the brain shows neuronal loss and demyelination of the cerebral cortex and cerebellum as well as the basal ganglia. The Purkinje cells manifest irregular swelling and fluoresce under UV light. There are diminished retinal ganglion cells. Low serum (normal 75–90 mg/dl), urine, brain, liver, and hair copper levels are found. Ceruloplasm is low to absent.

Differential Diagnosis The skeletal changes may suggest a *battered child, scurvy, rickets*, or other *rachitiform disorders. Kinky hair* may be an isolated finding or part of numerous syndromes (*arginosuccinicaciduria, Netherton syndrome, pili torti and hearing loss, tricho-dento-osseous syndrome*, etc.). Nutritional copper deficiency is distinguished by low erythrocyte copper which is normal in Menkes disease.

Prenatal Diagnosis Elevated incorporation of radioactive copper has been reported in cultured skin fibroblasts and in amniotic fetal cells.

Basic Defect, Genetics, and Other Considerations The basic defect appears to be one of copper transport within cells or across membranes. Low copper absorption results in enzyme dysfunction responsible for neurologic changes and for fragmentation of elastic fibers in various tissues. While mitochondrial or microsomal oxidative dysfunction has been suggested, the precise defect has not been identified. The disorder has X-linked recessive inheritance. There is genetic heterogeneity. About 50 cases have been reported. Perhaps the frequency is 1 per 35,000 live births. Obligate heterozygotes appear to be normal except for ultrastructural changes in the hair.

Prognosis and Treatment Death occurs by the age of two in almost 90%. The oldest known survivor has been about four years. Therapy consists only in anticonvulsant medication. There is no evidence of real improvement by copper supplementation either by diet or intravenously.

REFERENCES

Grover, W.D., Johnson, W.C., and Henkin, R.I. Clinical and biochemical aspects of trichopoliodystrophy. *Ann. Neurol. 5:* 65–71, 1979.

Wesenberg, R.L., Gwinn, J.L., and Barnes, G.R., Jr. Radiological findings in the kinky-hair syndrome. *Radiology 92:* 500–506, 1968.

Wheeler, E,M. and Roberts, P.F. Menkes's steely-hair disease. *Arch. Dis. Child. 51:* 269–274, 1976.

- **kinky scalp hair / eyebrows**
- **CNS degeneration**
- **short broad nose**
- **full cheeks**

Menkes Syndrome

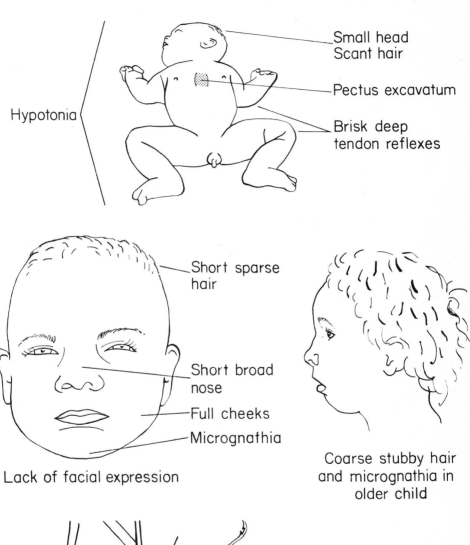

Small head
Scant hair

Pectus excavatum

Brisk deep
tendon reflexes

Hypotonia

Short sparse
hair

Short broad
nose

Full cheeks

Micrognathia

Lack of facial expression

Coarse stubby hair
and micrognathia in
older child

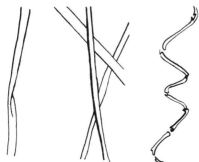

Spiral shape to hair,
points of fracture,
varying diameters
and twisting of
hair shafts

82. MUCOLIPIDOSIS II
(I cell disease)

Clinical Features Mucolipidosis II is characterized by severe psychomotor retardation, marked shortness of stature, pes equinovarus, coarse facies, and impressive gingival enlargement. Soon after birth, hypotonia, inguinal hernia in males, restricted joint mobility, and dislocated hips are noted. During the first year of life, there is a history of recurrent respiratory infections, failure to thrive, and marked lack of psychomotor development. The full clinical picture is reached by one year. The patient rarely is taller than 70 cm or weighs more than 8 kilos. Head circumference remains normal with respect to stature. The eyelids appear puffy with a mild degree of exophthalmos. There may be premature lightening of hair color. The supraorbital ridges are inapparent. The cheeks are full and may exhibit multiple fine telangiectasia. There is often intermittent copious nasal discharge. Corneal clouding can be detected as a late finding on slit-lamp examination in about 50%. The neck and thoracic cage are short. Umbilical and/or inguinal hernia is common. Restricted joint mobility, particularly in the shoulders and wrists, persists. The hands and fingers are stubby, the wrists widened, and the costochondral junctions knobby. Enlargement of gingiva and anterior alveolar process is present as early as four months and is slowly progressive, burying the teeth that rarely erupt.

Specific Diagnosis Numerous membrane-bound vacuolar coarse granular inclusions in the cytoplasm of cultured fibroblasts (I-cells) may be observed under phase-constrast microscopy. These granules represent altered lysosomes. Various lysosomal enzymes have been shown to be absent or considerably decreased in cultured fibroblasts, brain, or visceral organs, less so in leukocytes. However, the medium in which the fibroblasts are cultured or the serum, urine, cerebrospinal fluid, and tears of patients show an increased activity of several lysosomal enzymes, except for acid phosphatase and α-glucosidase: for some, 10-fold normal levels. Chorionic villi are edematous and there is extensive vacuolization of the syncytiotrophoblastic layer and of chorionic mesenchymal cells. Peripheral lymphocytes contain large cytoplasmic inclusions. There is neither splenomegaly nor excretion of AMPS in the urine. Radiographically, extensive periosteal cloaking of all bones can be observed from birth until four to six months of age. The bone structure appears coarse and there is no diaphyseal constriction. The metaphyses are widened or beaked or notched. Stippled epiphyses may be found up to the fourth month. Subsequently, the overgrowth becomes confluent with the underlying cortex and disappears entirely between the eighth and twelfth month of age. There is also, from that point, dysostosis multiplex (see MPS I-H). There may be minor thickening of the calvaria, premature suture synostosis, and a minor to moderate diaphyseal widening in long bones, especially in the lower limbs.

Differential Diagnosis The facies most closely resembles that of *MPS I-H*, but the gingivae are not enlarged in *Hurler syndrome*. Furthermore, children with MPS I-H grow normally during the first year of life. Dysostosis multiplex occurs in *MPS I-H, MPS II, MPS VI*, and *MPS VII*, but it is manifest within the first few months of life in ML II. Similar biochemical findings are seen in ML III but onset of clinical manifestations becomes evident between the second and fourth year of life and the course is much milder. Periosteal cloaking of long bones is also noted in G_M1 *gangliosidosis, Caffey disease, syphilis, osteomyelitis, battering*, etc. Bone stippling may be seen in a variety of disorders: *chondrodysplasia punctata, Zellweger syndrome, Neimann-Pick disease, Warfarin embryopathy*, and G_M1 *gangliosidosis*.

Prenatal Diagnosis Amniocytes exhibit coarse granulations under phase microscopy and amniotic fluid levels are elevated for lysosomal enzyme levels except for acid phosphatase and α-glucosidase. Prenatal diagnosis should be possible now that specific enzyme defect is known.

Basic Defect, Genetics, and Other Considerations The basic defect is deficiency of glycoprotein N-acetylglucosaminylphosphotransferase activity, necessary for proper intracellular processing of lysosomal enzymes. The disorder has autosomal recessive inheritance. Heterozygotes cannot yet be detected. Less than 50 cases have been reported. There appears to be genetic heterogeneity.

Prognosis and Treatment Death occurs prior to the age of six years. Therapy is supportive.

REFERENCES
Lemaitre, L., Remy, J., Farriaux, J.P. et al. Radiologic signs of mucolipidosis II or I-cell disease. *Pediatr. Radiol.* 7: 92–105, 1978.

Leroy, J.G. The oligosaccharidoses: proposal of a new name and classification for the mucolipidoses. *Birth Defects 18(3B):* 3–12, 1982.

Shapiro, L.J., Hickman, S., Hall, C.W. et al. Biochemical studies in mucolipidosis II and III. *Birth Defects 11(6):* 301–305, 1975.

- coarse facies / puffy eyelids
- gingival enlargement / thick tongue
- restricted joint movements
- thick, tight skin

Mucolipidosis II
[I cell disease]

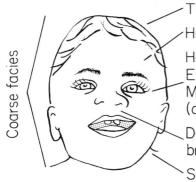

Coarse facies

Thick hair

High, narrow forehead

Heavy eyelashes
Epicanthal folds
Megalocornea
(at times)

Depressed nasal bridge

Short neck

Open mouth,
hyperplastic gums

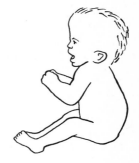

Scaphocephaly, rigid
posture, low-set ears,
anteverted nares,
short neck and gibbus

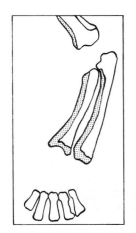

Irregularity in
metaphyseal outline
and cortical structures
in a newborn

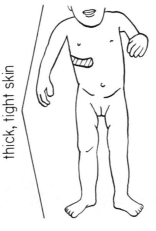

Short stature with thick, tight skin

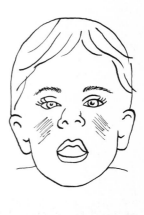

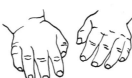

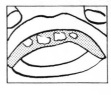

Hepatomegaly, contracture of fingers,
broad hands, telangiectasia
about face, thick upper lip
and gingival hypertrophy

83. MUCOLIPIDOSIS III

Clinical Features The most common features include growth retardation below the 3rd percentile by eight to ten years and onset of joint stiffness without pain especially in the hands and shoulders, by two to four years of age, which becomes progressive. There is no pain, swelling, or tenderness. Claw-hands are evident by six years of age. The stiffness seems to become stationary around puberty. During school years, the elbows and hips become involved. Carpal tunnel syndrome may be experienced even prior to puberty. The skin is tight and indurated. The facial features become somewhat coarse by six years. Progressive fine peripheral corneal opacity is noted in all patients under slit-lamp examination. Mental retardation of mild degree has been noted in most cases. Aortic and/or mitral regurgitation is common. Hepatosplenomegaly has late onset.

Specific Diagnosis There are normal levels of urinary acid mucopolysaccharides, deficient levels of multiple lysosomal hydrolases in cultured fibroblasts, but elevated levels in the culture medium, serum, and urine. Peripheral leukocytes are normal, but vacuolated plasma cells are found in the marrow. Radiographically the most striking changes are those of severe dysostosis multiplex. There is progressive flattening and irregularity of the capital femoral epiphyses and marked narrowing of the femoral neck with subluxation and coxa valga. The carpal bones undergo progressive dissolution. The vertebral bodies are ovoid and often there is odontoid hypoplasia. The iliac wings are low.

Differential Diagnosis This disorder must be differentiated from *MPS I-H, MPS I-S*, the milder forms of *MPS VI*, and *MPS VII* due to similar physical and radiographic findings. Separation from *ML II* is easy due to difference in clinical onset, and mild mental retardation in ML III, although they share the same enzyme defect. The corneal opacity is never as striking as in *MPS I* and *MPS VI*.

Prenatal Diagnosis We do not know of this disorder having been diagnosed prenatally, but it is theoretically possible now that the specific enzyme defect is known.

Basic Defect, Genetics, and Other Considerations The basic defect is deficiency or abnormality of glycoprotein N-acetylglucosaminylphosphotransferase activity. The same enzyme defect is that seen in I-cell disease. ML III has autosomal recessive inheritance. Because of this enzyme deficiency, multiple lysosomal enzymes are decreased in fibroblasts and elevated in cell culture medium.

Prognosis and Treatment Joint stiffness results in considerable handicap in the adult. Many suffer from the carpal tunnel syndrome which can be corrected surgically. The most disabling aspect is due to progressive destruction of the hip joints which may be evident even in the late teens, but survival to adult years is usual. Physical therapy has not been of great avail.

REFERENCES

Herd, J.K., Dvorak, A.D., Wiltse, H.E. et al. Mucolipidosis type III. *Am. J. Dis. Child. 132:* 1181–1186, 1978.

Kelly, T.E., Thomas, G., Taylor, H.A., Jr. et al. Mucolipidosis III (pseudo-Hurler polydystrophy). Clinical and laboratory studies in a series of 12 patients. *Johns Hopk. Med. J. 137:* 156–175, 1975.

Robinow, M. and Soukup, S.M. Mucolipidosis III: new studies. *Birth Defects 10(8):* 129–134, 1974.

- **coarse facies**
- **corneal opacity by slit lamp**
- **progressive joint stiffness**
- **claw-hand deformity**

Mucolipidosis III

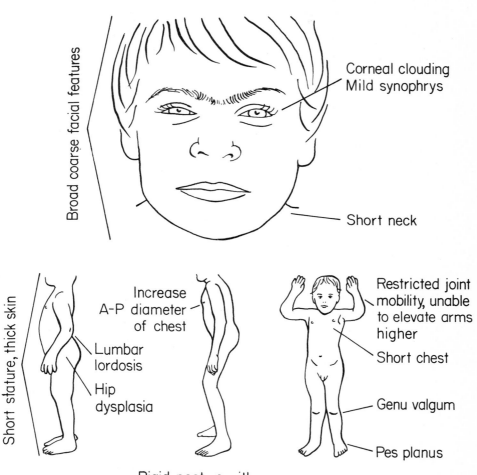

Broad coarse facial features

Corneal clouding
Mild synophrys

Short neck

Short stature, thick skin

Increase A-P diameter of chest

Lumbar lordosis

Hip dysplasia

Restricted joint mobility, unable to elevate arms higher

Short chest

Genu valgum

Pes planus

Rigid posture with age

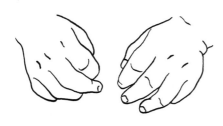

Claw hand deformity

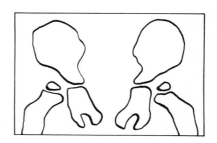

Flared iliac wings, shallow acetabula and coxa valga

84. MUCOPOLYSACCHARIDOSIS I-H
(Hurler syndrome)

Clinical Features Hurler syndrome, MPS I-H, is the classic prototype of the mucopolysaccharidoses, exhibiting growth failure after infancy, marked mental retardation, characteristic craniofacial dysmorphism, and physical habitus. In the first few months of life there are few, relatively nonspecific, findings such as macrocephaly, limited hip abduction, recurrent respiratory infections, and hernias. The full clinical picture usually does not develop until the second year. Slight coarsening of facial features may be noted at three to six months. The head is large with frontal bulging and occasionally scaphocephaly. Synophrys, depressed nasal bridge, broad nasal tip, and wide anteverted nostrils are common. Corneal clouding appears during the third year. Earlobes are thick, lips are enlarged, and the mouth is usually held open, especially after the age of three. Chronic nasal discharge is marked, even between the frequent bouts of upper respiratory infection. Nasal congestion with stertorous breathing through the mouth is severe. Increased growth is common until about 18 months, but growth usually ceases before two years of age. The neck is short. Pectus carinatum and excavatum are common and frequently there is lumbodorsal kyphosis and gibbus. Range of motion is limited in all joints, in the hands resulting in the claw-hand deformity. The abdomen protrudes because of hepatic and splenic enlargement, deformity of the chest, shortness of the spine, and laxity of the abdominal wall. These changes are manifest during the second year of life. Hepatomegaly may be detected as early as six to 12 months. Inguinal hernia present at birth or manifesting within the first three months is a constant feature in males. Mental retardation becomes more severe with age. Cardiomegaly due to deposition of AMPS in the myocardium and valves is common. Teeth become widely spaced and the alveolar ridges hyperplastic.

Specific Diagnosis Dermatan sulfate and heparan sulfate are excreted in the urine, the former about twice as much as the latter. A deficiency of α-L-iduronidase may be demonstrated in leukocytes or fibroblasts. Excessive storage of ^{35}S-labeled AMPS is found in cultured fibroblasts. From 30 to 50% of peripheral leukocytes, bone marrow cells, or cultured fibroblasts exhibit metachromatic granules. The most popular rapid screening tests are the toluidine blue spot test and the gross albumin turbidity test, the latter being far more accurate. Radiographically, in infancy, bone trabeculation is coarse. In late infancy and early childhood, changes of dysostosis multiplex emerge. There is often premature closure of the sagittal, lambdoidal, and metopic sutures. The skull is large and scaphocephalic, the sella J-shaped. The ribs are wide, the vertebral bodies dysplastic with bi-convex endplates and hook-shaped configuration of the lower thoracic and upper lumbar bodies after 12 to 18 months. The basilar portions of the ilia are underdeveloped with flaring of the wings. Long tubular bones show marked diaphyseal widening and distortion with small and deformed epiphyses. The shafts of short tubular bones are underconstricted, becoming bullet-shaped.

Differential Diagnosis Dermatan sulfate and heparan sulfate are also excreted in *MPS II*, while only the former is elevated in *MPS VI*. Gross corneal clouding is present in *MPS I-H* but not in *MPS VI*. Intelligence is normal in MPS VI in contrast to *MPS I-H* and *MPS II*, except for the mild form of *MPS II*. Dysostosis multiplex occurs in *MPS I-H*, *MPS II*, *MPS VI*, *ML II*, and to a lesser extent in *MPS VII*. The bone changes are as severe in *MPS I-H* as in the severe form of *MPS VI*. The same enzyme defect is present in *MPS I-H*, *MPS I-S*, and *MPS I-H-S*, but the phenotype is different, those with the Hurler-Scheie compound being intermediate in type.

Prenatal Diagnosis Levels of α-L-iduronidase or sulfate incorporation studies may be carried out in cultured amniotic cells.

Basic Defect, Genetics, and Other Considerations The basic defect is absence of α-L-iduronidase activity which inhibits intralysosomal degradation of α-L-iduronide-containing mucopolysaccharides. This interferes with normal function of affected cells and leads to characteristic clinical signs and symptoms. The disorder has autosomal recessive inheritance. Heterozygotes exhibit intermediate enzyme activity. The frequency has been estimated at about 1 in 100,000 live births.

Prognosis and Treatment In MPS I-H, mental and motor deterioration and loss of vision and hearing occur after two years of age and death usually occurs before ten years from pneumonia and/or heart failure. Treatment is supportive.

REFERENCES

Kaibara, N., Eguchi, M., Shibata, K. et al. Hurler-Scheie phenotype: a report of two pairs of inbred sibs. *Hum. Genet. 53:* 37–41, 1979.

Spranger, J. The systemic mucopolysaccharidoses. *Ergeb. Inn. Med. Kinderheilkd. 32:* 165–265, 1972.

Stevenson, R.E., Howell, R.R., McKusick, V.A. et al. The iduronidase-deficient mucopolysaccharidoses: clinical and roentgenographic features. *Pediatrics* 57: 111–122, 1976.

- **macrocephaly / frontal bossing**
- **coarse facies / thick ear lobes and lips**
- **hepatosplenomegaly**
- **chest and spine deformities**

Mucopolysaccharidosis I-H
[Hurler syndrome]

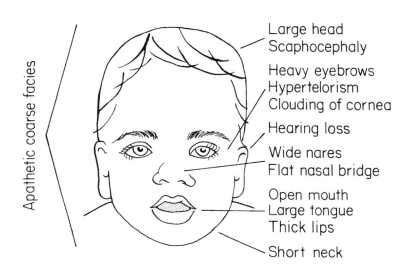

Apathetic coarse facies

Large head
Scaphocephaly

Heavy eyebrows
Hypertelorism
Clouding of cornea

Hearing loss

Wide nares
Flat nasal bridge

Open mouth
Large tongue
Thick lips

Short neck

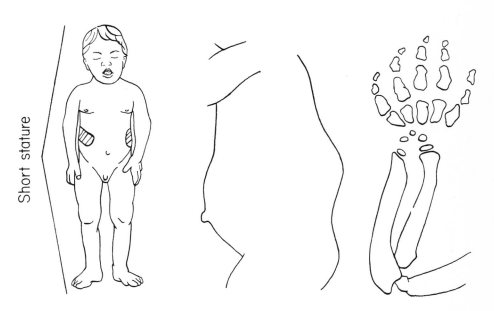

Short stature

Protuberant abdomen with hepatosplenomegaly, umbilical hernia, gibbus deformity, joint limitation, claw-hand deformity and long bones are broad and short

85. MUCOPOLYSACCHARIDOSIS II
(Hunter syndrome)

Clinical Features There appear to be at least two forms, a severe (MPS IIA) and a mild type (MPS IIB) and possibly a severe autosomal recessively inherited type based on intellectual impairment and longevity. During the first year of life, there is little reason to suspect that something is wrong. Occasionally radiographic investigation of a gibbus at this time may reveal the characteristic vertebral changes. Stertorous breathing and rhinorrhea are usually the first signs. The liver and spleen become clinically enlarged at about two years of age and continue to enlarge. The lips, tongue, and nostrils become thick, producing a characteristic facies. Growth failure becomes evident during the third year of life. The skin becomes thick and hirsute and hearing loss may be evident and gradually progresses. Patients may exhibit nodular skin lesions of the posterior upper thorax or arms. Joint stiffness (especially claw hands) becomes evident. Inguinal and umbilical hernia are common. The corneas are nearly always clear. Destructive behavior and mental retardation become evident in the severe forms.

Specific Diagnosis There is marked deficiency of iduronate sulfatase in the hemizygotes and reduced levels in female heterozygotes. Radiographically, the skeletal changes are those of dysostosis multiplex. As with MPS I-H and MPS VI, cystic changes are noted around unerupted permanent molar teeth.

Differential Diagnosis Hunter syndrome (MPS II) most closely resembles *Hurler syndrome* (*MPS I-H*) and while they excrete the same acid mucopolysaccharides, they are due to different enzyme defects. Both MPS I-H and MPS I-S (Scheie syndrome) are caused by α-L-iduronidase deficiency, while MPS II is related to a deficiency of iduronate sulfatase. Clinically, MPS II is milder than MPS I-H. The skeletal alterations are less marked and longevity is greater. The phenotype of *MPS I-S* does not resemble that of *MPS I-H*. Patients with the autosomal recessive form of MPS II are more severely affected than those with the severe X-linked recessive form.

Prenatal Diagnosis Iduronate sulfatase assay on amniotic fluid or cultured amniotic cells can be performed at 16 weeks' gestation. Sulfate incorporation studies may also be performed but female heterozygotic fetuses may also exhibit abnormal AMPS metabolism.

Basic Defect, Genetics, and Other Considerations The basic defect is a deficiency of iduronate sulfatase with consequent storage of undegraded AMPS in the lysosomes. Usually this has X-linked recessive inheritance. The mild and severe forms share the same enzyme defect and are possibly allelic. The female heterozygote can be determined by enzyme assay or by sulfate incorporation studies of cloned skin fibroblasts or from hair-root analysis. The frequency of MPS II has been estimated to be approximately 1 in 150,000 live births with the division between mild and severe forms being about equal.

Prognosis and Treatment Prognosis depends on whether the patient has the mild form (MPS II B), in which mentation is often normal and deterioration is very slow; or the severe form (MPS II A), in which mental retardation is profound becoming severe by the fifth or sixth year of life. Patients with the mild form survive beyond the age of 20 years. However, most of those with the severe form die prior to the end of the second decade of pneumonia, or more often congestive heart failure. Adults with the mild type reach 120–140 cm in height, exceeding that of patients with the severe form by about 20 cm. Treatment is supportive.

REFERENCES

Neufeld, E.F., Liebaers, I., Epstein, C.J. et al. The Hunter syndrome in females: is there an autosomal recessive form of iduronate sulfatase deficiency? *Am. J. Hum. Genet. 29:* 455–461, 1977.

Spranger, J. The systemic mucopolysaccharidoses. *Ergeb. Inn. Med. Kinderheilkd. 32:* 165–265, 1972.

Wiesmann, U.N. and Rampini, S. Mild form of the Hunter syndrome: identification of the biochemical defect with the severe type. *Helv. Paediat. Acta 29:* 73–78, 1974.

M.R. [+ / all,
severe form]

• **coarse facies /
thick lips and nose**
• **thick, hirsute skin**
• **joint-stiffness /
claw hand deformity**
• **hepatosplenomegaly**

Mucopolysaccharidosis II
[Hunter syndrome]

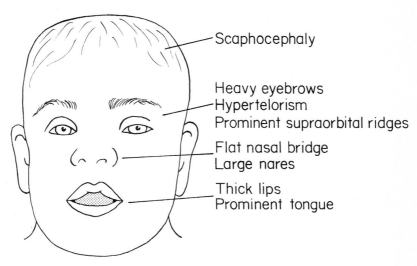

- Scaphocephaly

- Heavy eyebrows
- Hypertelorism
- Prominent supraorbital ridges

- Flat nasal bridge
- Large nares

- Thick lips
- Prominent tongue

Coarse facies, short neck and progressive deafness

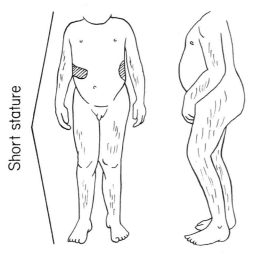

Short stature

Hepatosplenomegaly, hypertrichosis,
claw hand, stiff joints, pes cavus

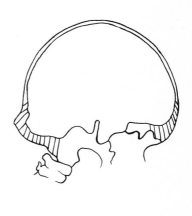

Large sella turcica, frontal
and occipital hyperostosis

189

86. MUCOPOLYSACCHARIDOSIS III
(Sanfilippo syndrome)

Clinical Features Genetic heterogeneity is present in this disorder, there being four known types which are difficult to distinguish clinically. There is considerable intertype and intrafamilial variability. In the young child, no abnormalities are usually noted. As the child grows older, the facies becomes mildly coarse. There is mild scaphocephaly and moderate enlargement of the head, somewhat sunken nasal bridge, and abundant coarse scalp hair. The corneas are clear. Height may be slightly reduced and joint mobility may be mildly restricted at the elbow and knee. Behavioral problems such as restlessness, aggressiveness, diminished attention span, and sleep disturbances usually become evident between the second and fifth year of life and frequently constitute the parents' reason for seeking medical help. Subsequently during adolescence there is progressive loss of mental and motor skills. Loss of environmental contact is evident prior to a vegetative state which may eventuate in spastic diplegia. Hepatosplenomegaly is mild.

Specific Diagnosis Coarse granulations are seen in the cytoplasm of at least 35% of peripheral lymphocytes. The inclusions stain metachromatically with toluidine blue. Excessive amounts of heparan sulfate are excreted in the urine and there is abnormal intracellular accumulation of ^{35}S-labeled acid mucopolysaccharide in cultured fibroblasts. Enzyme levels may be determined in cultured fibroblasts and leukocytes. Radiographic changes are relatively mild. The calvaria is thickened. The ribs and clavicles are somewhat broadened. Vertebral changes are mild. Pulp chambers and root canals of the deciduous teeth are largely obliterated.

Differential Diagnosis Unlike other forms of mucopolysaccharidoses, MPS III is characterized by early onset of severe mental retardation in the absence of marked skeletal and somatic manifestations and growth is generally not retarded. Leukocyte inclusions may also be found in *MPS I-H, MPS II,* and *MPS VII.* Hepatosplenomegaly and joint limitation in MPS III is milder than in *MPS I, II,* or *VI.*

Prenatal Diagnosis MPS III may be diagnosed in utero by enzyme assay or by labeled sulfate incorporation by cultured amniocytes.

Basic Defect, Genetics, and Other Considerations MPS III represents a group of defects in heparan sulfate catabolism, characterized by intralysosomal storage and increased urinary excretion of this glycosaminoglycan. MPS III is genetically heterogeneous, but all forms have autosomal recessive inheritance. MPS III-A is caused by deficient activity of heparan sulfate-N-sulfatase, MPS III-B by deficient activity of α-N-acetylglucosaminidase, while in MPS III-C there is deficient activity of acetyl-CoA:α-glucosaminide N-acetyltransferase and in MPS III-D, a heparan-specific N-acetylglucosamine 6-sulfate sulfatase. The four genetically different forms of MPS III cannot be differentiated clinically. They are the result of nonallelic mutations. Type B may be heterogeneous.

Prognosis and Treatment There is progressive deterioration to a vegetative state. While many die during adolescence, possibly one-third may exceed 30 years of age. Type A has earlier onset, severe course, and earlier death than Type B, which is relatively mild. Type C is somewhat less severe than Type A. Treatment is supportive.

REFERENCES

Bartsocas, C., Gröbe, H., van de Kamp, J.J.P. et al. Sanfilippo type C disease: clinical findings in four patients with a new variant of mucopolysaccharidosis III. *Eur. J. Pediatr. 130:* 251–258, 1979.

Kresse, H., Paschke, E., von Figura, K. et al. Sanfilippo disease type D: deficiency of N-acetylglucosamine 6-sulfate sulfatase required for heparan degradation. *Proc. Nat. Acad. Sci. (Wash.)* 77: 6822–6826, 1980.

Van de Kamp, J.J.P., Niermeijer, M.F., von Figura, K., Genetic heterogeneity and clinical variability in the Sanfilippo syndrome (types A, B, and C). *Clin. Genet. 20:* 152–160, 1981.

M.R. [+ / all]

- **coarse facies**
- **abundant coarse scalp hair**
- **mild hepato-splenomegaly**
- **behavioral problems**

Mucopolysaccharidosis III
[Sanfilippo syndrome]

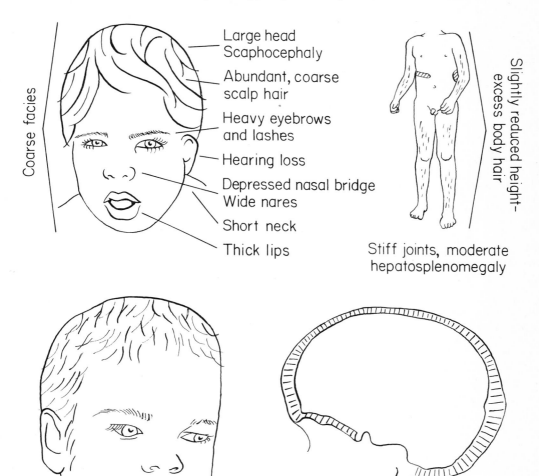

Coarse facies

Large head
Scaphocephaly

Abundant, coarse
scalp hair

Heavy eyebrows
and lashes

Hearing loss

Depressed nasal bridge
Wide nares

Short neck

Thick lips

Slightly reduced height –
excess body hair

Stiff joints, moderate
hepatosplenomegaly

More coarse facies in older child – thick calvaria

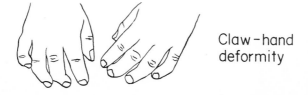

Claw – hand
deformity

87. MUCOPOLYSACCHARIDOSIS IV
(Morquio syndrome)

Clinical Features The Morquio syndromes represent a genetic heterogeneity characterized by marked growth failure, progressive spinal deformity, short neck, pectus carinatum, various typical skeletal anomalies (including platyspondyly, odontoid hypoplasia, genu valgum, pes planus), waddling gait, and normal intelligence. There are severe (MPS IV A) and mild (MPS IV B) forms. The affected child appears normal at birth, but usually by two years of age retarded growth and genu valgum are noted. The facies is not specific, but the lower half of the face is often outstanding because of shortness and hyperextension of the neck. Reduced body height results from shortened neck and trunk and to a lesser extent from shortened extremities. Adult height rarely exceeds 100 cm. The head seems to rest directly on the shoulders with exaggerated cervical curvature and restricted movement of the neck. Kyphosis or kyphoscoliosis becomes marked after the second year. There is characteristic pectus carinatum, the sternum extending almost horizontally from its clavicular junction. The lumbar spine frequently exhibits a gibbus-like kyphosis, or less often hyperlordosis, at or about the first lumbar vertebra. Extremities appear disproportionately long. There may be excessive joint mobility. The wrists are often enlarged. Genu valgum, enlarged knee joints, and pes planus/valgus are common. The stance is often semicrouching. Aortic regurgitation occurs with increased frequency. The corneas become slowly but diffusely opacified with a filmy haze, especially after the tenth year. Progressive hearing loss begins in adolescence. The enamel of the teeth is remarkably thinned in the severe MPS IV A form. Recurrent respiratory infections are common in infancy.

Specific Diagnosis Marked excretion of keratan sulfate and chondroitin sulfate A in the urine in childhood can be detected by two-dimensional electrophoresis or thin-layer chromatography. Specific enzyme assays in serum, leukocytes, or fibroblasts may be carried out; however, they slowly decrease, reaching normal levels in adults. Increased amounts of chondroitin sulfate C are also excreted. Abnormal granules may be detected in peripheral neutrophilic leukocytes. Radiographically, there are initially ovoid deformities of the vertebrae with tongue-like protrusions which eventuate in generalized platyspondyly.

Hypoplasia of the last thoracic and first lumbar vertebrae, widened ribs, coxa valga, flared ilia, osteoporosis, and progressive femoral head flattening and fragmentation are common. In the young child, the vertebral bodies are ovoid and the superior acetabula deficiently ossified. The odontoid is hypoplastic or absent. The metaphyses of long bones are widened. The bases of the second to fifth metacarpals are conical. The distal ends of the radius and ulna are inclined toward one another.

Differential Diagnosis One must exclude various *spondyloepiphyseal dysplasias* and *multiple epiphyseal dysplasias*. These disorders can be separated from the Morquio syndrome (MPS IV) by absence of keratan sulfate excretion in the urine. Patients with G_{M1}-gangliosidosis also are β-galactosidase deficient but exhibit motor and mental retardation. Patients having the *mild form (MPS IV B)* exhibit odontoid hypoplasia, platyspondyly, and thoracolumbar kyphosis, but the bone changes in the limbs are less severe. *Dyggve-Melchior-Clausen disease* resemble MPS IV but the corneas are clear, there is usually mental retardation, the iliac crest is lacy, the proximal metacarpals are not conical, and keratan sulfate is not excreted.

Prenatal Diagnosis Can be carried out for either variant on cultured amniocytes by showing a deficiency of N-acetyl galactosamine-6-sulfate sulfatase.

Basic Defect, Genetics, and Other Considerations The disorder in MPS IV A is a deficiency of N-acetyl galactosamine-6-sulfate sulfatase. MPS IV B shows a deficiency in acid β-galactosidase. However, in both type A and B, keratan sulfate is excreted in the urine. All types are transmitted in an autosomal recessive manner.

Prognosis and Treatment Spinal cord compression is common. Orthopedic management consists of spinal bracing for the thoracolumbar kyphosis, centering osteotomies of the hips to correct the subluxation of the femoral heads, alignment osteotomies of the lower limbs to correct the knock-knee deformity, and occipitocervical fusion when indicated by neurologic signs or progressive upper cervical instability.

REFERENCES

Hollister, D.W., Cohen, A.H., Rimoin, D.L. et al. The Morquio syndrome (MPS IV): morphologic and biochemical studies. *Johns Hopk. Med. J. 137:* 176–183, 1975.

Holzgreve, W., Gröbe, H., von Figura, K. et al. Morquio syndrome: clinical findings in 11 patients with MPS IV A and 2 patients with MPS IV B. *Hum. Genet. 57:* 360–365, 1981.

Trojak, J.E., Ho, C.K., Roesel, R.A. et al. Morquio-like syndrome (MPS IV B) associated with deficiency of β-galactosidase. *Johns Hopk. Med. J. 146:* 75–79, 1980.

- **genu valgum**
- **pectus carinatum**
- **short neck / kyphoscoliosis**
- **marked growth failure**

Mucopolysaccharidosis IV
[Morquio syndrome]

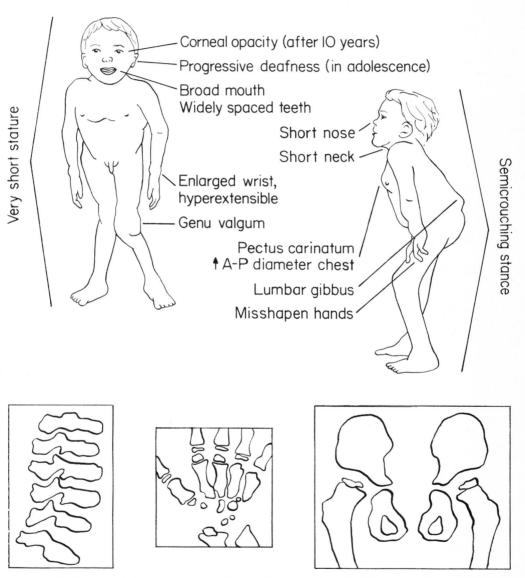

Very short stature

Corneal opacity (after 10 years)

Progressive deafness (in adolescence)

Broad mouth
Widely spaced teeth

Short nose

Short neck

Enlarged wrist,
hyperextensible

Genu valgum

Pectus carinatum
↑A-P diameter chest

Lumbar gibbus

Misshapen hands

Semicrouching stance

Platyspondyly, tapering of proximal ends of metacarpals, coxa valga, hypoplasia of femoral heads and widening of acetabula

88. MUCOPOLYSACCHARIDOSIS VI
(Maroteaux-Lamy syndrome)

Clinical Features There appear to be three forms of MPS VI: severe, intermediate, and mild types. In none of the forms is there mental retardation. Those with the mild type develop reasonably well until the age of about six years when small stature (adult height 158–168 cm) and spinal deformities are noted. With age, signs of cervical and lumbar radiculopathy and cervical myelopathy (tetraspastic syndrome) develop. In those with the severe type, changes are noted in early childhood and the disease progresses more rapidly to a state of severe disability with striking short stature (adult height 110–140 cm), marked facial and skeletal abnormalities, severely impaired vision and hearing, and prominent cardiac defects. In the severe form the facies is rather similar to that in MPS I-H, with depressed nasal bridge, full cheeks and lips, large cranium, and abundant eyebrows and scalp hair. Marked corneal clouding is regularly present. Stature is short. The chest is deformed with a prominent sternum and there are multiple joint contractures, claw deformities noted after the first year of life, lumbar kyphosis, and genu valgum. Hepatomegaly is almost invariably present. The spleen is enlarged in about half the cases and hernias are common. Cardiovascular involvement with valvular incompetence and narrowing of the coronary and other arteries is often noted. Mixed hearing loss is frequent. While mentation is normal, impaired vision and hearing, restricted mobility, and secondary psychological reaction may impede intellectual performance. Neurologic deficits include hydrocephalus and peripheral nerve compression. The tongue is large and the teeth widely spaced. Eruption of permanent molars is retarded and some of them may be completely buried and angulated in the mandible.

Specific Diagnosis Radiographically, the changes are similar to those in MPS I-H. Ossification of the superior portion of the capital femoral epiphysis may be markedly defective. Cysts are present around the crowns of unerupted molar teeth. In the mild type there are cranial changes, wide ribs, and pelvic dysplasia but few changes in the spine and fibulae. Numerous coarse dense inclusions are noted in granulocytes, monocytes, and a large proportion of lymphocytes in peripheral blood smears. Large quantities of dermatan sulfate are excreted in the urine, but the level decreases with age. Deficient arylsulfatase B (about 10–15% of normal activity) and increased amounts of ^{35}S-labeled MPS are found in cultured fibroblasts. Obligate heterozygotes have about 35–47% of normal arylsulfatase B activity.

Differential Diagnosis The mild and severe forms can be distinguished on the basis of height, increased longevity, lack of cardiac insufficiency, absence of herniae or severe splenomegaly or marked corneal opacities. The severe form of MPS VI is most often confused with *MPS I-H* or *MPS IV*, but normal mentation and severely clouded corneas should clinically separate the disorders. The mild form of MPS VI may be confused with *MPS I-S*.

Prenatal Diagnosis Arylsulfatase B can be shown to be deficient in amniotic fluid cell cultures or in ^{35}S-sulfate studies. Residual enzyme activity in the affected homozygote makes interpretation difficult.

Basic Defect, Genetics, and Other Considerations The basis defect is deficient activity of arylsulfatase B. All forms exhibit autosomal recessive inheritance.

Prognosis and Treatment The mild form apparently is associated with a normal life span, although there are complications such as cervical and lumbar radiculopathy and cervical myelopathy. In the severe form, few survive the second decade, due to cardiorespiratory problems. Surgical correction of hernias and physical therapy for correction of contractures, and hearing aids, are of benefit.

REFERENCES

Pilz, H., von Figura, K., and Goebel, H.H. Deficiency of arylsulfatase B in 2 brothers aged 40 and 38 years (Maroteaux-Lamy syndrome, type B). *Ann. Neurol. 6:* 315–325, 1979.

Stumpf, D.A., Austin, J.H., Crocker, A.C. et al. Mucopolysaccharidosis type VI (Maroteaux-Lamy syndrome). *Am. J. Dis. Child. 126:* 747–755, 1973.

Van Dyke, D.L., Fluharty, A.L., Shafer, I.A., Shapiro, L.H. et al. Prenatal diagnosis of Maroteaux-Lamy syndrome. *Am. J. Med. Genet. 8:* 235–242, 1981.

- **macrocephaly**
- **coarse facies /
  full cheeks and lips**
- **corneal clouding**
- **prominent sternum and
  skeletal deformities**

Mucopolysaccharidosis VI
[Maroteaux-Lamy syndrome]

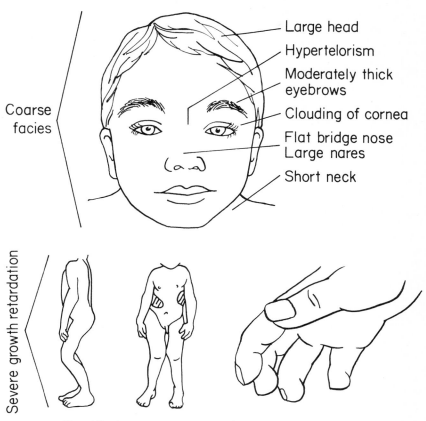

Coarse facies

Large head
Hypertelorism
Moderately thick eyebrows
Clouding of cornea
Flat bridge nose
Large nares
Short neck

Severe growth retardation

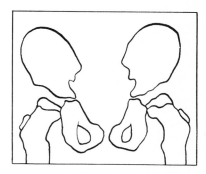

Semiflexion stance, protruding sternum, hepato-splenomegaly, genu valgum and clawhand deformity

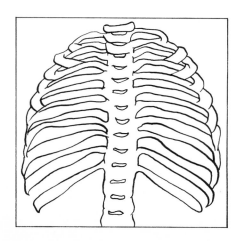

Broad ribs, dysplastic femoral head, coxa valga and widened acetabula

195

89. PENDRED SYNDROME

Clinical Features Pendred syndrome consists of goiter (usually euthyroid) and congenital sensorineural hearing loss. Preservation of hearing in the low tones is variable. The thyroid enlargement is usually evident before puberty. While the average age at which it becomes evident is approximately eight years, in some cases it may be observed at birth. The goiter is diffuse and soft without a bruit and tends to remain small, but with time tends to become nodular. While variations in hearing loss occur in this syndrome, audiometric testing usually shows a congenital bilateral 40–100 dB sensorineural hearing loss, more severe in the higher frequencies. It is severe in over half of the cases. The average age at which deafness is detected has been about two years. The hearing loss progresses slightly during childhood.

Specific Diagnosis Diagnosis is based on audiometric assessment of hearing loss. Positive recruitment has been found in most cases, suggesting that the auditory defect is in the organ of Corti. Caloric tests have generally shown depressed vestibular function. Tomographic studies of the cochlea have shown malformation of the bony inner ear with enlarged bony semicircular canals and only two cochlear turns in the membranous labyrinth (Mondini defect); hair cells are absent in the tectorial membrane in about 50%. Critical is demonstration of organic binding of iodine demonstrable by the perchlorate or thiocyanate test, which releases pooled or unbound iodine as shown by a sharp decline in the thyroid counting rate when isotopically labelled iodine is employed. In patients with Pendred syndrome, the iodine is variably discharged (15–80%) from the thyroid by perchlorate, resulting in a rapid decrease in radioactivity in the thyroid. The intravenous, rather than the oral, perchlorate test appears to be more reliable.

Differential Diagnosis One must exclude cases of *endemic cretinism with deafness,* which occurs in certain isolated areas (Alps, Andes, Himalayas) where iodine is deficient. This is demonstrated by absence of cretinoid signs in Pendred syndrome and by a negative perchlorate test in cretinism. However, the perchlorate test may be positive in

Hashimoto thyroiditis, in *sporadic goitrous cretinism,* in *nontoxic goiter,* and in *congenital deafness without goiter.* Impaired hearing is seen in about half of *adult myxedematous patients.* Microscopically, the cells lining the thyroid follicles are tall and active and colloid is scanty. At times, nuclear pleomorphism and papillary infoldings are noted, leading to the erroneous diagnosis of *adenocarcinoma.*

Prenatal Diagnosis There is no test for the prenatal diagnosis of this disorder.

Basic Defect, Genetics, and Other Considerations The basic defect lies in thyroxin synthesis at the level of incorporation of iodine into organic forms in the thyroglobulin molecule. The block is incomplete and of variable degree. The thyroid changes thus are extremely variable. Although euthyroidism is the rule, hypothyroidism may occur in infancy or follow surgical removal of the thyroid. The hyperplasia of the thyroid is a response to the difficulty in hormone synthesis, especially in females. The growth of the thyroid remnant may involve many operations. In the event of pronounced hypothyroidism, there may be mental and/or physical retardation and occasionally death may occur due to respiratory obstruction due to thyroid enlargement. The disorder clearly has autosomal recessive inheritance. The frequency of Pendred syndrome varies in different parts of the world from about 1 per 100,000 to 8 per 100,000. It may account for as much as 10% of cases of profound congenital hearing loss.

Prognosis and Treatment Patients with Pendred syndrome have been subjected to a large number of surgical procedures for removal of the goiter, which invariably returns following continued stimulation by thyroid-stimulating hormone. The goiter is best treated by exogenous hormone which causes a decrease in production of TSH and thyroid stimulation. If therapy is started early, the goiter may regress. Hearing does not improve, however; the hearing loss remains stable with little change over the years. If there is some residual hearing, a hearing aid may be of help.

REFERENCES

Batsakis, J.G. and Nishiyama, R.H. Deafness with sporadic goiter. Pendred's syndrome. *Arch. Otolaryngol. 76:* 401–406, 1962.

Fraser, G.R. Association of congenital deafness with goiter (Pendred's syndrome). A study of 207 families. *Ann. Hum. Genet. 28:* 201–249, 1965.

Illum, P., Kiaer, H.W., Hvidberg-Hansen, J. et al. Fifteen cases of Pendred's syndrome. *Arch. Otolaryngol. 96:* 297–304, 1972.

- goiter
- sensorineural hearing loss

Pendred Syndrome

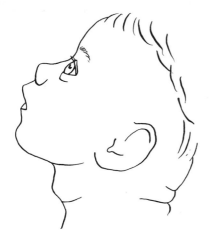

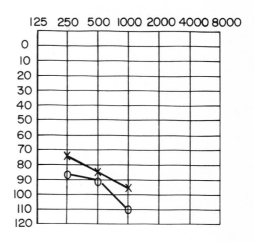

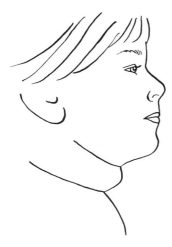

Diffuse, soft goiter which later becomes nodular – typical audiogram showing remaining hearing in the lowest frequencies – right ear = O, left ear = X

Uptake of radioactive iodine in the thyroid gland with subsequent perchlorate test – a, administration I 131, 8.1 microcuries; b = I 131, 16 microcuries; c potassium perchlorate, I gram – perchlorate test showed a fall in activity of 80 per cent

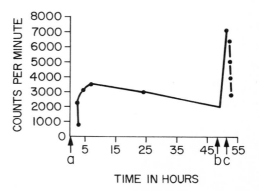

90. PITUITARY DWARFISM SYNDROMES

Clinical Features We shall briefly consider (a) panhypopituitarism, (b) congenital absence of the pituitary, (c) isolated HGH deficiency, and (d) Laron-type dwarfism. Common to all forms are essentially normal growth for the first six months to two years, hypoglycemic episodes with or without coma (except in autosomal dominant isolated HGH deficiency), truncal obesity, and highpitched voice. The forehead is broad with hypoplastic maxilla and mandible creating craniofacial disproportion. Usually by age 30 the facial skin becomes wrinkled and soft with increased subcutaneous adipose tissue giving the young individual an older appearance (except in autosomal dominant isolated HGH deficiency). If gonadotropins are deficient, pubertal changes never occur. *Familial panhypopituitary dwarfism* refers to HGH deficiency with lack of one or more pituitary tropic hormones, most frequently gonadotropin, ACTH, and TSH in that order, the clinical features depending on the specific tropic hormone deficiency, e.g., deficiency of gonadotropin results in sexual immaturity, primary amenorrhea, and lack of secondary sexual characteristics in the female, with small testes and penis and lack of beard in the male. TSH deficiency usually does not result in severe thyroid deficiency. ACTH deficiency may be manifest as severe hypoglycemia. In so-called *congenital absence of the pituitary* there is relative deficiency of HGH, TSH, and ACTH. Motor and mental retardation occur. *Isolated HGH deficiency* is characterized by normal sexual development and thyroid and adrenal function. In the autosomal recessive form, the patient exhibits wrinkled skin, hypoglycemic attacks, and insulin hypersensitivity, while these are normal in the autosomal dominant form. The *Laron-type* patient is proportionately but severely dwarfed. In contrast to those with panhypopituitarism, there are high plasma concentrations of immunoreactive HGH and females mature sexually, but males have delayed puberty. Borderline intelligence with distinct deficiencies in visuomotor performance is common. HGH levels rise following insulin or arginine stimulation.

Specific Diagnosis The HGH deficiency of pituitary dwarfism (except in the case of Laron-type dwarfism) can be demonstrated by radioimmunoassay. Since plasma levels are normally low, this may be demonstrated by failure to respond to various stimuli (insulin-induced hypoglycemia,

arginine infusion). Pituitary responsiveness may be indirectly measured by the metapyrone test. TSH, ACTH, and gonadotropin levels should be determined if tropic hormone deficiency is suspected. Sulfation factor is low in probably all forms. There is insulin hypersensitivity and decreased insulin secretion (save for autosomal dominant isolated HGH deficiency). In response to HGH therapy, plasma-free fatty acids are decreased both in Laron-type dwarfism and autosomal dominant HGH deficiency. Radiologically, bone age is retarded in all types. A mild caveat: those with isolated HGH deficiency may not exhibit puberty until late teens or early twenties; thus, separation from HGH with those who lack gonadotropin may require gonadotropin assays.

Differential Diagnosis One should rule out *emotional deprivation* and pituitary lesions such as *craniopharyngioma* that may produce growth retardation in middle childhood or preadolescence.

Prenatal Diagnosis Currently not possible, although a deficiency of prolactin has been reported in the amniotic fluid of those with primary pituitary dysgenesis.

Basic Defect, Genetics, and Other Considerations The basic defect is not known, but abnormal HGH receptor sites are suspected. Familial panhypopituitary dwarfism (asexual ateleosis) is more often nongenetic than genetic, but there are autosomal recessive or less often X-linked recessive types which are otherwise indistinguishable. So-called congenital absence of the pituitary exhibits autosomal recessive inheritance. Isolated HGH deficiency can have either autosomal recessive or autosomal dominant transmission. The Laron-type exhibits autosomal recessive inheritance.

Prognosis and Treatment Life span is normal. In most patients, greatly accelerated growth rates can be produced by the administration of HGH. In those who lack other tropic hormones, administration of thyroxin, cortisone, and/or testosterone should be given appropriately. Individuals with isolated HGH deficiency tend to have spontaneous hypoglycemia and may require frequent feedings but such episodes tend to disappear in mid-childhood.

REFERENCES

Rona, R.J. and Tanner, J.M. Aetiology of idiopathic growth hormone deficiency in England and Wales. *Arch. Dis. Child.* 52: 197–208, 1977.

Sadeghi-Nejad, A., and Senior, B. A familial syndrome of isolated "aplasia" of the anterior pituitary. *J. Pediatr.* 84: 79–84, 1974.

Saldanha, P.H. and Toledo, S.P.A. Familial dwarfism with high IR-GH: report of two affected sibs with genetic and epidemiologic considerations. *Hum. Genet.* 59: 367–372, 1981.

M.R. [+ / few,
depending on type]

- **craniofacial disproportion**
- **dwarfism**
- **truncal obesity**
- **high-pitched voice**

Pituitary Dwarfism Syndromes

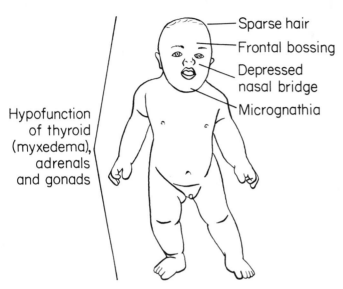

Sparse hair
Frontal bossing
Depressed nasal bridge
Micrognathia

Hypofunction of thyroid (myxedema), adrenals and gonads

Congenital absence of pituitary in a 14 year old boy—height 81 cm

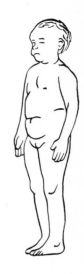

Laron type—12 year old boy, small face, height 93 cm

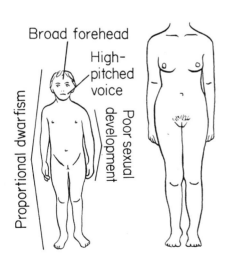

Broad forehead
High-pitched voice

Proportional dwarfism

Poor sexual development

Panhypopituitarism in 15 year old female, height 116 cm—normal girl of same age

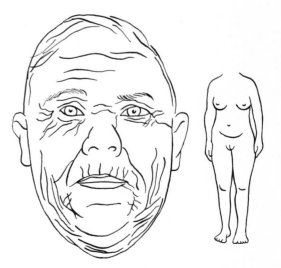

Isolated HGH deficiency with premature and excessive facial wrinkling—normal sexual development, age 20 years, height 135 cm

91. PRADER-WILLI SYNDROME

Clinical Features Hypotonia, hypomentia, hypogonadism, and obesity characterize the syndrome. Short stature, the tendency to develop diabetes mellitus, and small hands and feet should be added as distinctive features. There is often decreased fetal movement in the last trimester of pregnancy. Delivery, breach in about 30% of the cases, usually occurs at term, with birth weight usually below 3000 g. In the newborn period, there is marked hypotonia associated with poor sucking and swallowing reflexes, a weak cry, and sometimes episodes of asphyxia. Congenitally dislocated hips are not uncommon. The Moro response and tendon reflexes are decreased or absent. The child sits, stands, and walks late. Intellectual impairment is quite variable (30–85 IQ). Speech is especially retarded. In general, the child is happy, friendly, and cooperative but may exhibit extreme frustration, negativism, and temper tantrums when denied unlimited food.

Specific Diagnosis Generalized obesity does not become apparent until the second and third year of life, when patients begin to exhibit uncontrolled appetite. The accumulation of fat on the lower part of the trunk, proximal limbs, and buttocks is particularly marked. However, the hands and feet remain small (acromicria). The face is often characteristic. Bifrontal diameter is reduced and there is marked obesity around the cheeks and under the chin. The mouth is often fishlike with a triangular-shaped upper lip. In males, the penis is small, the testes ectopic or infantile, and the scrotum rudimentary. Pubertal changes are delayed and diminished. The voice in males usually remains high-pitched. During childhood and adolescence diabetes mellitus frequently is manifest, but differs from the usual form by the absence of weight loss and acidosis, the presence of insulin resistance, and the good response to oral hypoglycemic drugs.

Differential Diagnosis During the neonatal period, because of the hypotonia, *severe congenital muscular dystrophy, neonatal myasthenia, Werdnig-Hoffman disease* with prenatal onset, *traumatic brain injuries, intracranial hemorrhage,* and *cerebral malformations* must be distinguished from the Prader-Willi syndrome. As the individual grows older, one must rule out *Laurence-Moon syndrome, Bardet-Biedl syndrome, obesity* with feminine habitus and small genitalia sometimes observed in prepubertal boys, the *Summitt syndrome* (which may possibly be the *Carpenter syndrome*), and *Alstrom syndrome* (retinal degeneration combined with obesity, diabetes mellitus, and neurogenic deafness).

Prenatal Diagnosis Not currently available.

Basic Defect, Genetics, and Other Considerations The basic defect is not known. Studies of the hypothalamus-pituitary-gonadal complex have yielded inconsistent results. Almost all cases have been sporadic. Karyotypes have been abnormal in about half of the cases. Most of these have exhibited del(15q), especially bands 15q11-q12. Various other chromosomal abnormalities have been reported. The syndrome is rather common and over 200 cases have been reported. The preponderance of reported males probably reflects the early recognition of the rudimentary scrotum and the micropenis.

Prognosis and Treatment Life expectancy is shortened due to cardiorespiratory embarrassment (Pickwickian syndrome) or occasionally diabetic glomerulosclerosis. Most adults with the disorder have been able to carry out simple tasks under a protected environment. The caloric intake must be severely restricted. One may have to reinforce this with locking the refrigerator. Appetite suppressants such as dexedrine sulfate in very small amounts may be used. In some cases, gastric bypass has been employed, with considerable success. Orchiopexy should be carried out if possible.

REFERENCES

Bistrian, B.R., Blackburn, G.L., and Stanbury, J.B. Metabolic aspects of a protein-sparing modified fast in the dietary management of Prader-Willi obesity. *N. Engl. J. Med. 296:* 774–779, 1977.

Hall, B.D. and Smith, D.W. Prader-Willi syndrome. *J. Pediatr. 81:* 286–293, 1972.

Ledbetter, D.H., Mascarello, J.T., Riccardi, V.M. et al. Chromosome 15 abnormalities and the Prader-Willi syndrome: a follow-up report of 40 cases. *Am. J. Hum. Genet. 34:* 278–285, 1982.

- **hypotonia**
- **obesity**
- **small hands/feet**
- **hypogonadism**

Prader-Willi Syndrome

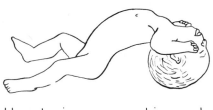

Hypotonia, poor sucking and swallowing reflexes at birth

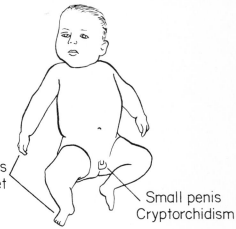

Small hands and feet

Small penis
Cryptorchidism

After first year
polyphagia with obesity

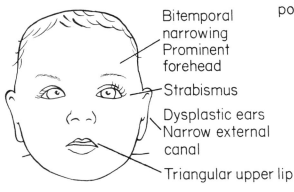

Bitemporal narrowing
Prominent forehead

Strabismus

Dysplastic ears
Narrow external canal

Triangular upper lip

Fat face with micrognathia

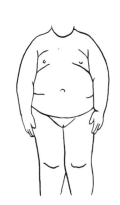

Short stature, decreased muscle with increased adipose tissue

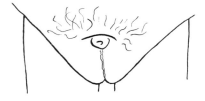

Atrophic scrotum, small testes and penis

92. PROGERIA

Clinical Features Progeria is a combination of growth retardation and pseudosenility. Birth weight is usually less than 2500 g. Growth is normal until the first year, when it essentially plateaus until puberty. During the second year, scalp hair is lost and replaced by downy fuzz. Eyebrows and eyelashes are also lost. The voice is high and squeaky. By the end of the first decade, the height of the patient is approximately that of a three-year-old. Only rarely does an adult exceed 110 cm (43.5 inches) in height or 15 kg in weight. Intelligence is normal. The face is disproportionately small, giving a hydrocephalic appearance, although in fact head circumference is somewhat smaller than normal. Scalp veins are prominent. There is frontal and parietal bossing. There is poor midface development and mandibular hypoplasia. Because of the small jaw size, the teeth, usually of normal size, are crowded. The nose is thin and rather beaked. Dentition is delayed. There is mild flexion of the knees, producing a "horse-riding" stance. The bones are delicate but the joints appear prominent. There is loss of muscular and subcutaneous fat with age. Cardiac murmurs appear after the age of five years. This is followed by diastolic systemic hypertension and cardiomegaly. Atherosclerosis is early and severe and anginal attacks and cerebrovascular accidents have been experienced as early as seven years of age. Skin is thin, atrophic, and often pigmented. The nails are short and often dystrophic. Failure of sexual maturation is a constant feature.

Specific Diagnosis Diagnosis is essentially clinical. Roentgenographic alterations include osteoporosis, although there is normal bone maturation. The small joints of the extremities become thickened because of periarticular fibrosis. The terminal phalanges are abnormally short and taper abruptly to a pointed end. There is thinning of the calvaria. The anterior fontanel tends to remain open and often there are no frontal sinuses. Coxa valga is a constant finding. Terminal phalanges and clavicles undergo progressive osteolysis.

Differential Diagnosis Because the appearance is so characteristic, differential diagnosis is limited. A number of cases of *Hallermann-Streiff syndrome* have been erroneously labeled progeria. Patients with *Seckel syndrome, Bloom syndrome,* and *Cockayne syndrome* have also been mistaken to have progeria.

Prenatal Diagnosis As yet there is none.

Basic Defect, Genetics, and Other Considerations There are over 100 case reports. Almost all cases have been sporadic. Although there have been a few cases in sibs, autosomal recessive inheritance does not appear likely. Its frequency in the United States is about 1 per 250,000 births. Numerous biochemical studies have been carried out, but there are no consistent findings.

Prognosis and Treatment These patients frequently have psychological problems due to their appearance. Mean age at death is about 14 years, but some have survived to their late twenties. Death has resulted most often from myocardial infarcts with congestive heart failure, less often cerebrovascular accidents. Treatment is symptomatic.

REFERENCES

De Busk, F.L. The Hutchinson-Gilford progeria syndrome. *J. Pediatr. 80:* 697–724, 1972.

Margolin, F.R. and Steinbach, H.L. Progeria: Hutchinson-Gilford syndrome. *Am. J. Roentgenol. 103:* 173–178, 1968.

Reichel, W. and Garcia-Bunuel, R. Pathologic findings in progeria. *Am. J. Clin. Pathol. 53:* 243–253, 1970.

- **frontal, parietal bossing / prominent scalp veins**
- **small face / beaked nose**
- **loss of body hair**
- **flexion of knees**

Progeria

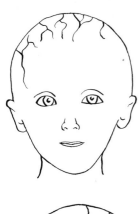
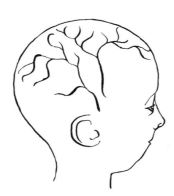
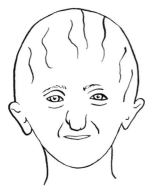
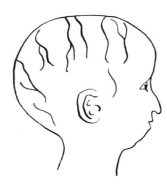

Young and older child showing prominent cranium, eyes, scalp veins, beak-like nose, micrognathia, sparse hair, premature aging, and small facies

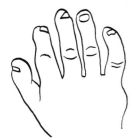
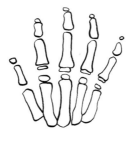
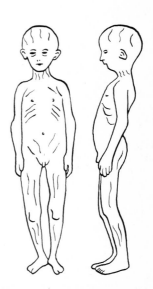

Dry skin, short fingers, enlarged joints, dry, brittle nails and short terminal phalanges

Cachetic, stooped posture, protruding abdomen, small external genitalia and senile appearance

93. TESTICULAR FEMINIZATION SYNDROME
(complete androgen insensitivity)

Clinical Features Patients having complete testicular feminization syndrome have a female external genital phenotype and hence the condition is usually not recognized in the infant. Most often the patient presents because of primary amenorrhea. The external genitalia have a normal appearance. Without close examination, the shallow vagina is usually not noted. Internally there are no uterus or Fallopian tubes. Testicles, while present, not uncommonly are intraabdominal or they may present as hernias in the inguinal area or in the labia. Following puberty, cells present within the seminiferous tubules are Sertoli cells. There is a deficiency of spermatogonia and spermatozoa. The interstitial cells of Leydig are hyperplastic. About 50% of affected patients have inguinal hernias. Any female child with an inguinal hernia should be investigated but less than 1% have the syndrome. Normal female breast development occurs at puberty and apart from a paucity of pubic and other body hair, the individual has a quite normal female habitus. Risk of gonadal neoplasia (tubular adenomas, seminomas) is approximately 5%, being similar to that seen in males with undescended testes.

Specific Diagnosis The condition is rarely diagnosed until puberty unless one has an affected sib, since the patient has a normal female phenotype except for the absence of pubic and/or other body hair. Neither Mullerian nor Wolffian duct derivatives are present. There is primary amenorrhea, the presence of testicles, feminization at puberty, and a 46,XY karyotype. Testosterone biosynthesis is not deficient, nor is there any abnormality in conversion of testosterone to dihydrotestosterone. Virilization does not follow administration of androgen, nor is there failure of nitrogen retention.

Differential Diagnosis To be excluded are a host of disorders which include *incomplete androgen insensitivity, Reifenstein syndrome, pseudovaginal peroneoscrotal hypospadias,* and *various forms of male pseudohermaphroditism* producing a female genital phenotype. There are various biochemical defects in which testosterone is inhibited such as

20-α-hydroxylase deficiency, 22R-hydroxylase deficiency, and *20,22-desmolase deficiency.* These enzyme defects involve failure of conversion of cholesterol to delta-t-pregnenolone. One must also exclude steroid *17-α-hydroxylase deficiency* and steroid *17,20-desmolase deficiency.*

Prenatal Diagnosis This has not been done, but the condition could be detected by noting a defect of androgen cytosol-binding protein in amniocytes. Furthermore, the diagnosis would be suggested from a normal male fetal karyotype but no penis and scrotum on sonography.

Basic Defect, Genetics, and Other Considerations The basic defect is due to an abnormality in androgen cytosol-binding protein. This specific binding protein is required for the attachment of testosterone and dihydrotestosterone to the plasma membrane and for transportation of the androgen to the nucleus where it carries out its inductive functions. The estrogen elaborated by the testes is responsible for the normal breast development. Thus, there is target tissue unresponsiveness to testosterone, whether synthesized within the body or administered externally. This can be demonstrated in cultured genital skin fibroblasts from most affected patients. The disorder has X-linked recessive inheritance. Perhaps the disorder occurs in one in each 70,000 liveborn males.

Prognosis and Treatment Life span and intellect are normal. Surgical treatment involves removal of the testes, hernia repair, and plastic surgical correction of the reduced size of the vagina. If removal of the testes is delayed until after puberty, no therapy is needed to effect feminization. This has psychological advantage. Estrogen therapy is initiated following removal of the testes to avoid menopausal signs and/or symptoms. Nothing, of course, can be done to correct the sterility. We would suggest that patients not be informed of their true genetic sex as they are well oriented as females except for the problem of sterility, which in itself, is not uncommon in normal genetic females.

REFERENCES

Amrhein, J.A., Meyer, W.J. III, Jones, J.W., Jr. et al. Androgen insensitivity in man: evidence for genetic heterogeneity. *Proc. Nat. Acad. Sci. 73:* 891–894, 1976.

Rosenfeld, R.L., Lawrence, A.M., Liao, S. et al. Androgens and androgen responsiveness in the feminizing testis syndrome. Comparison of complete and "incomplete" forms. *J. Clin. Endocrinol. Metab. 32:* 625–632, 1971.

Simpson, J.L. Male pseudohermaphroditism: genetics and clinical delineation. *Human Genetics 44:* 1–49, 1978.

- **female appearance**
- **shallow vagina**
- **intra or extra abdominal testes**
- **inguinal hernia**

Testicular Feminization Syndrome
[complete androgen insensitivity]

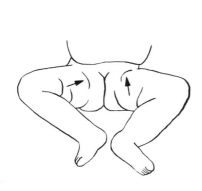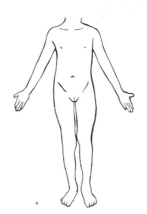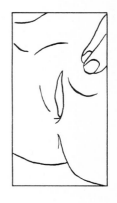

Affected infant with female external genitalia and testes in inguinal canal (arrows), prepuberal affected child with female phenotype, no external malformations, finger over left testis

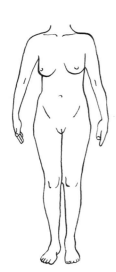

A   B

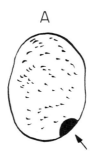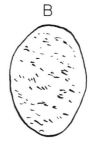

Well proportioned female appearing affected adult, A) one sex chromatin body (arrow) in normal female, B) absence of sex chromatin body in the patient, like that in a normal male

205

C. Genetic Syndromes
d. Facial / Skeletal

94. Aarskog Syndrome
    (facial-digital-genital syndrome)
95. Aniridia and Related Syndromes
96. Apert Syndrome
97. Asymmetric Crying Facies
98. Ataxia-Telangiectasia
99. Beckwith-Wiedemann Syndrome
100. Blepharophimosis-Ptosis Syndrome
101. Branchio-Oto-Renal Syndrome
102. Carpenter Syndrome
103. Cerebral Gigantism
104. Cerebrocostomandibular Syndrome
105. Cerebrohepatorenal Syndrome
106. Cherubism
107. Cleft Lip/Palate with Paramedian Pits
    of Lower Lip
108. Cockayne Syndrome
109. Coffin-Lowry Syndrome
110. Coffin-Siris Syndrome
111. Congenital Indifference to Pain
112. Craniocarpotarsal Dysplasia
113. Crouzon Syndrome
114. Cryptophthalmos Syndrome
115. de Lange Syndrome
116. Dubowitz Syndrome
117. Ectrodactyly-Ectodermal Dysplasia-
    Clefting Syndrome
118. Familial Dysautonomia
119. Fanconi Pancytopenia Syndrome
120. Fetal Face Syndrome
    (Robinow syndrome)
121. Frontonasal Dysplasia
    (median cleft face syndrome)
122. G-Syndrome (hypertelorism with
    esophageal abnormality and hypospadias)
123. Infantile Cortical Hyperostosis
    (Caffey disease)
124. Lenz Microphthalmia Syndrome
125. Leprechaunism
    (Donohue syndrome)
126. Mandibulofacial Dysostosis
    (Treacher Collins syndrome)
127. Meckel Syndrome
128. Multiple Endocrine Adenomatosis
    (multiple mucosal neuromas; MEA, type
    III)
129. Myotonic Dystrophy
    (Steinert disease)
130. Nager Syndrome
    (acrofacial dysostosis)
131. Noonan Syndrome
132. Oculoauriculovertebral Dysplasia
    (Goldenhar syndrome)
133. Oculocerebrorenal Syndrome
    (Lowe syndrome)
134. Oculodentoosseous Dysplasia
135. Oculomandibulofacial Syndrome
    (Hallermann-Streiff syndrome)
136. Oral-Facial-Digital Syndrome I
137. Oral-Facial-Digital Syndrome II
    (Mohr syndrome)
138. Otopalatodigital Syndrome
139. Pfeiffer Syndrome
140. Progressive Hemifacial Atrophy
    (Parry-Romberg syndrome)
141. Rieger Syndrome
142. Roberts Syndrome
143. Rubinstein-Taybi Syndrome
144. Russell-Silver Syndrome
145. Saethre-Chotzen Syndrome
146. Schwartz-Jampel Syndrome
147. Smith-Lemli-Opitz Syndrome
148. Trichorhinophalangeal Syndromes
149. Williams Syndrome

94. AARSKOG SYNDROME
(facial-digital-genital syndrome)

Clinical Features The disorder is characterized by short stature, genital anomalies, and unusual facies. Birth size is usually normal, growth retardation not usually becoming evident until the age of two to four years. Most patients are below the third percentile in height, adults rarely exceeding the third percentile. The facies is especially characteristic. Often there is a widow's peak. The forehead is broad and the metopic ridge prominent. Ocular hypertelorism, mild antimongoloid obliquity of palpebral fissures, and ptosis of one or both upper eyelids are found in about half the patients, often combined with a short, broad, somewhat stubby nose with anteverted nostrils. The philtrum is long and the midface somewhat flattened. Frequently there is a broad upper lip with a linear dimple below the lower lip. The earlobes are often thick, and the upper helices malformed. The hands are short and wide with hypermobile fingers and hyperextensibility of the proximal interphalangeal joints and mild flexion deformity at the distal interphalangeal joints. There may be mild cutaneous syndactyly. Bilateral simian creases and a single crease in the fifth fingers are frequent. The feet are broad, with bulbous toes. The joints in the hands, knees, and feet are lax. Distal axial triradii appear to be relatively common. The genital anomalies are striking. The scrotal fold extends ventrally around the base of the penis, causing the scrotum to appear bifid and somewhat resembling a shawl thrown around the neck; hence the term "shawl scrotum." Often there are unilateral or bilateral cryptorchidism and inguinal hernia. There are various orthopedic problems: mild cubitus valgus, internal tibial torsion, metatarsus varus, pigeon-toed gait, pes planus, pectus excavatum, and hypermobility of interphalangeal joints. Bone age is retarded.

Specific Diagnosis The diagnosis is made clinically. Radiographic changes are usually not striking. They are generally limited to hypoplasia of the first cervical vertebra with resultant subluxation or fusion of the first few cervical vertebrae. The terminal phalanges of the fingers and the middle phalanx of the fifth finger are often hypoplastic.

Differential Diagnosis Aarskog syndrome should be differentiated from *Noonan syndrome* and from the *LEOPARD syndrome* (*multiple lentigines syndrome*). All three syndromes share such features as short stature, ocular hypertelorism, ptosis of upper eyelids, and hypogonadism. There is some similarity in phenotype with the *2p- syndrome,* but in the latter, mental retardation is relatively severe. Certain facial features are also seen in the *fetal face syndrome.*

Prenatal Diagnosis Not currently possible.

Basic Defect, Genetics, and Other Considerations The basic defect in this relatively rare X-linked recessive disorder is not known. The female heterozygote tends to be short and may exhibit minor stigmata. There is no evidence to indicate that the disorder is limited to any ethnic group. About 50 cases have been reported.

Prognosis and Treatment Puberty is often delayed, and as indicated earlier, adult height rarely exceeds 160 cm. Mild mental retardation is relatively frequent. Treatment is limited, consisting of correction of the possible cryptorchidism and/or inguinal hernia.

REFERENCES

Aarskog, D. A familial syndrome of short stature associated with facial dysplasia and genital anomalies. *J. Pediatr. 77:* 856–861, 1970.

Berman, P., Desjardins, C., and Fraser, F.C. The inheritance of the Aarskog facial-digital-genital syndrome. *J. Pediatr. 86:* 885–891, 1975.

Sugarman, G.I., Rimoin, D.L., and Lachman, R.S. The facial-digital-genital (Aarskog) syndrome. *Am. J. Dis. Child. 126:* 248–252, 1973.

M.R. [+ / some]

- **broad forehead / widow's peak**
- **ptosis eyelids**
- **short nose / anteverted nares**
- **scrotal folds around base of penis**

Aarskog Syndrome
[facial-digital-genital syndrome]

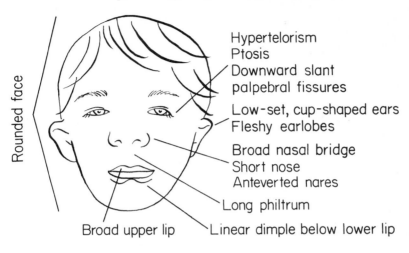

Rounded face

Hypertelorism
Ptosis
Downward slant
palpebral fissures

Low-set, cup-shaped ears
Fleshy earlobes

Broad nasal bridge
Short nose
Anteverted nares

Long philtrum

Broad upper lip

Linear dimple below lower lip

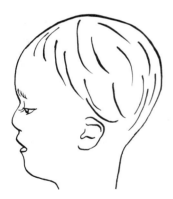

Low-set, thick, cup-shaped ear

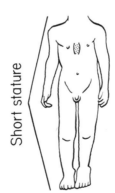

Short stature

Pectus excavatum, broad flat feet

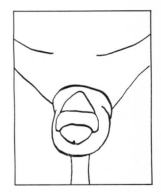

Scrotal folds encircles penis ventrally and cryptorchidism

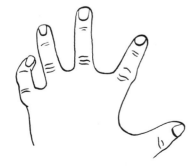

Short thumb, syndactyly, clinodactyly, brachydactyly, camptodactyly and hypermobility of fingers

95. ANIRIDIA AND RELATED SYNDROMES

Clinical Features Aniridia may occur by itself or in combination with various syndromes. Aniridia as an isolated finding is inherited as an autosomal dominant disorder with variable expressivity. There may be variable iris thinning, typical or atypical colobomas and relatively complete aniridia within families. Absence of the iris is frequently associated with nystagmus, corneal pannus, amblyopia, glaucoma, ectopia lentis, macular hypoplasia, optic nerve hypoplasia, and/ or cataract. Aniridia has been seen with absent or hypoplastic patellae as a possible autosomal dominant disorder, and with cerebellar ataxia, mental deficiency, hypotonia, and scanning speech as a possible autosomal recessive disorder. Partial aniridia has also been reported with unilateral renal agenesis, telecanthus, frontal bossing, and psychomotor retardation in which the genetic pattern is uncertain, but may be autosomal recessive. So-called sporadic non-familial aniridia which forms a triad of aniridia, genitourinary abnormalities (Wilms tumor) in the male, and mental retardation (AGR triad) has been shown to be associated with interstitial deletion of the short arm of chromosome 11. While the interstitial deletion of 11p has been of different size, all cases have in common the deletion of band 11p13. The Wilms tumor in these patients usually develops before the age of four years. The craniofacial alterations involve a long narrow face, high nasal root, ptosis of eyelids, small palpebral fissures, and low-set poorly lobulated ears.

Specific Diagnosis The degree of iris hypoplasia is variable. It varies from being merely thinned to being completely absent. Some patients have colobomas. Fluorescein angiographs of the iris demonstrate early filling of vascular loops followed by leakage of dye at the pupillary margin. Macular hypoplasia may be noted in those patients with poor visual acuity. Fluorescein angiography demonstrates capillaries in the usually avascular macular zones and electroretinograms exhibit abnormal amplitudes.

Differential Diagnosis To be excluded from aniridia and/or its syndromes are *simple iris colobomas* and *colobomatous microphthalmia*. Various *anterior cleavage syndromes* may be differentiated from aniridia by having prominent Schwalbe lines and iris adhesions to the Schwalbe line and to the posterior cornea.

Prenatal Diagnosis Theoretically possible in those where aniridia is associated with Wilms tumor and an interstitial deletion of the short arm of chromosome 11.

Basic Defect, Genetics, and Other Considerations The basic defect producing the various forms of iris hypoplasia is not known. As mentioned previously, aniridia by itself is usually inherited as an autosomal dominant disorder. When associated with various syndromes it may be transmitted as an autosomal dominant or recessive trait, or be usually sporadic when found with Wilms tumor and 11p chromosomal deletion. Isolated aniridia has been estimated to have a frequency of 1 in 50,000 in the general population.

Prognosis and Treatment The prognosis and treatment depend on the associated components.

REFERENCES

Hittner, H.M., Riccardi, V.M., Ferrell, R.E. et al. Variable expression in autosomal dominant aniridia by clinical, electrophysiologic and angiographic criteria. *Am. J. Ophthalmol. 89:* 531–539, 1980.

Mirkinson, A.E. and Mirkinson, N.K. A familial syndrome of aniridia and absence of the patella. *Birth Defects 11(5):* 129–131, 1975.

Sarsfield, J.K. The syndrome of congenital cerebellar ataxia, aniridia and mental retardation. *Develop. Med. Child. Neurol. 13:* 508–511, 1971.

Sommer, A., Rathbun, M.A., and Battles, M.L. A syndrome of partial aniridia, unilateral renal agenesis and mild psychomotor retardation in siblings. *J. Pediatr. 85:* 870–872, 1974.

Yunis, J.J. and Ramsay, N.K.C. Familial occurrence of the aniridia-Wilms tumor syndrome with deletion of 11p13–14.1 *J. Pediatr. 96:* 1027–1030, 1980.

- **hypoplasia or
  absence of iris**
- **other eye anomalies**
- **see findings
  in each syndrome**

Aniridia and Related Syndromes

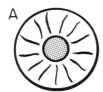 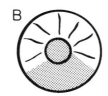 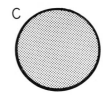

(A) normal iris and pupil, (B) partial aniridia, (C) aniridia,
absence of iris-often with nystagmus, cataract and glaucoma

SYNDROMES

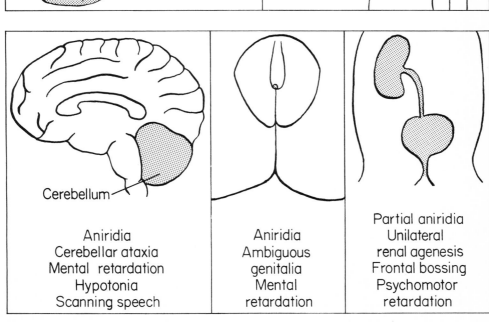

Kidney

Aniridia
Wilms tumor
Hemihypertrophy
Congenital
anomalies
Deletion short
arm chromo-
some 11

Wilms tumor

Small
patella

Aniridia
Absent
or hypo-
plastic
patella

Cerebellum

Aniridia
Cerebellar ataxia
Mental retardation
Hypotonia
Scanning speech

Aniridia
Ambiguous
genitalia
Mental
retardation

Partial aniridia
Unilateral
renal agenesis
Frontal bossing
Psychomotor
retardation

96. APERT SYNDROME

Clinical Features Apert syndrome is characterized by congenital craniosynostosis leading to turribrachycephaly, syndactyly of the hands and feet, various ankyloses, and progressive synostoses of the hands, feet, and cervical spine. Most patients with the disorder are mentally retarded. Acne vulgaris is commonly noted, with extension to the forearm. Facial variability is remarkably pronounced. The orbits are quite hyperteloric. The midface is usually underdeveloped, lending prominence to the mandible. The skull is malformed with the frontal and occipital bones being flattened and the apex of the cranium located near or anterior to the bregma. Irregular early obliteration of the cranial sutures is common, especially the coronal. Digital markings are often accentuated. The palate is highly arched, constricted, and may have a median furrow. Cleft of the soft palate has been observed in approximately one-third of the cases. Malocclusion is common, due to the midfacial hypoplasia.

Specific Diagnosis The hands and feet are symmetrically deformed. A mid-digital hand-mass with bony and soft-tissue syndactyly of digits two, three, and four is found. Digits one and five are often incompletely attached to the mid-digital hand mass. In the feet, the hallux is frequently partially separated from the rest of the toes, which have complete soft tissue syndactyly and usually have a common nail. Six metatarsals have been noted in several cases. With age, the interphalangeal joints of the fingers become stiff. The upper extremities are shortened and there may be ankylosis of joints, especially those of the elbow, shoulder, and hip. The bones of the hands, feet, and cervical spine become progressively synostosed.

Differential Diagnosis This disorder should be differentiated from *Pfeiffer syndrome, Crouzon syndrome,* and *Carpenter syndrome.* It is likely that *Summitt syndrome* is the same as Carpenter syndrome. Marked syndactyly resembling that in the Apert syndrome may be seen in *cryptophthalmos syndrome.*

Prenatal Diagnosis Prenatal diagnosis has been made by fetoscopy noting the hand and foot alterations.

Basic Defect, Genetics, and Other Considerations The basic defect is not known. There is autosomal dominant inheritance. Increased paternal age at the time of conception has been found. Although most cases are sporadic, there are several examples in which females with the disorder have given birth to an affected child. Over 250 cases have been reported. It is thought to occur approximately 1 in 160,000 births. However, due to the high mortality rate in the neonatal period, there is approximately 1 case per 2,000,000 in the general population. There does not appear to be genetic heterogeneity.

Prognosis and Treatment Prognosis in large part depends on the degree of mental retardation manifested. Although nothing is ordinarily done for treatment of the syndactyly of the toes, considerable orthopedic surgery is usually carried out for correction of the syndactyly in the hands, with separation of the thumb and little finger from the rest of the digits so that objects may be grasped. Major maxillofacial surgery may be done for correction of the midface deformity to bring the maxilla forward and to reduce the exophthalmos.

REFERENCES

Buchanan, R.C. Acrocephalosyndactyly or Apert's syndrome. *Br. J. Plast. Surg. 21:* 406–418, 1968.
Cohen, M.M., Jr. An etiologic and nosologic overview of craniosynostosis syndromes. *Birth Defects 11(2):* 137–189, 1973.

Schauerte, E.W. and St. Aubin, P.M. Progressive synosteosis in Apert's syndrome (acrocephalosyndactyly). *Am. J. Roentgenol. 97:* 67–73, 1966.

- **turribrachycephaly**
- **syndactyly of hands and feet**
- **hypertelorism**
- **midface hypoplasia / prominent mandible**

Apert Syndrome

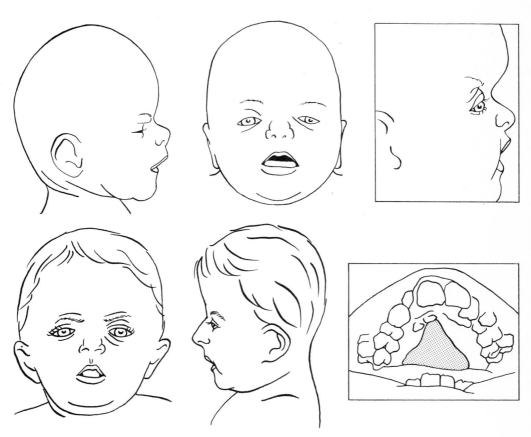

Turribrachycephaly with high, steep, flat frontal bones, small pinched nose, strabismus, proptosis of eyes, downward slant to fissures, flat midface-narrow, high arched palate with dental malocclusion

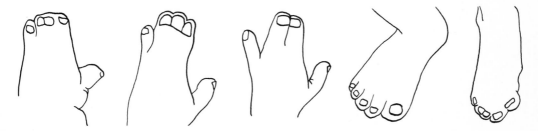

Varying degrees of syndactyly of fingers and toes

213

97. ASYMMETRIC CRYING FACIES

Clinical Features Unilateral weakness of the lower lip depressor muscles causes the appearance of asymmetric face when crying. This trait was originally thought to be a valuable index of congenital anomalies, especially of cardiovascular, genitourinary, and respiratory systems. Enthusiasm for the sign has waned, some authors indicating that it is without any significance, while others suggest an association only with congenital heart disease. We do not regard asymmetric crying facies as a specific sign. While cardiovascular defects predominate (1–5%), a host of minor anomalies is seen in perhaps 20%. Because the muscles involved act only to depress the lower lip margin, the defect does not interfere with feeding or smiling and does not foster drooling. At rest, the lips are symmetric, the sign becoming apparent only during crying. There may be a left-sided predilection. Approximately 10% have either cleft lip/palate or cleft palate.

Specific Diagnosis Diagnosis is purely clinical. Cardiovascular anomalies have included VSD, PDA, tetralogy of Fallot, right aortic arch, double aortic arch, pulmonary stenosis, coarctation of aorta, ASD, AV communis, tricuspid atresia, single ventricle, hypoplastic right ventricle, hypoplastic pulmonary arteries, and bicuspid aortic valve. Radiographically, various minor skeletal anomalies have been noted such as hemivertebrae, fused vertebrae, sternal and rib anomalies, hypoplastic or absent radius and thumb. Genitourinary anomalies have included absent kidney, hypoplastic kidney, ectopic kidney, bifid kidney, polycystic kidneys, bifid scrotum, hypogonadism, cryptorchidism, and hypospadias. Tracheoesophageal fistula or atresia, laryngeal malacia, bronchial stenosis, absent bronchus, absent lung lobe, anal stenosis, imperforate anus, absent thymus, and a variety of other defects have been noted. Electromyographic studies have shown normal activity of the facial nerves except for absence of motor unit activity in the depressor anguli oris muscle.

Differential Diagnosis The disorder should be distinguished from *facial palsy secondary to birth trauma* (injury to facial nerve, intracranial hemorrhage). Facial palsy may be seen in association with *oculo-auriculo-vertebral syndrome* or very rarely due to *agenesis of the 7th nerve nucleus.*

Prenatal Diagnosis This is not possible.

Basic Defect, Genetics, and Other Considerations Asymmetric crying facies results from unilateral hypoplasia or absence of the depressor anguli oris muscle of the lower lip. There is no evidence that either intrauterine molding or forcep injury during delivery is responsible for the disorder. Its frequency would appear to be about 6–8 per 1000 infants. There appears to be familial constellation and autosomal dominant inheritance has been suggested. If this is true, penetrance must be considerably reduced.

Prognosis and Treatment Lower facial weakness persists in most cases, but it may diminish to some degree with time. Minor plastic surgery may be employed to improve the appearance if desired.

REFERENCES

Alexiou, D., Manolidis, C., Papaevangeliou, G. et al. Frequency of other malformations in congenital hypoplasia of depressor anguli oris muscle syndrome. *Arch. Dis. Childh. 51:* 891–893, 1976.

Levin, S.E., Silverman, N.H., and Milner, S. Hypoplasia or absence of the depressor anguli oris muscle and congenital abnormalities, with specific reference to the cardiofacial syndrome. *S. Afr. Med. J. 61:* 227–231, 1982.

Miller, M. and Hall, J.G. Familial asymmetric crying facies. *Am. J. Dis. Child. 133:* 743–746, 1979.

- asymmetric face on crying
- left-sided predilection
- cardiac and minor anomalies in some

Asymmetric Crying Facies

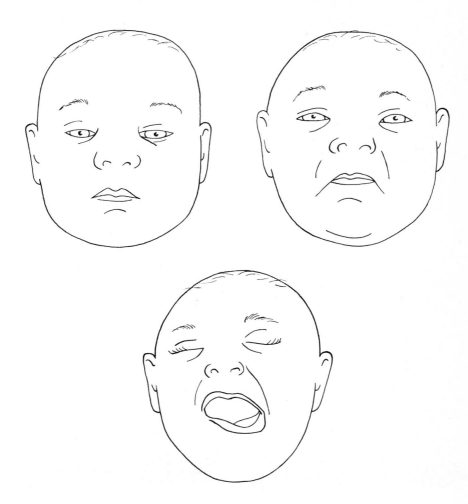

Drooping of the left corner of
the mouth as the child cries

215

98. ATAXIA-TELANGIECTASIA

Clinical Features The syndrome consists of progressive cerebellar ataxia, oculocutaneous telangiectasia, and sinopulmonary infections. Growth is markedly diminished in over 65% of patients. The face is thin, the expression relaxed, dull, or sad. The patient often stoops with the shoulders drooped and the head held to one side. Truncal ataxia becomes slowly progressive. Eventually there may be intention tremor of the upper extremities. General muscle weakness due in part to a peripheral neuropathy and diminished or absent deep tendon reflexes eventuate. Speech is invariably dysarthric. Mental deficiency, seen in about 30%, is usually not apparent until the child reaches the age of nine. Drooling is noted in about half the patients. At about five years of age, fine symmetric venous telangiectases are noted in the temporal and nasal areas of the conjunctiva. Strabismus, oculomotor apraxia, and nystagmus are common. Fixation nystagmus is present in over 80%. The cutaneous telangiectasia is first noted on the ears, eyelids, butterfly area of face, nasal bridge, and periorbitally, that is, in areas receiving the greatest sun exposure. With time, it extends to the neck, antecubital and popliteal areas, and dorsum of hands and feet. There is heightened sensitivity to radiation and to radiomimetic drugs. With continued sun exposure and/or aging, the skin tends to become sclerodermatous with mottled hyperpigmentation and hypopigmentation. Diffuse graying of the scalp hair is frequent, even in young patients. Seborrheic dermatitis, follicular keratosis, and hirsutism of the arms and legs are constant features. Ovarian agenesis with germ-cell deficiency and testicular hypoplasia are common. Recurrent sinopulmonary infections occur in about 75%. About 10–15% exhibit lymphoreticular malignancy (lymphosarcoma, histiocytic lymphoma, lymphocytic leukemia).

Specific Diagnosis CT scans show cerebellar atrophy. At necropsy, there is thinning of the granular layer of the cerebellum with diminished numbers of Purkinje cells. The thymus is abnormal with absent corticomedullary differentiation, vestigial lobular structure, and absent Hassall corpuscles. The ovaries and uterus are often hypoplastic. An increased number of chromosome breaks, gaps, dicentrics, and multiradial configurations and mutant clones of translocation chromosomes (especially involving 14q12 and bands p14 and q35 of chromosome 7), have been found in about 25%. Progressive abnormal humoral and cell-mediated immunities are found. Lymphocyte transformation is impaired and there is abnormal T-helper lymphocyte function. There are decreased levels of serum and salivary IgA and serum IgE in 60–80% and serum IgA2 and IgA4 are deficient in most patients. Over 50% have abnormal glucose tolerance, but glycosuria is rare and there is never ketosis. Insulin output is low. Alpha-fetoprotein levels are elevated in nearly all patients.

Differential Diagnosis *Cerebral palsy, neoplasm of the posterior fossa,* or any of several degenerative or metabolic disorders such as *Friedreich ataxia, hepatolenticular degeneration, Pelizaeus-Merzbacher disease,* or *Hallevorden-Spatz disease* must be excluded. The telangiectases in *Osler-Rendu syndrome* are larger and tend to bleed.

Prenatal Diagnosis Possible to do by evaluation of radiosensitivity (clastogenic factor) in cultured cells obtained at amniocentesis.

Basic Defect, Genetics, and Other Considerations The basic defect appears to be an alteration in DNA repair in which there is a reduced cell capacity to remove bases and nucleotides damaged by ionizing radiation. The ability to scavenge free radicals and to rejoin breaks in sugar-phosphate backbones is intact, however. The IgA and IgE are probably deficient due to reduced rate of synthesis. The disorder has autosomal recessive inheritance. There is probably genetic heterogeneity. The parental consanguinity rate of approximately 4% suggests that the gene is far more frequent in the population than imagined. Over 300 cases have been reported. Its frequency has been estimated as 3 per 100,000; thus carriers constitute about 1% of the population. Carriers may be identified by altered DNA repair ability and apparently have a five-fold increase in tumors of all types.

Prognosis and Treatment Rarely does an affected person live past 20 years of age. Death results from either infection or, less often, malignancy. Diagnostic X-rays should be minimized because of risk of tumors. Therapeutic radiation is often accompanied by severe cutaneous toxicity.

REFERENCES

Boder, E. Ataxia-telangiectasia: some historic, clinical and pathologic observations. *Birth Defects 11(1):* 255–270, 1975.

Hvang, P.C. and Sheridan, R.B. III. Genetic and biochemical studies in ataxia telangiectasia. *Hum. Genet. 59:* 1–9, 1981.

McFarlin, D.E., Strober, W., and Waldmann, T.A. Ataxia-telangiectasia. *Medicine 51:* 281–314, 1972.

- **cutaneous telangiectasia about face**
- **thin, sad facies**
- **cerebellar ataxia**
- **graying of scalp hair**

Ataxia-Telangiectasia

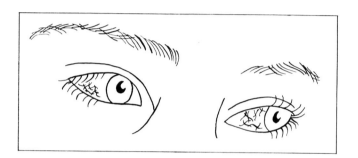

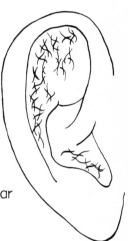

Telangiectasia in temporal and nasal areas of conjunctiva and external ear

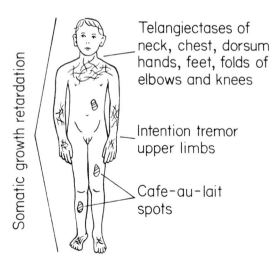

Telangiectases of neck, chest, dorsum hands, feet, folds of elbows and knees

Intention tremor upper limbs

Cafe-au-lait spots

Somatic growth retardation

Slowly progressive truncal ataxia

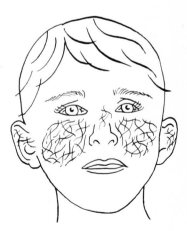

Thin face, dull or sad expression with telangiectases about face, nose, ears and conjunctiva

99. BECKWITH-WIEDEMANN SYNDROME

Clinical Features The classic features include macroglossia, omphalocele, postnatal somatic gigantism, and neonatal hypoglycemia. Mean birth weight is about 3900 g, although prematurity occurs in about 25%. Eventually height and weight are above the 90th percentile and most exhibit advanced bone age. Hemihypertrophy has been noted in about 15%. Mild to moderate mental retardation is frequent and mild microcephaly occurs in about 50%. The tongue, which extrudes from the mouth, eventually is included within the dental arch. The macroglossia is associated with anterior open bite. Facial birthmarks, principally in the glabellar area and over the upper eyelids, are seen in over 90% of the patients. They tend to become less prominent during the first year of life. Asymmetric earlobe grooves and pits and circular depressions on the posterior helix are noted in over half the patients. Omphalocele and umbilical hernia or malrotation are present in most cases. Inguinal hernia is common and diaphragmatic eventration occurs in about 30%. Some patients have diastasis recti. Hepatomegaly is common. General visceromegaly (nephromegaly, pancreatomegaly, hyperplasia of bladder, uterus, liver, and thymus) is frequent. Clitoromegaly has increased frequency.

Specific Diagnosis Advanced bone age is present in most and there is widening of the metaphyses and cortical thickening of long bones. Medullary dysplasia of the kidney and nodular renal blastoma are characteristic. Cytomegaly and nucleomegaly of the fetal zone of the adrenal cortex is a constant feature. Gonadal interstitial cells are hyperplastic and the pancreatic islands are hyperplastic and mixed irregularly with acinar and ductal tissue (nesidioblastosis). Symptomatic neonatal hypoglycemia is seen in 30–50% of the infants. It rarely persists for a year or more.

Differential Diagnosis It is important to realize that neither macroglossia nor omphalocele are obligatory findings. The coarse facies may suggest *hypothyroidism* or a *mucopolysaccharidosis* or *mucolipidosis*. Infants of *diabetic mothers* are often large and hypoglycemic. *Earlobe grooves* can be inherited as an isolated trait. *Hemihypertophy* must also be ruled out. Adrenal cytomegaly occurs with *congenital* and *primary cytotoxic adrenocortical hypoplasia*.

Prenatal Diagnosis Ultrasonography and elevated α-fetoprotein levels may detect the disorder if an omphalocele is present.

Basic Defect, Genetics, and Other Considerations The basic defect is unknown, but it may be that the fetal adrenal cortex is either overactive or underactive with excessive stimulation by a feedback mechanism. The hypoglycemia may be due to hyperinsulinism or to glycogen deficiency. Most cases are sporadic; however familial occurrence has been found in about 5%. It has been suggested that these cases are due to delayed mutation of an unstable premutated gene. There is no significant sex difference. An estimate of frequency is approximately 1 per 15,000 births. It occurs in approximately 15% of infants presenting with omphalocele.

Prognosis and Treatment Most have mild mental retardation and a few die during the neonatal period from complications. The hypoglycemia may be corrected with a high caloric, nonketogenic diet, intravenous glucose, or it may require sterner measures. There is a 5% chance of developing nephroblastoma or adrenal cortical carcinoma. Surgery is indicated for correction of omphalocele, intestinal rotation, and macroglossia.

REFERENCES

Cohen, M.M., Jr. Macroglossia, omphalocele, visceromegaly, cytomegaly of the adrenal cortex and neonatal hypoglycemia. *Birth Defects 7(7):* 226–232, 1971.

Kosseff, A.L., Herrmann, J., Gilbert, E.F. et al. The Wiedemann-Beckwith syndrome. Clinical, genetic and pathogenetic studies of 12 cases. *Eur. J. Pediatr. 123:* 139–166, 1976.

Roe, T.F., Kershnar, A.K., Weitzman, J.J. et al. Beckwith syndrome with extreme organ hyperplasia. *Pediatrics 52:* 372–381, 1973.

- **omphalocele**
- **macroglossia**
- **earlobe grooves / depressions on posterior helix**
- **visceromegaly**

Beckwith-Wiedemann Syndrome

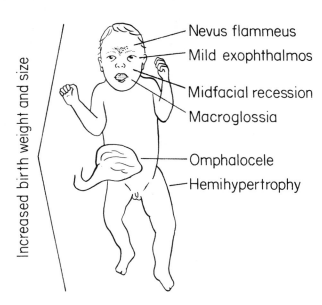

Increased birth weight and size

- Nevus flammeus
- Mild exophthalmos
- Midfacial recession
- Macroglossia
- Omphalocele
- Hemihypertrophy

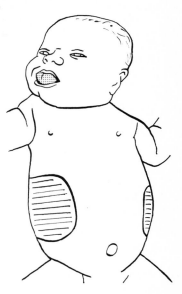

Enlarged kidneys and adrenals
with umbilical hernia

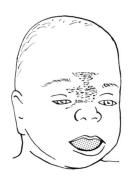 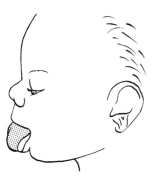 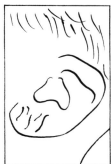 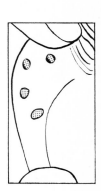

Nevus flammeus, macroglossia, linear fissures on
earlobe and punched–out depressions on posterior pinna

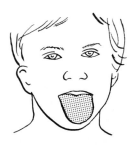 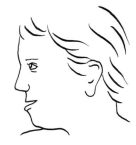

Older child –
large tongue
and prognathism

100. BLEPHAROPHIMOSIS-PTOSIS SYNDROME

Clinical Features Blepharophimosis-ptosis consists of four components: short palpebral fissures, upper eyelid ptosis, inverse epicanthus, and protruding dysmorphic ears. Dystopia canthorum is also a common feature. The eye abnormalities lend a special quality to the facies. The levator palpebrae superioris is hypoactive and there is hypoplasia of the upper tarsal plates. To compensate for the blepharoptosis, the patients assume a characteristic posture with the head tilted backward and the chin arched upward. The eyelids are covered by remarkably smooth skin without eyelid folds. There is vertically increased eyebrow height. The margin of the upper eyelid is often S-shaped, while the lower has a downward concavity, especially laterally, with or without mild ectropion. Various anomalies of the lacrimal punctae (lateral displacement, elongation, reduplication) have been noted. The ears often exhibit an overhanging helix (lop ears) or are cupped. Often the philtrum is long. Perhaps there is primary amenorrhea or at least lowered fertility in females with the disorder (see below).

Specific Diagnosis The diagnosis of this disorder is a clinical one based on the above clinical findings. Normal palpebral length and width vary with age. From 1 to 10 years, normal length ranges from 19 to 29 mm (av. 25 mm) with width from 8.5 to 9.0 mm. Those 11 years or older range from 23 to 33 mm (av. 28 mm) in length and 8–11 mm (av. 9 mm) in width. In one kindred in which primary amenorrhea was manifested, there were elevated gonadotropins, suggesting the absence of ovarian follicles.

Differential Diagnosis While ptosis and blepharophimosis may be seen either singly or in combination in a number of disorders, this specific combination is so unique that it should not be confused. A number of other conditions such as *Schwartz-Jampel syndrome, myotonic dystrophy, Dubowitz syndrome,* and *Smith-Lemli-Opitz syndrome* exhibit some facial features noted in blepharophimosis-ptosis syndrome. Blepharophimosis is seen in the *whistling-face syndrome* and in *fetal alcohol syndrome.*

Prenatal Diagnosis This is not presently possible.

Basic Defect, Genetics, and Other Considerations It has been suggested that the primary ocular defects represent embryonic developmental fixation during the third month of fetal life. The disorder clearly has autosomal dominant inheritance. It represents only about 5% of those with genetic ptosis of the upper lids. More than 125 cases have been reported. Several authors have noted that it seems to be transmitted by affected males, rarely by affected females (6M:1F). Whether this can be explained by the occurrence of primary amenorrhea is not currently known, since it has been mentioned in only one pedigree in spite of the marked male predilection for transmission.

Prognosis and Treatment Psychological problems may result from the unusual facial appearance and surgical correction is often necessary. The surgery should be carried out early to prevent deprivation amblyopia.

REFERENCES

Kohn, R. and Romano, P.E. Blepharoptosis, blepharophimosis, epicanthus inversus and telecanthus: a syndrome with no name. *Am. J. Ophthalmol. 72:* 625–632, 1971.

Owens, N., Hadley, R., and Kloepfer, H. Hereditary blepharophimosis, ptosis and epicanthus inversus. *J. Int. Coll. Surg. 33:* 558–574, 1960.

Townes, P.L. and Muechler, E.K. Blepharophimosis, ptosis, epicanthus inversus and primary amenorrhea. A dominant trait. *Arch. Ophthalmol. 97:* 1664–1666, 1979.

- short palpebral fissures
- ptosis upper eyelid
- inversus epicanthus
- prominent dysplastic ears

Blepharophimosis-Ptosis Syndrome

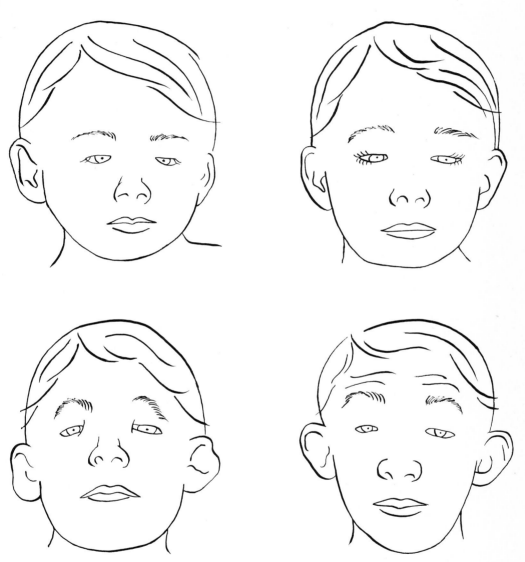

Short palpebral fissures, ptosis upper
eyelids, prominent and malformed ears

101. BRANCHIO-OTO-RENAL SYNDROME

Clinical Features The syndrome is characterized by ear malformations, cervical fistulae, hearing loss, and renal anomalies. More specifically the ear deformities may be unilateral or bilateral—one ear frequently being more affected than the other. The helix is usually thickened (cup-shaped) and the auricle is small. In the more deformed ears, the entire auricle is very small and thickened with the alterations being more marked in the dorsal portion of the helix. Preauricular pits, either unilateral or bilateral, are present in 75%. A few patients have a preauricular appendage or atresia of the external auditory canal. Low-set ears have occasionally been noted. The hearing loss is variable and of a conductive, mixed, or sensorineural cause, usually being more marked in the lower frequencies (ranging from 20 to 100 dB). The more severely deformed auricle usually has the greater degree of hearing loss. Most patients have bilateral symmetrical cervical fistulas or nodules located anterior to the sternocleidomastoid muscle. Renal anomalies have included: bilateral renal dysplasia, bilateral polycystic kidneys in a child who died at age five months, and various malformations of the collecting system. Other reported findings are facial paralysis, asthenic habitus with a long narrow face, constricted palate, deep overbite, aplasia of the lacrimal ducts, and myopia.

Specific Diagnosis Diagnosis is clinical, based on the above features. An intravenous pyelogram and other renal studies should be considered in all suspected cases, along with an audiologic evaluation. Sonography and tomography are useful in demonstrating anomalies of the auditory ossicles (shortened lenticular process of the incus, enlarged and misplaced incus, fixation of footplate of the stapes and hypoplastic ossicles) which have been observed in this condition. Histologic studies of the temporal bone have shown some patients to have a Mondini type cochlear malformation (narrowing of the cochlear canal and endolymphatic sac with atrophy of the hair cells).

Differential Diagnosis There are various other *branchio-dysplasia syndromes (Types I–III)* along with *branchio-oto-dysplasia,* and *oto-renal dysplasia* all showing autosomal dominant transmission and overlapping in some of their clinical features, making the differential diagnosis at times difficult. Further studies are needed to better understand this group of branchial arch syndromes. Several families have been reported with congenital dominantly inherited *cup-shaped ears* without hearing loss.

Prenatal Diagnosis This has not yet been achieved, but in a fetus at risk ultrasonography could possibly detect the more severe renal abnormalities.

Basic Defect, Genetics, and Other Considerations The basic defect is not known, but the association of ear and renal malformations has long been recognized. Recent animal studies provide evidence for a shared antigen between the kidney and cochlea. This relationship appears to be particularly strong between the stria vascularis of the inner ear and the renal glomeruli. Autopsy findings in one affected child showed that the stria vascularis was dysplastic and atrophic, and the cochlear cavity was hypoplastic with a reduced number of cochlear neurons. Several families with this syndrome have been reported and all show autosomal dominant transmission with marked variability in expression.

Prognosis and Treatment Approximately 50% suffer from hearing loss. Middle ear exploration should be considered where the conductive hearing loss is severe. Plastic surgery may be helpful in the correction of auricular deformities, preauricular appendages, and cervical fistulas or nodules.

REFERENCES

Fraser, F.C., Ling, D., Clogg, D. et al. Genetic aspects of the BOR syndrome—branchial fistulas, earpits, hearing loss, and renal anomalies. *Am. J. Med. Genet. 2:* 241–252, 1978.

Melnick, M., Bixler, D., Nance, W.E., Silk, K., and Yune, H. Familial branchio-oto-renal dysplasia: a new addition to branchial arch syndromes. *Clin. Genet. 9:* 25–34, 1976.

Melnick, M., Hodes, M.E., Nance, W.E. et al. Branchio-oto-renal dysplasia and branchio-oto dysplasia: two distinct autosomal dominant disorders. *Clin. Genet. 13:* 425–442, 1978.

- **cervical fistulae / nodules**
- **small, thick ears / preauricular pits**
- **hearing loss**
- **renal anomalies**

Branchio-Oto-Renal Syndrome

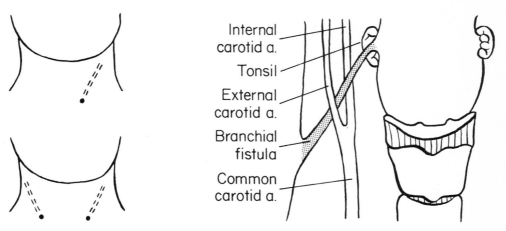

Internal carotid a.
Tonsil
External carotid a.
Branchial fistula
Common carotid a.

Unilateral or bilateral branchial fistula(s) opening in lower part of neck–tract begins in the pharynx posterior to the tonsil and descends in the neck between the internal and external carotid arteries

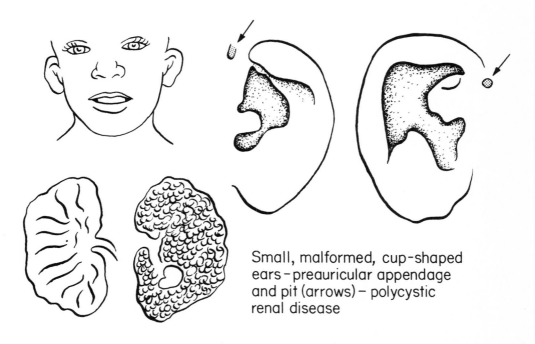

Small, malformed, cup-shaped ears–preauricular appendage and pit (arrows) – polycystic renal disease

102. CARPENTER SYNDROME

Clinical Features Acrocephaly, soft tissue syndactyly of the third and fourth fingers associated with brachymesophalangy, preaxial polydactyly and syndactyly of the toes, congenital heart disease, hypogenitalism, mild obesity, and frequently mental retardation characterize the disorder. A number of the children have had associated hernia and postminimal polydactyly of the hands. The obesity largely involves the trunk, proximal portions of the limbs, face, and nape. Height is usually below the 25th percentile.

Specific Diagnosis Asymmetric premature synostosis of all cranial sutures produces a distorted calvaria. The nasal bridge is often flat and there may be dystopia canthorum. The hands are short with stubby fingers with syndactyly most marked between the third and fourth fingers. Several fingers have but a single flexion crease. Congenital heart disease has been reported in several cases, most often ventricular and/or atrial septal defect. Omphalocele, undescended testes, and variable mental retardation complete the picture. Radiographically, the proximal phalanx of the thumb has two ossification centers. Often there is brachymesophalangy of all digits or agenesis of some middle phalanges of the second and fifth digits. Usually there is bilateral varus deformity of the feet and preaxial polydactyly with duplication of the first or second toe. Not uncommonly the toes will exhibit soft tissue syndactyly. Metatarsus varus and reduplication of the second toe, and to a lesser extent replication of the second metacarpal, are seen. The first metacarpal is short and remarkably broad. Only two phalanges are present in each toe. In nearly all cases there has been genu valgum with lateral displacement of the patellae.

Differential Diagnosis The *Apert syndrome* and *Bardet-Biedl syndrome* must be excluded. In *Apert syndrome* there is no obesity or hypogenitalism. Complete soft tissue syndactyly of the fingers and often bony fusion in the hands and usually complete syndactyly of the toes, with no preaxial or postaxial polydactyly or syndactyly of the toes clearly separates that disorder from Carpenter syndrome. It is inherited as an autosomal dominant characteristic. *Bardet-Biedl syndrome* usually does not exhibit significant alteration in the skull, but it is characterized by obesity and hypogenitalism and retinitis pigmentosa. There may be postaxial polydactyly of the hands and feet. It also has autosomal recessive inheritance. Patients with normal mentation have been artificially separated from Carpenter syndrome. We believe that they do not represent a separate entity.

Prenatal Diagnosis While conceivably one might be able to see the polydactyly on fetoscopy or by sonographic means, this has not been done to date.

Basic Defect, Genetics, and Other Considerations The basic defect of this rare autosomal recessive disorder is not known. Approximately 35 cases have been reported to date.

Prognosis and Treatment The prognosis depends on the degree of mental retardation present or the severity of the congenital heart anomalies. Orthopedic and cardiac surgical correction should be considered when indicated.

REFERENCES

der Kaloustian, V., Sinno, A.A., and Nassar, S.I. Acrocephalopolysyndactyly, Type II—Carpenter's syndrome. *Am. J. Dis. Child. 124:* 716–718, 1972.
Eaton, A.P., Sommer, A., Kontras, S.B., and Sayers, M.P. Carpenter syndrome—acrocephalopolysyn-

dactyly Type II. *Birth Defects 10(9):* 249–260, 1974.
Temtamy, S.A. Carpenter's syndrome: acrocephalopolysyndactyly. An autosomal recessive syndrome. *J. Pediatr. 69:* 111–120, 1966.

- acrocephaly
- flat nasal bridge
- syndactyly fingers / polysyndactyly toes
- obesity

Carpenter Syndrome

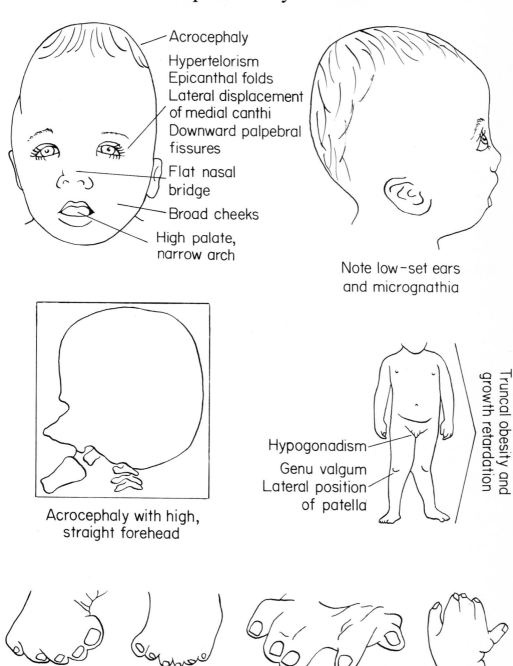

Acrocephaly

Hypertelorism
Epicanthal folds
Lateral displacement
of medial canthi
Downward palpebral
fissures

Flat nasal
bridge

Broad cheeks

High palate,
narrow arch

Note low-set ears
and micrognathia

Acrocephaly with high,
straight forehead

Hypogonadism
Genu valgum
Lateral position
of patella

Truncal obesity and
growth retardation

Pes varus, broad hallux, polydactyly, syndactyly and brachydactyly

103. CEREBRAL GIGANTISM

Clinical Features This disorder, sometimes called Sotos syndrome, presents at birth with a distinct craniofacial appearance and increased birth weight, height, and bone maturation. The facies is characterized by macrocrania with dolichocephaly, prominent forehead with a receding hairline, hypertelorism, antimongoloid obliquity of palpebral fissures, anteverted nares, and mandibular prognathism with a pointed chin. A high-arched palate is very common and precocious dentition is present in more than half the patients. Most infants are large at birth, the mean weight and height being 4250 g and 55 cm, respectively. Head circumference and height are usually well above the 97th percentile for age. The span is greater than the height in most patients. Bone age is usually two to three years in advance of the chronologic age. Hands and feet are frequently disproportionately large.

Specific Diagnosis The diagnosis is mainly a clinical one to be suspected in any infant born with increased birth weight and size, and having the facial and other features described above. Dermatoglyphic findings are abnormal with vertical alignment, an *A* line in the thenar area, and a loop in the fourth interdigital area. Levels of 17-ketosteroids and gonadotropins have been elevated in several patients; however, extensive endocrinologic studies including growth hormone, adrenopituitary interrelationships, and glucose and fatty acid metabolism have shown no consistent abnormalities. Fifteen percent may have an abnormal glucose tolerance test. Over 80% of the patients have dilatation of the cerebral ventricles. Frequently EEG studies show abnormal nonspecific changes.

Differential Diagnosis This disorder should be differentiated from *generalized lipodystrophy, gigantism* due to a *hypophyseal tumor* and the *XYY syndrome. Macrocephaly* may be inherited as an autosomal dominant trait. Enlarged brain ventricles may be seen in *familial megalencephaly, achondroplasia, lipodystrophic diabetes, neurofibromatosis, aqueductal stenosis, Arnold-Chiari malformation,* and *Dandy-Walker syndrome.* Various laboratory studies make possible the differentiation of these disorders from that of cerebral gigantism.

Prenatal Diagnosis An accurate prenatal diagnosis of this syndrome is not yet possible. It could be suspected in a pregnancy at risk based on ultrasound evidence for increased size for date.

Basic Defect, Genetics, and Other Considerations The basic defect is not known. Most cases have been sporadic, although the disorder has been reported concordant in identical twins and there are a few families described with affected individuals in two generations. In one family a brother and sister were reported affected with the parents normal and consanguineous, but since these patients are known to us there is doubt as to the accuracy of the diagnosis. At present the genetics of this syndrome is not well understood. Over 125 examples have been reported, about two-thirds of them being male.

Prognosis and Treatment Most patients exhibit a nonprogressive neurologic dysfunction manifested by unusual clumsiness, mental deficiency (mean IQ 60), and at times aggressive behavior. Delay in walking until after fifteen months, and in speech development until after two and one-half years are usual. Seizures, respiratory and feeding problems are common during infancy. Although growth is rapid in the first years of life, final height may not be excessive. Treatment is supportive.

REFERENCES

Milunsky, A., Cowie, V., and Donoghue, E.C. Cerebral gigantism in childhood and a review of the literature. *Pediatrics, 40:* 395–402, 1967.

Motohashi, N., Pruzansky, S., and Kawata, T. Roentgenocephalometric analysis of cerebral gigantism: report of four patients. *J. Craniofacial Genet. Devel. Biol. 1:* 73–94, 1981.

Sotos, J.F., Cutler, E.A., and Dodge, P. Cerebral gigantism. *Am. J. Dis. Child. 131:* 625–627, 1977.

- increased birth weight
- macrocrania / dolichocephaly
- prominent forehead / receding hairline
- anteverted nares

Cerebral Gigantism

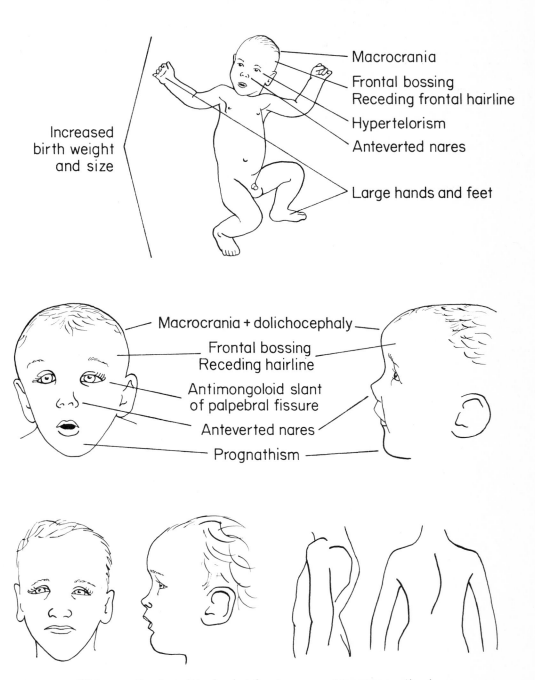

Increased birth weight and size

Macrocrania
Frontal bossing
Receding frontal hairline
Hypertelorism
Anteverted nares

Large hands and feet

Macrocrania + dolichocephaly
Frontal bossing
Receding hairline
Antimongoloid slant of palpebral fissure
Anteverted nares
Prognathism

Older patients with facial features and kyphoscoliosis

227

104. CEREBROCOSTOMANDIBULAR SYNDROME
(rib-gap syndrome)

Clinical Features An affected infant usually presents at birth with severe respiratory distress due to a flail chest. Characteristic clinical findings include severe micrognathia, glossoptosis, cleft palate, posterior rib-gap defects, microcephaly, and mental retardation. In addition various anomalies of the hair, tracheal cartilage, skin (pterygium colli), skeleton, heart, and kidneys have been reported. The number of ribs involved in the reported cases has varied from a few to almost all. Both sides have always been involved, although not necessarily symmetrically. The extent of involvement has varied from a very short defect resembling pseudoarthrosis to complete absence of the anterior three-fourths of the ribs.

Specific Diagnosis The association of severe rib defects with micrognathia makes for relative ease in the recognition of this syndrome. Roentgenographic findings show multiple rib defects (rib gaps, hypoplastic or absent ribs), bizarre vertebral anomalies, and hypoplasia of the mandible. One case showed an unusual internal rotation of the iliac bones producing a flask-shaped configuration of the ilia.

Differential Diagnosis This syndrome must be differentiated from all those in which the *Robin anomaly* (micrognathia plus cleft palate) has been associated (see p. 78).

Prenatal Diagnosis In some cases (if the rib anomalies are severe) this condition should theoretically be detectable early in pregnancy by means of ultrasound. Late in pregnancy roentgenographic studies could make diagnosis possible.

Basic Defect, Genetics, and Other Considerations The basic defect in this condition is not known. Microscopic studies have shown that the defective areas (the rib gaps) contain undifferentiated fibrous connective tissue, striated muscle, and small foci of cartilage undergoing calcification, which suggests a defect in the transition of primitive mesenchyme to cartilage. Almost all cases of this rare syndrome have been isolated examples. While it has been reported in sibs and in two generations, there is little reason to assume single gene inheritance.

Prognosis and Treatment Most infants die during the neonatal period from multiple bouts of respiratory distress, however, vigorous treatment has resulted in the survival of some patients. The overall prognosis must be guarded depending on the presence and severity of other anomalies. Most of those who have survived have been mildly mentally retarded.

REFERENCES

Harris, D.J. and Fellows, R.A. The course of the cerebrocostomandibular syndrome. *Birth Defects 13(3C):* 117–130, 1977.

Silverman, F.N., Strefling, A.M., Stevenson, D.K., and Lazarus, J. Cerebro-costo-mandibular syndrome. *J. Pediatr. 97:* 406–416, 1980.

Williams, H.J. & Sane, S.M.: Cerebro-costo-mandibular syndrome: Long term follow-up of a patient and review of the literature. *Am. J. Roentgenol. 126:* 1223–1228, 1976.

- **microcephaly**
- **micrognathia**
- **deformed chest**
- **glossoptosis**

Cerebrocostomandibular Syndrome
[rib-gap syndrome]

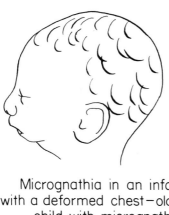

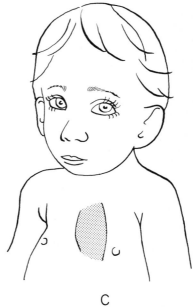

Micrognathia in an infant with a deformed chest—older child with micrognathia, microcephaly and narrow upper thorax

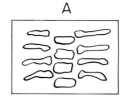

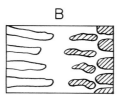

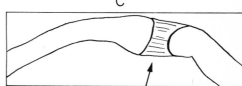

(A) short ribs, (B) gap between cartilaginous lateral ribs and proximal ossified ribs, (C) rib gap traversed by primitive mesenchymal tissue (arrow)

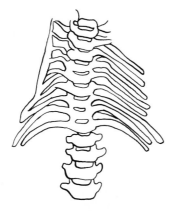

Multiple rib and vertebral anomalies

105. CEREBROHEPATORENAL SYNDROME

Clinical Features Prenatal history is usually uneventful, however, during in utero development growth failure is common and despite normal gestation, half the affected infants are born with a birth weight below 3000 g. At birth they show marked muscular hypotonia with a weak or absent Moro response and tendon, suck, and swallowing reflexes. These patients show characteristic physical findings: high and bulging forehead, widely patent sutures and fontanels, puffy eyelids, poorly developed supraorbital ridges, ocular hypertelorism, mongoloid slant to palpebral fissures, epicanthal folds, Brushfield spots, glaucoma, corneal clouding, cataracts, anteverted nares, low-set and posteriorly rotated ears, high-arched palate, round face with micrognathia. Hepatomegaly is usually present as well as cryptorchidism in the male, and clitoral hypertrophy in the female. Flexion contractures of fingers and knees, ulnar deviation of the fingers, and talipes equinovarus are the more common associated limb abnormalities. Psychomotor development is extremely limited. Seizures are common.

Specific Diagnosis The diagnosis of this disorder is mainly a clinical one based on the characteristic clinical features described. Autopsy findings have shown developmental malformations of the CNS resulting in pachygyria, micropolygyria, olfactory hypoplasia, absent corpus callosum, disorganized neuronal migration, and gliosis. Cardiac malformations, renal cortical cysts, partial malrotation of the colon, pancreatic islet cell hyperplasia, and hypoplasia of the thymus gland along with other internal organ malformations have been reported. Radiographic changes in the skeleton are many and may include bone age retardation, hypomineralization, presence of Wormian bones, calcific stippling in the acetabular cartilages and about the inferior medial margin of the patellae, and stippled epiphyses in the long bones. Calcification of the hyoid bone and thyroid cartilage has been noted. A variety of nonspecific laboratory findings have been recorded and these include abnormal EEG, elevated serum iron and copper, high iron-binding capacity, hypoglycemia, hyperbilirubinemia, hypothrombinemia with bleeding, nonspecific aminoaciduria, altered pipecolic acid metabolism, mitochondrial dysfunction in certain organs, and absence of the peroxisomes in liver cells and renal tubular epithelia.

Differential Diagnosis Certain eye findings and flat facial features may suggest trisomy 21 while other eye abnormalities in the presence of severe hypotonia and psychomotor retardation in affected males may resemble features of the *oculocerebrorenal syndrome* (*Lowe syndrome*). Calcific stippling, cataracts and limb deformities could be confused with *chondrodysplasia punctata*. However, each of the above disorders can be easily distinguished from this syndrome when all its features are considered.

Prenatal Diagnosis Although this disorder has not yet been diagnosed prenatally, certain serum findings described above could be considered for use in selective instances for possible prenatal diagnosis providing that a fetal blood sample could be obtained.

Basic Defect, Genetics, and Other Considerations The basic defect in this autosomal recessive disorder is not known. Evidence has been presented for an abnormality in peroxisomes and mitochondria, the two organelles principally concerned with cellular respiration. Electronmicroscopy from liver biopsies have shown mitochondrial abnormalities. Approximately 65 cases have been reported. Parental consanguinity and multiple affected sibs have been noted in some families. The sex ratio of affected infants seems to be altered (M1:F2).

Prognosis and Treatment This is considered to be a fatal disorder since infants succumb to pneumonia in the early neonatal period or before the age of six months.

REFERENCES

Gilchrist, K.W., Gilbert, E.F., Shahidi, N.T., et al. The evaluation of infants with the Zellweger (cerebro-hepato-renal) syndrome. *Clin. Genet. 7:* 413–416, 1975.

Goldfischer, S., Moore, C.L., Johnson, A.B. et al. Peroxisomal and mitochondrial defects in the cerebral-hepato-renal syndrome. *Science 182:* 62–64, 1973.

Poznanski, A.K., Nosanchuk, J.S., Baublis, J. et al. The cerebro-hepato-renal syndrome (CHRS) (Zellweger's syndrome). *Am. J. Roentgenol. 109:* 313–322, 1970.

- **severe hypotonia / poor reflexes**
- **high, bulging forehead**
- **round face / micrognathia**
- **hepatomegaly**

Cerebrohepatorenal Syndrome

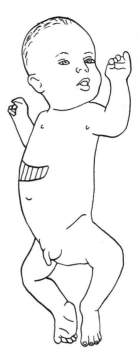

Severe hypotonia, brachycephaly,
fontanels and sutures widely
patent, hepatomegaly, hypospadias
and cryptorchidism

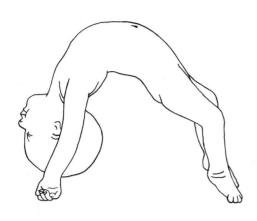

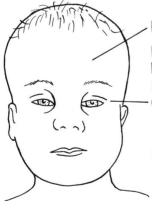

Prominent forehead

Hypertelorism
Puffy eyelids
Epicanthal folds
Glaucoma
Cataracts
Corneal clouding
Brushfield spots

Round face

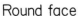

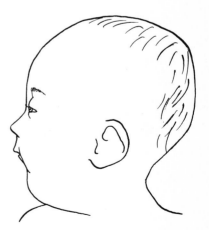

Micrognathia, anteverted nares,
low-set dysplastic ears
and flat occiput

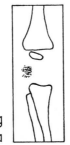

Calcified stippling
of patella

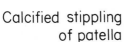

231

106. CHERUBISM

Clinical Features Affected children are normal at birth but painless swelling of the face usually becomes apparent between the ages of two and four years. Exaggerated fullness occurs mainly over the angles of the mandible, and in more severe cases there may be extensive maxillary swelling with involvement of the orbital floor producing an upward displacement of the globe and exposure of scleral rims, creating a "cherubic" appearance. The process seems to plateau at about puberty but in our experience it may remain radiographically "active" until 20–35 years of age. The palate may be diffusely enlarged. In extreme instances the swellings may result in grotesque facial deformity with associated difficulty in jaw movement and in speech, deglutition, and respiration. Irregularly placed deciduous teeth and absent secondary second and third molars are common findings. Lymphadenopathy of the submandibular and cervical nodes is observed in approximately half of the patients during the active phase of the disease. While bilateral lesions at the angles of the mandible are necessary for the diagnosis, a child may first present with unilateral swelling but later develop bilateral involvement. Other bone lesions involving ribs, humerus, femur, and phalanges have been reported, but it is not certain that such are associated findings. Multiple warty nevi and/or cafe-au-lait spots have been observed in some patients.

Specific Diagnosis Radiographically the bony lesions are bilaterally symmetric, radiolucent, and usually multilocular ("soap bubble" appearance). Adjacent tooth roots may be aplastic or deformed. On biopsy the tissue may resemble that of giant cell granuloma of the jaw or there may be few multinucleated giant cells in loose, pale, edematous ground substance and a few mature fibroblasts. Alkaline phosphatase may be slightly elevated during the active phase of the disorder.

Differential Diagnosis. This disorder should be differentiated from the *nevoid basal cell carcinoma syndrome, pseudohypoparathyroidism, giant cell tumor of jaws,* and *odontogenic keratocysts.*

Prenatal Diagnosis This is not currently possible.

Basic Defect Genetics and Other Considerations The basic defect is not known. The disorder has autosomal dominant inheritance with variable expressivity and possibly reduced penetrance in females. Commonly, one parent will give only a history of having facial swellings but will not be affected at the time the affected offspring is being evaluated. Over 200 cases have been reported.

Prognosis and Treatment Facial swellings may account for psychological problems. Usually there is regression of the lesion by the time of early adult life so that in most cases, no residual findings are present in adulthood. In general, no treatment is indicated. When treatment is being considered, most suggest delay of therapy until late adolescence or early adult life when operative reduction of the expanded bone may be carried out.

REFERENCES

Anderson, D.E. and McClendon, J.L. Cherubism—hereditary fibrous dysplasia of the jaws. Part II: Genetic considerations. *Oral Surg. 15 (suppl. 2):* 5–16, 1962.

Peters, W.J. Cherubism: a study of twenty cases from one family. *Oral Surg. 47:* 307–311, 1979.

Wayman, J.B. Cherubism: a report on three cases. *Br. J. Oral Surg. 16:* 47–56, 1978.

- **painless swelling face / mandible**
- **mainly bilateral involvement**
- **hypertelorism**
- **rim of sclera visible**

Cherubism

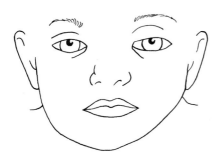

Unilateral submandibular swelling

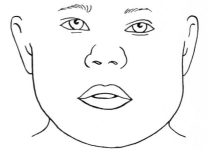

Bilateral fullness of cheeks and hypertelorism

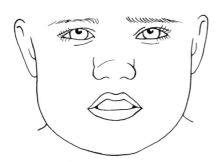

More severe involvement

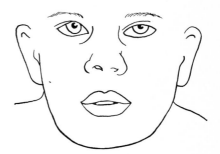

Rim of sclera visible

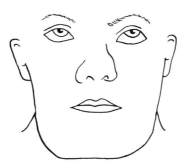

Both maxilla and mandible involved, rim of sclera more visible

107. CLEFT LIP / PALATE WITH PARAMEDIAN
PITS OF LOWER LIP

Clinical Features The oral findings in this syndrome consist usually of bilateral symmetrical depressions on the vermilion portion of the lower lip—one on each side of the midline. These dimples are either circular or appear as transverse slits. Occasionally they may be located at the apex of nipplelike elevations which may rarely fuse in the midline, resembling a snoutlike structure. These fistulas frequently excrete a viscous saliva either spontaneously or upon pressure. Variations may include an asymmetric or central single pit. About 20–35% of the patients have associated cleft lip, cleft palate, or both. Adhesions between maxilla and mandible have been described, as well as absence of maxillary and mandibular second premolars. Other findings occasionally observed are talipes equinovarus, syndactyly, ankyloblepharon, symblepharon, accessory nipples, and (more recently) congenital heart disease.

Specific Diagnosis This condition is diagnosed clinically based on the main features described above. It is noteworthy that because of the variable expressivity, some affected family members may have only pits, clefts without pits, or both.

Differential Diagnosis Lip pits also may be seen as part of the *popliteal pterygium syndrome* and the *orofaciodigital syndrome,* but both have other features that make differentiation easy.

Prenatal Diagnosis This disorder has not yet been diagnosed prenatally.

Basic Defect, Genetics, and Other Considerations The basic defect in this condition is not known, but it has been suggested that these fistulas arise from arrested development, i.e. persistence of a median and/or lateral sulcus or sulci which are evanescent embryological structures. These median and lateral grooves appear in the 5 to 6 mm embryo and disappear at the 10 to 16 mm stage. The grooves disappear at approximately the same time that fusion occurs between several facial processes and may account for the simultaneous occurrence of pits and facial clefts. The condition is transmitted as an autosomal dominant trait with variable expressivity; penetrance is estimated to be close to 100%. This rare syndrome has an incidence of about 1 : 85,000 in the white population or about 1% of those with cleft lip and/or cleft palate.

Prognosis and Treatment Life span is not affected. Orthodontic treatment, speech therapy, and plastic surgery on the lip pits and clefts should be considered depending on the severity of the case.

REFERENCES

Cervenka, J., Gorlin, R.J., and Anderson, V.E. The syndrome of pits of the lower lip and cleft lip and/or palate: genetic considerations. *Am. J. Hum. Genet. 19:* 416–432, 1967.

Janku, P., Robinow, M., Kelly, T. et al. The Van der Woude syndrome in a large kindred: variability, penetrance, genetic risks. *Am. J. Med. Genet. 5:* 117–123, 1980.

Shprintzen, R.J., Goldberg, R.B., and Sidoti, E.J. The penetrance and variable expression of the Van der Woude syndrome: implications of genetic counseling. *Cleft Palate J. 17:* 52–57, 1980.

• depressions /
  pits on lower lip
• cleft lip / palate
• agenesis of second
  premolar teeth

Cleft Lip / Palate with Paramedian Pits of Lower Lip

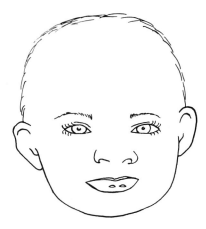

Bilateral depressions on vermilion portion
of lower lip in infant

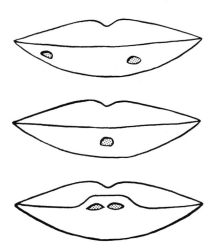

Variations in pit location with
asymmetry, single and
snout-like lower lip

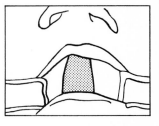

Cleft palate in an
affected child

235

108. COCKAYNE SYNDROME

Clinical Features At birth affected infants usually appear normal, but during early childhood they begin to develop distinct facial features characterized by loss of subcutaneous fat about the cheeks giving a prominence to the facial bones. This feature combined with microcephaly, sunken eyes, thin beaklike nose, large ears, and jutting chin accounts for the distinct facial appearance. In addition to enophthalmos these patients have pigmentary retinal degeneration, optic atrophy, and frequently have cataracts by adolescence. Corneal dystrophy, nystagmus, photophobia, lack of tearing, and a poor response to mydriatic drugs are other eye findings that may be present. Oral manifestations include: congenital absence of some permanent teeth, an increase in dental caries, atrophy of the alveolar processes, and condylar hypoplasia. Dwarfism is a prominent feature of this syndrome and growth retardation becomes evident during the second year of life. The limbs are disproportionately long while the hands and feet are disproportionately large. Dorsal kyphosis is common. Flexion contractures may involve the ankles, knees, and elbows. Neurologic findings tend to be progressive and consist of cerebellar ataxia, choreoathetosis, moderate to severe mental retardation, sensorineural deafness, and blindness. Dermatitis appears on the exposed parts of the body by the second year of life with a butterfly configuration on the face. The ears and chin are frequently involved. Frequently the photodermatitis results in scarring and pigmentary changes in older patients. Scalp hair and eyebrows may be sparse. Subcutaneous fat tends to be decreased throughout the body except for the suprapubic region. Females do not develop normal breasts. Males may have cryptorchidism, small testes, and a female pubic hair pattern.

Specific Diagnosis The diagnosis is essentially clinical based on the above features. Cultured skin fibroblasts exhibit marked sensitivity to ultraviolet light. Roentgenographic studies may show thickened calvaria, anterior notching of the thoracic vertebrae, intracranial calcifications in the area of the basal ganglia, and osteoporosis.

Differential Diagnosis The infant with *Seckel syndrome* has markedly retarded birth weight. *Bloom syndrome* has many features of the Cockayne syndrome except for neurologic and ophthalmologic findings and also the latter is not associated with an increase in neoplasia and chromosomal breakage. Other disorders to consider include the *Rothmund-Thomson syndrome, xerodermic idiocy, progeria,* and *erythropoietic porphyria. Cerebro-oculo-facio-skeletal (COFS)* syndrome has a similar facies. There is severe microcephaly, microphthalmos, blepharophimosis, cataracts, large pinnae, long philtrum with overlapping upper lip, micrognathia, flexion contractures, camptodactyly, and rocker-bottom feet. Birth weight is low. There is severe failure to thrive with marked somatic and mental retardation. The disorder has autosomal recessive inheritance.

Prenatal Diagnosis This has not yet been achieved.

Basic Defect, Genetics, and Other Considerations The basic defect in the Cockayne syndrome is not known, but there is some evidence to suggest that there may be an abnormality in DNA metabolism related to a late step in excision repair. Collagen synthesis and growth hormone production have been shown to be normal. Affected sibs and parental consanguinity have been observed and autosomal recessive inheritance has been established. Identification of the heterozygous carrier is not yet possible. An unexplained male sex predilection (3M:1F) has been noted. Fewer than 60 cases of this rare syndrome have been reported in the literature.

Prognosis and Treatment By the late teens these individuals are usually unable to care for themselves. Death frequently occurs in early adulthood from inanition and respiratory infections. Treatment is supportive.

REFERENCES

Keren, G., Duksin, D., Cohen, B.E., et al. Collagen synthesis by fibroblasts in a patient with the Cockayne syndrome. *Europ. J. Pediatr. 137:* 339–342, 1981.

Macdonald, W.B., Fitch, K.L., and Lewis, I.C. Cockayne's syndrome. An heredofamilial disorder of growth and development. *Pediatrics 25:* 997–1007, 1960.

Sofer, D., Grotsky, H.W., Rapin, I. et al. Cockayne syndrome: unusual neuropathological findings and review of the literature. *Ann Neurol. 6:* 340–348, 1979.

- **microcephaly / progressive CNS degeneration**
- **thin facies / beaked nose**
- **eye anomalies**
- **photodermatitis**

Cockayne Syndrome

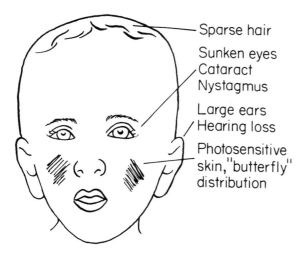

Sparse hair

Sunken eyes
Cataract
Nystagmus

Large ears
Hearing loss

Photosensitive skin, "butterfly" distribution

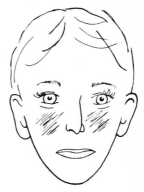

Pinched facies,
loss of subcutaneous
fat with age

Retinal pigmentation
and optic atrophy

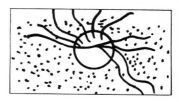

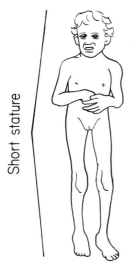

Short stature

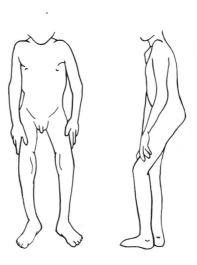

Loss of subcutaneous fat,
poor muscular development,
cyanotic digits, pinched
facies giving senile appearance

Disproportionally long limbs with
large hands and feet, semi-crouching
stance, kyphoscoliosis

109. COFFIN-LOWRY SYNDROME

Clinical Features Characteristic craniofacial anomalies along with severe mental retardation, short stature, and hand findings are common to most affected males while such features are more variable and less severe in females with this disorder. Although the facies becomes progressively marked with age, affected males in early childhood show a square forehead with bitemporal narrowing, prominent supraorbital ridges, hypertelorism, antimongoloid slant to palpebral fissures, thickened upper eyelids, midfacial hypoplasia, relative mandibular prognathism, thick pouting lips, open mouth, deep midline tongue groove, anteverted nares, and large prominent ears. Dental malocclusion with an overbite is very common, while oligodontia with absent or cone-shaped lower central incisors, winging of upper central incisors, peg-shaped upper lateral incisors, and diastema can be observed in affected males. Torus palatinus may also be present. The hands frequently appear large and soft with hyperextensible thick fingers that taper distally. The hallux is often short. Other musculoskeletal changes include short stature, clumsy broad-based gait, hypotonia, lax ligaments, pes planus, inguinal hernia, large anterior fontanel with delayed suture closure, pectus carinatum or excavatum, and kyphoscoliosis in affected males. Affected females tend to be obese. Males usually have coarse, straight hair, while their skin is frequently loose and easily stretched. Cutis marmorata, dependent acrocyanosis, and varicose veins are common.

Specific Diagnosis Since males show the full syndrome and affected females have much milder findings it is logical that the diagnosis will be more readily made in the male. The clinical features in conjunction with roentgenologic findings such as thickened facial bones, hyperostosis frontalis interna, narrowed intervertebral spaces, short distal phalanges with prominent tufting, shortening of long bones of legs and of metacarpals and great toe, kyphoscoliosis, and sternal defects allow for ease in the diagnosis of this condition. Abnormal dermatoglyphic changes have been observed with a transverse hypothenar crease, Sydney line, and increased *atd* angle.

Differential Diagnosis In the past this disorder has been confused during infancy and early childhood with *trisomy 21, cretinism,* and *idiopathic hypercalcemia.* With age the coarse facial features should be differentiated from those seen in the *mucopolysaccharidoses* and *acromegaly.*

Prenatal Diagnosis Although prenatal diagnosis is not yet possible in this syndrome, the changes in a skin biopsy on electron microscopy (see below) suggest that the examination of a fetal skin biopsy may be informative.

Basic Defect, Genetics, and Other Considerations The basic defect in this disorder is not known, however, ultrastructural studies from conjunctival and skin biopsy specimens have shown cells filled with small intracytoplasmic inclusions suggestive of a lysosomal storage disease. The severity of expression in males and transmission of this condition through mildly affected females supports X-linked dominant inheritance. Male-to-male transmission has not been observed. Autosomal sex-influenced inheritance cannot be excluded. This syndrome should be considered relatively rare since fewer than 50 cases have been reported.

Prognosis and Treatment In most cases life span is probably normal although there is some evidence to suggest that this condition is lethal in severely affected males. Mental and motor deterioration is progressive, especially in males. Most affected males are severely mentally deficient with an IQ of less than 50. The majority of affected females have mild mental retardation. Treatment is presently symptomatic with supportive care.

REFERENCES

Lowry, R.B., Miller, J.R., and Fraser, F.C. A new dominant gene mental retardation syndrome: associated with small stature, tapering fingers, characteristic facies and possible hydrocephalus. *Am. J. Dis. Child., 121:* 496–500, 1971.

Temtamy, S.A., Miller, J.D., and Hussels-Maumenee,

I. The Coffin-Lowry syndrome: an inherited faciodigital mental retardation syndrome. *J. Pediatr. 86:* 724–731, 1975.

Wilson, W.G. and Kelly, T. Early recognition of the Coffin-Lowry syndrome. *Am. J. Med. Genet. 8:* 215–220, 1981.

- square forehead /
  bitemporal narrowing
- thick lips
- prominent ears
- prognathism

Coffin-Lowry Syndrome

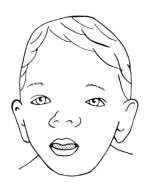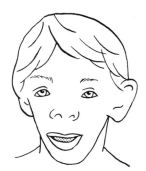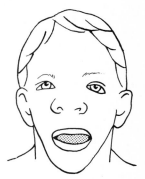

Progressive coarsening of facial features with hypertelorism,
downward slant of palpebral fissures, broad nasal bridge,
thick nasal septum, anteverted nares, thick lips, pouting
lower lip, prominent chin and large protruding ears

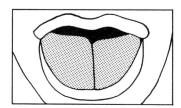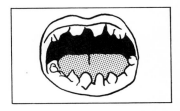

Deep tongue groove

Hypodontia and conical
crowned incisors

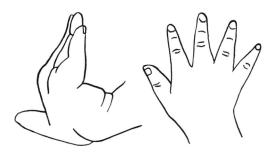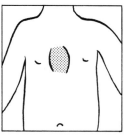

Hyperextensible fingers,
hand broad and thick,
fingers taper distally

Pectus excavatum
and kyphoscoliosis

110. COFFIN-SIRIS SYNDROME

Clinical Features At birth an affected infant usually presents with short distal phalanges of fingers and toes along with hypoplasia or absence of the nails of the fifth fingers and toes. The nails and distal phalanges of the other toes may also be hypoplastic. Associated anomalies consist of abnormal facies with coarse facial features, wide nose with anteverted nares, thick lips, heavy eyebrows, sparse scalp hair, hirsutism on back and limbs, and joint laxity. Less frequently observed features include cleft palate, microcephaly, hypotelorism, ptosis of eyelids, esotropia, preauricular skin tags, hemangioma, hernias, cryptorchidism, congenital heart disease, short sternum and forearm, and Dandy-Walker malformation. There is usually mild to moderate growth deficiency with retardation in psychomotor development. Moderate to severe hypotonia has been noted in some affected infants at birth.

Specific Diagnosis The diagnosis of this syndrome is a clinical one based on the digital findings in combination with the previously described anomalies. Various roentgenographic findings have been noted and these include hypoplastic or absent patellas, unilateral or bilateral dislocation of head of radius, narrowed intervertebral discs, block vertebrae, six lumbar vertebrae, and retarded bone age.

Differential Diagnosis Similar hypoplastic nail findings are noted in the *fetal hydantoin syndrome* which can be excluded by case history. Coarse facial features can be seen in a number of syndromes such as the *Coffin-Lowry syndrome,* the *mucopolysaccharidoses* and *mucolipidoses, generalized gangliosidosis,* and *leprechaunism.* Hypoplasia or absence of patellas along with nail changes are also found in the *nail-patella syndrome.*

Prenatal Diagnosis This syndrome has not yet been diagnosed prenatally.

Basic Defect, Genetics, and Other Considerations The basic defect is not known. No biochemical or chromosomal aberration has been observed. This is a relatively rare syndrome and with the exception of one family with affected sibs, all the other cases have been sporadic. Thus, the etiology remains unknown.

Prognosis and Treatment Feeding problems and recurrent respiratory infections are common during infancy. The degree of mental retardation is usually the limiting factor in these children. Treatment is supportive.

REFERENCES

Coffin, G.S. and Siris, E. Mental retardation with absent fifth fingernail and terminal phalanx. *Am. J. Dis. Child. 119:* 433–439, 1970.

Mace, J.W. and Gotlin, R.W. Short stature and onychodysplasia. Report of a case resembling Senior syndrome. *Am. J. Dis. Child. 125:* 114–116, 1973.

Senior, B. Impaired growth and onychodysplasia. Short children with tiny toenails. *Am. J. Dis. Child. 122:* 7–9, 1971.

- **coarse facies**
- **anteverted nares**
- **sparse scalp hair**
- **hypoplasia of nails and digits**

Coffin-Siris Syndrome

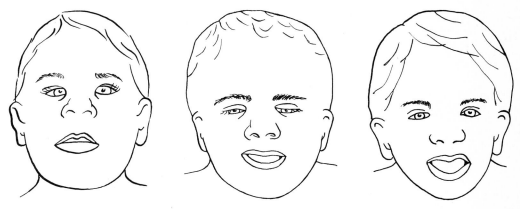

Sparse scalp hair, coarse facies, heavy eyebrows,
ptosis of eyelids, strabismus, wide nose and full lips

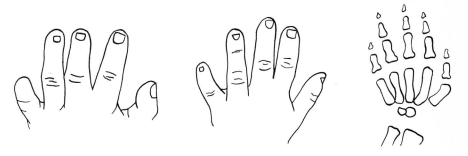

Hypoplasia and partial absence of 5th
finger—hypoplasia of other distal phalanges

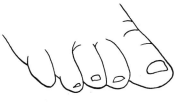

Hypoplasia of 5th toe with
lesser involvement of others

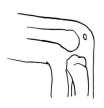

Hypoplasia of
patella

111. CONGENITAL INDIFFERENCE TO PAIN

Clinical features These patients have a total absence of reaction to painful stimuli over the entire body and as a result they sustain severe injury with scarring to soft and hard tissues. Oral mutilation involving the tongue and lips is common. This usually manifests itself as soon as teeth appear and may lead to early diagnosis. Extensive tooth decay is not accompanied by pain and patients may extract their own teeth. Osteomyelitis, aseptic necrosis, fracture, Charcot joint, and distal necrosis with spontaneous resorption of fingers and toes are constant features. Hyperextensible joints have been reported in some patients. The corneal reflex is often absent or diminished. Anosmia has been noted in some cases. Intelligence ranges from normal to dull. Deep-tendon reflexes, taste, touch, temperature, and vibration senses are usually normal.

Specific Diagnosis The diagnosis of this syndrome is a clinical one based on the above features. Various abnormal laboratory findings have been reported such as mosaicism of cells with normal karyotype and cells trisomic for a chromosome in the 13–15 group and an unidentified metabolite in the urine, but these observations have not been further substantiated.

Differential Diagnosis Indifference to pain can occur in a number of disorders, but in children the following conditions should be ruled out: *familial dysautonomia, radicular sensory neuropathy, sensory neuropathy with anhidrosis, congenital sensory neuropathy,* and *Lesch-Nyhan syndrome.* In the *Lesch-Nyhan syndrome* self-mutilation of the hands and lips is common, but these patients have severe mental retardation, choreoathetosis, and hyperuricemia.

Prenatal Diagnosis Not yet possible for this condition.

Basic Defect, Genetics, and Other Considerations The basic defect is not known. It has been shown that there is a reduction in large myelinated fibers but abundant normal unmyelinated fibers. Affected sibs and parental consanguinity have been reported, compatible with autosomal recessive transmission.

Prognosis and Treatment Although these patients do not react to painful stimuli, they are for the most part otherwise neurologically normal. Prognosis depends on protection of the child from trauma. Thought should be given to the possible extraction of teeth or use of cemented mouth guards to prevent destruction of lips, tongue, fingers, and toes.

REFERENCES

Baxter, D.W. and Olszewski, J. Congenital universal insensitivity to pain. *Brain 83:* 381–393, 1960.

Thompson, C.C., Park, R.I., and Prescott, G.H. Oral manifestations of the congenital insensitivity to pain syndrome. *Oral Surg. 50:* 220–225, 1980.

Thrush, D.C. Congenital insensitivity to pain. *Brain 96:* 369–386, 1973.

- **no reaction to painful stimuli**
- **mutilation of face / body**
- **joint complications**

Congenital Indifference to Pain

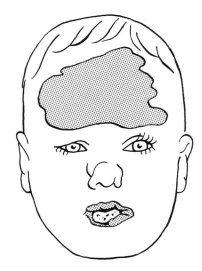 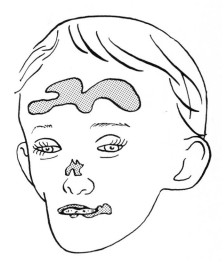

Degrees of self-mutilation of lips, nose
and forehead with scarring and loss of tissue

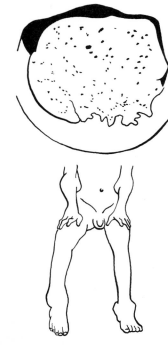 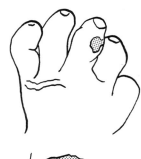 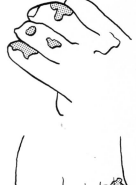 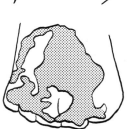

Destruction of tissues of tongue, hands,
feet and Charcot joints

243

112. CRANIOCARPOTARSAL DYSPLASIA

Clinical Features The characteristic features in this disorder, sometimes called the Freeman-Sheldon syndrome, are present at birth and consist of microstomia and flat midface, talipes equinovarus, and ulnar deviation of the fingers. The facies is distinct, appearing immobile with a flat midface, long philtrum, and puckered mouth. The palate is highly arched and mandible and tongue tend to be small. Extending from the middle of the lower lip to the chin is a fibrous band or elevation which is demarcated by two paramedian grooves forming an H- or V-shaped structure. The eyes have a sunken appearance and may exhibit hypertelorism, epicanthal folds, convergent strabismus, blepharophimosis, ptosis of the upper eyelids, and antimongoloid slant of the palpebral fissures. The nose is small and the philtrum long. The nares are narrow with the alae often bent, simulating colobomas. Near the tip, the alae are of normal thickness, but they thin dorsally to be inserted close to the columella. The nasolabial folds are evident only near the side of the nose. The upper limbs show small muscle mass, limited mobility of shoulders, decreased pronation and supination of forearms, and contracture deformities of the fingers, especially of the thumbs at the metacarpophalangeal joints. There is ulnar deviation of the fingers without bony abnormalities. The lower limbs show bilateral talipes equinovarus (rarely unilateral) and tightly contracted toes. Less frequent findings include short, broad neck with pterygium colli, moderate to severe scoliosis, spina bifida occulta, and inguinal hernia.

Specific Diagnosis The facial and limb findings in this syndrome are quite characteristic and allow for ease in diagnosis. Radiographs of the skull show an abnormal appearance of the floor of the anterior cranial fossa. Biopsy of the buccinator muscle reveals fibrous connective tissue replacement of muscle bundles. Electromyographic studies show reduced activity most pronounced in the muscles of facial expression.

Differential Diagnosis This syndrome should not be confused with either autosomal dominant disorders characterized by *inability to open the mouth fully, pseudocamptodactyly,* and *short stature* or *recessive osteochondro-muscular dystrophy (Schwartz-Jampel syndrome).* The deformities in craniocarpotarsal dysplasia, when combined with talipes equinovarus, have at times been mistaken for *arthrogryposis multiplex congenita.*

Prenatal Diagnosis Has not yet been achieved, but in a pregnancy at risk where fetal skeletal changes are destined to be severe, ultrasonography and also fetoscopy may be used in an effort to make an early prenatal diagnosis.

Basic Defect, Genetics, and Other Considerations The basic defect is not known. Although most cases are sporadic, there is good evidence for autosomal dominant inheritance with variable expressivity. Genetic heterogeneity may be present since an autosomal recessive form has been reported.

Prognosis and Treatment Intelligence as well as life span are normal in this disorder. Vomiting and swallowing difficulties may lead to failure to thrive in infancy. Plastic and orthopedic surgical procedures may be indicated for improvement of facial appearance and functions of hands and feet.

REFERENCES

Alves, A.F. and Azevedo, E.S. Recessive form of Freeman-Sheldon's syndrome or "whistling face." *J. Med. Genet. 14:* 139–141, 1977.

Antley, R.M., Uga, N., and Burzynski, N.J. Diagnostic criteria for the whistling face syndrome. *Birth Defects 11 (5):* 161–168, 1975.

O'Connell, D.J. and Hall, C.M. Cranio-carpo-tarsal dysplasia. A report of seven cases. *Radiology 123:* 719–722, 1977.

- **microstomia / puckered mouth**
- **H or V groove on chin**
- **flat midface**
- **talipes equinovarus / ulnar deviation of fingers**

Craniocarpotarsal Dysplasia

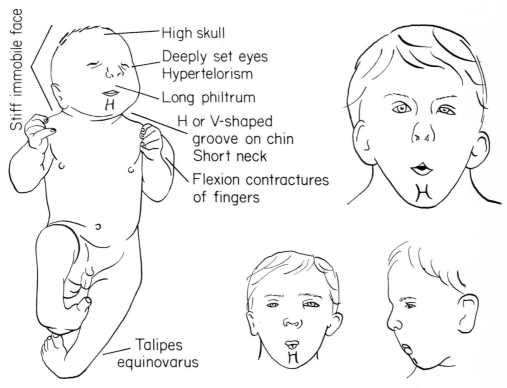

Stiff immobile face

High skull
Deeply set eyes
Hypertelorism
Long philtrum
H or V-shaped groove on chin
Short neck
Flexion contractures of fingers

Talipes equinovarus

Note blepharophimosis, mild ptosis, convergent strabismus, downward slant to palpebral fissures, small nose with bent alae, whistling shape to lips, receding chin, asymmetric protruding ears and pterygium colli

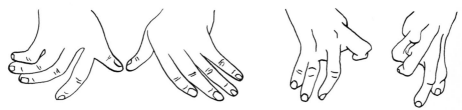

Ulnar deviation and flexion contractures of fingers

245

113. CROUZON SYNDROME

Clinical Features The disorder is characterized by premature craniosynostosis, midface hypoplasia with shallow orbits, and ocular proptosis. Premature and progressive craniosynostosis usually begins during the first year of life and is usually complete by two to three years of age. Headache has been documented in 30% and seizures in 10%. Midface hypoplasia with relative mandibular prognathism, drooping lower lip, and short upper lip are hallmarks. The nasal bridge is often flat and the tip of the nose may appear beak-like. Oral findings include narrow high-arched palate due to lateral palatal swellings, crowding of upper teeth due to hypoplastic maxilla, and open bite. Ectopic eruption of maxillary first molars occurs in about half the patients. About 35% are obligate mouth-breathers. Bifid uvula occurs in about 10% and cleft palate in 3%. Exophthalmos is a constant finding which is secondary to shallow orbits. Exotropia (75%), exposure conjunctivitis (50%) or keratitis (10%), poor vision (45%), optic atrophy (25%), hypertelorism, and nystagmus are noted. Rarely there is spontaneous luxation of the globes. Atretic auditory canals (15%) and malformed ear ossicles are associated with the conductive hearing loss noted in over 50% of patients. Stiffness of joints, especially the elbows, has been reported in about 15%. Head circumference and body height are generally smaller than normal.

Specific Diagnosis The cranial and facial findings, though variable, tend to be distinct, and in combination with the features noted in skull radiography usually lead to easy diagnosis. Radiographically, the coronal and sagittal sutures are nearly always fused, the lambdoidal in 80%. Other findings include digital markings (90%),

calcification of stylohyoid ligament (85%), deviation of nasal septum (35%), obstruction of nasopharynx (30%), and cervical spine anomalies (30%). Cephalometric studies show the calvaria short, the forehead steep, and the occiput flattened. Usually there is protrusion in the region of the anterior fontanel. Cranial base is short and narrow with the clivus especially shortened.

Differential Diagnosis This disorder should be differentiated from *simple craniosynostosis, Apert, Pfeiffer,* and *Saethre-Chotzen* syndromes.

Prenatal Diagnosis When skull and facial anomalies are severe, the syndrome should be theoretically diagnosable utilizing fetoscopy and possibly sonography.

Basic Defect, Genetics, and Other Considerations The basic defect is not known. The disorder has autosomal dominant transmission. Sporadic cases representing new mutations constitute about 50% of cases. Increased paternal age effect probably accounts for the new mutations in this disorder.

Prognosis and Treatment Increased intracranial pressure and mental deficiency have been noted occasionally. If the skull deformity is severe, correction in early infancy is recommended. Maxillofacial surgery may be helpful in improving the facial appearance of the patient. In general these patients have a normal life span. However, cor pulmonale from upper airway obstruction has been described. Progressive loss of vision is an indication for neurosurgical intervention.

REFERENCES

Jones, K.L., Smith, D.W., Harvey, M.A.S. et al. Older paternal age and fresh gene mutation: data on additional disorders. *J. Pediatr.* 86: 84–88, 1975.

Kreiborg, S. Crouzon syndrome: a clinical and roentgencephalometric study. *Scand. J. Plast. Reconstr. Surg. (suppl.) 18:* 1–198, 1981.

Turvy, T.A., Long, R.E., Jr., and Hall, J.D. Multidisciplinary management of Crouzon syndrome. *J. Am. Dent. Assoc. 99:* 205–209, 1979.

M.R. [+ / few]

- craniosynostosis
- midface hypoplasia
- short upper lip / drooping lower lip
- exophthalmos

Crouzon Syndrome

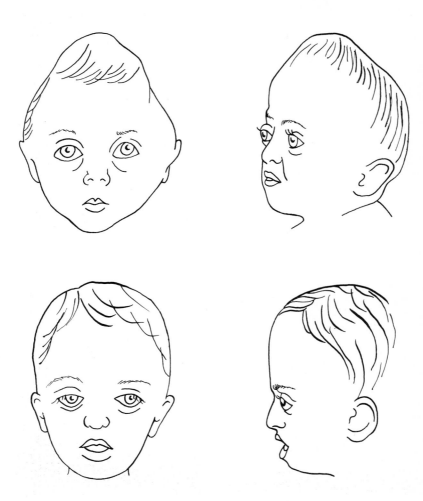

Variable cranial form with exophthalmos,
divergent strabismus, hypertelorism, short
upper lip, relative prognathism and midfacial
hypoplasia with beak—like nose

114. CRYPTOPHTHALMOS SYNDROME

Clinical Features The key features of this syndrome are extension of the skin of the forehead over one or both eyes, total or partial cutaneous syndactyly of fingers and toes, coloboma of nasal alae, bizarre hairline, and various urogenital anomalies. The facial features are so distorted that this condition can easily be recognized at birth. Findings include various combinations of the following: facial asymmetry, partially or completely missing eyebrows, skin from the forehead covering one or both globes of the eye, partially or completely obliterated conjunctival sac, absent or sparse eyelashes, absent lacrimal glands, hypoplastic, absent, or calcified and displaced lens; hairline tends to extend over the entire temple area tapering to a point overlying the eyes, nasal anomalies consisting of malformed conchas, colobomas of the nasal alae with a groove extending to the nasal tip, and low-set small external ears with a narrowed external auditory meatus. Conduction loss and malformed ossicles have been described. Marked cutaneous syndactyly has been observed in approximately half the cases. This usually involves both fingers and toes. Other anomalies less frequently observed include small penis, cryptorchidism, hypospadias, hypertrophy of clitoris, vaginal atresia, incomplete labial development, anal atresia, umbilical hernia, renal anomalies, skull malformations, calcification of falx cerebri, cleft lip and/or palate, ankyloglossia, and laryngeal atresia or hypoplasia.

Specific Diagnosis The diagnosis of this condition is a clinical one based on the above features involving primarily one or both eyes. In approximately 65% of the cases the cryptophthalmos is bilateral.

Differential Diagnosis The eye and facial features in this syndrome are so distinct that they would not be confused with other conditions. The syndactyly resembles that seen in *Apert syndrome*.

Prenatal Diagnosis This disorder has not yet been diagnosed prenatally but it is conceivable that efforts in this direction will be made using fetoscopy.

Basic Defect, Genetics, and Other Considerations The basic defect is not known in this relatively rare autosomal recessive syndrome. Parental consanguinity has been reported in several affected families.

Prognosis and Treatment Life expectancy is related to the severity of the associated anomalies. Mild mental retardation is a common finding. If both eyes are affected the prognosis for vision is poor. Detection of laryngeal atresia at birth requires immediate tracheotomy. Treatment consists of surgical restoration of existing eyelids in partial cases, and cosmetic and functional repair of other anomalies as indicated.

REFERENCES

Howard, R.O., Fineman, R.M., Anderson, B. Jr., Moseley, N., Gilman, M., and Rothman, S. Unilateral cryptophthalmia. *Am. J. Ophthalmol.* 87: 556–560, 1979.

Ide, C.H. and Wollschlaeger, P.B. Multiple congenital abnormalities associated with cryptophthalmia. *Arch. Ophthalmol. 81:* 640–644, 1969.

Sugar, H.S. The cryptophthalmos-syndactyly syndrome. *Am. J. Ophthalmol. 66:* 897–899, 1968.

M.R. [+ / most, mild]

- skin covering eyes / bizarre hairline
- absent lids / eyelashes
- nasal anomalies
- contractures of fingers

Cryptophthalmos Syndrome

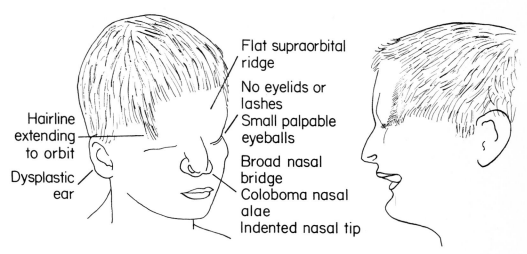

Flat supraorbital ridge

No eyelids or lashes

Small palpable eyeballs

Broad nasal bridge

Coloboma nasal alae

Indented nasal tip

Hairline extending to orbit

Dysplastic ear

Abnormal hairline into orbit, dysplastic ear with atretic external canal

Widely spaced nipples

Pectus carinatum

Flexion deformity of hands

Aberrant umbilicus

Hypospadias Cryptorchidism

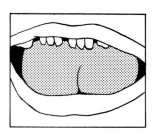

Ankyloglossia and teeth deformities

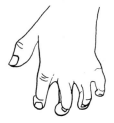

Syndactyly and camptodactyly of fingers

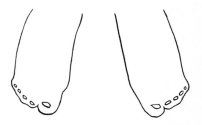

Marked syndactyly of feet

115. de LANGE SYNDROME

Clinical Features de Lange syndrome consists of primordial growth deficiency, severe mental retardation, anomalies of the extremities, and characteristic facies. Birth weight is usually less than 2500 g and both height and weight remain below the third percentile for age. Recurrent respiratory infections and gastrointestinal upsets are extremely common. Sucking and swallowing ability are diminished. Seizures are observed in less than 25% of the cases. The IQ is usually below 50 and speech maturation is especially defective. The skull is microbrachycephalic and there is characteristic synophrys. The eyelashes are long and curly and the hairline is low. The nose is small with a flat bridge and anteverted nostrils. There is a long philtrum. The lips are thin, and the corners of the mouth downturned (carpmouth). The cry is usually low-pitched and growling. The typical facies may not be evident during the first year of life. In about one-third of cases there is initial hypertonia. Generally the hands and feet are small, fingers being short and tapering with clinodactyly of the fifth digits which have only a single flexion crease. The thumbs are characteristically proximally placed. Perhaps 15 to 20% exhibit oligodactyly or absence or deformity of the bones of the upper limbs. Flexure contractures of the elbow are present in at least 80% of cases. Often there are hair whorls over the shoulders, lower back, and extremities. The nipples and umbilicus are frequently hypoplastic. Cutis marmorata is present in at least half the patients. The kidneys are often hypoplastic, dysplastic, or cystic. The testes are undescended in over 70% of males. Female patients commonly have a bicornuate or septate uterus.

Specific Diagnosis Diagnosis is clinical. Roentgenographic examination shows the skull to be small with the dorsum sellae enlarged. Bone age is delayed and not uncommonly there is a discrepancy in the sequence of development of the various centers of ossification. The humerus, radius, and ulna are commonly shortened and often there is hypoplasia or dorsal dislocation of the radial head. In some cases the forearm bones are absent. The first metacarpal and middle phalanx of the fifth fingers are often hypoplastic. The sternum is short with a reduced number of ossification centers. Dermatoglyphic changes include hypoplastic ridge patterns, transverse palmar creases and increased *atd* palmar angle.

Differential Diagnosis The overall clinical findings are generally diagnostic. In the relatively uncommon child with blond hair, diagnosis may be more difficult. The *3q+ syndrome* has considerable overlap.

Prenatal Diagnosis At present there is no known method of prenatal diagnosis.

Basic Defect, Genetics, and Other Considerations The basic defect is not known. Most cases have been sporadic. The frequency of affected sibs among reported cases is probably on the order of about 2%. No increased rate of parental consanguinity has been demonstrated. The disorder has been reported in identical twins. While chromosomal abnormalities have been reported in approximately 10% of the cases, it appears that these are aleatory. The frequency of the disorder in the population is about 1 in 20,000 live births.

Prognosis and Treatment The prognosis is poor. There is diminished life expectancy largely due to increased susceptibility to infections. Treatment consists essentially of anticonvulsants for those with seizures and tranquilizers for those having behavior disorders.

REFERENCES

McArthur, R.G. and Edwards, J.H. DeLange syndrome: report of 20 cases. *Can. Med. Assoc. J. 96:* 1185–1198, 1967.

Motl, M.L. and Opitz, J.M. Studies of malformation syndromes XXVA. Phenotypic and genetic studies of the Brachmann-deLange syndrome. *Hum. Hered. 21:* 1–16, 1971.

Pashayan, H. Variability of the deLange syndrome: report of three cases and genetic analysis of 54 families. *J. Pediatr. 75:* 853–858, 1969.

- **microbrachycephaly**
- **synophrys /
  long eyelashes**
- **thin lips /
  downturned mouth**
- **hand and limb
  anomalies**

deLange Syndrome

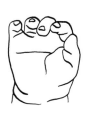

Short stature with digital anomalies

Microcephaly

Heavy eyebrows
Long eyelashes
Strabismus

Small nose
Anteverted nares
Long philtrum

Flexion contracture
of elbows

Hypoplastic
nipples / umbilicus

Micromelia

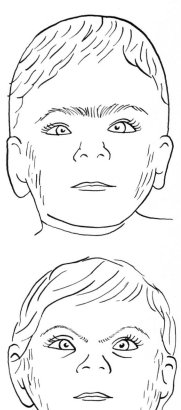

Similar facies with thin
lips, small nose, long philtrum,
facial hirsutism with
heavy eyebrows, long lashes
and low-set ears

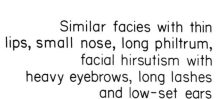

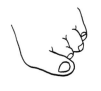

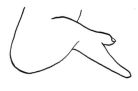

Low-set thumb, brachydactyly,
severe hypoplasia and
ectrodactyly, syndactyly
toes (2–3), hallux valgus
and absent 3rd toe

116. DUBOWITZ SYNDROME

Clinical Features The disorder is characterized by low birth weight, postnatal growth retardation, microcephaly, and a distinct facial appearance. The dysmorphic facial features include: sparse hair, high sloping forehead, flat supraorbital ridges, relatively high nasal bridge, facial asymmetry, telecanthus, ptosis, blepharophimosis with short palpebral fissures, epicanthal folds, micrognathia, and prominent or low-set ears. The lateral portions of the eyebrows may be hypoplastic. Oral manifestations consist of submucous cleft palate, high arched palate, bifid uvula, delayed dental eruption, and severe dental caries. The voice is usually high-pitched and hoarse. An eczematous skin eruption about the face and extremities has been observed during infancy in some patients. Chronic rhinorrhea and serous otitis media have also been reported. Other findings observed in some patients are diarrhea in infancy, pilonidal dimples, hypospadias, cryptorchidism, preaxial polydactyly, clinodactyly, megalocornea, retinal malformation, vascular abnormalities, migraine headaches, metatarsus varus, pes planus, and pes planovalgus.

Specific Diagnosis The characteristic clinical features mentioned above allow for an early diagnosis of this syndrome in infancy. Roentgenographically, slightly retarded bone age, periosteal hyperostosis of the long bones, and rib anomalies have been reported. Microcytic, normochromic, or mildly hypochromic anemia has been described.

Differential Diagnosis This syndrome should be differentiated from *Bloom syndrome* and *fetal alcohol syndrome*. Chromosomal findings in Bloom syndrome and a history of alcoholism in the mother during pregnancy are helpful discriminating features.

Prenatal Diagnosis This syndrome has not yet been diagnosed prenatally.

Basic Defect, Genetics, and Other Considerations The basic defect in this rare autosomal recessive disorder is not known. Approximately 30 cases of this syndrome have been reported. Parental consanguinity and multiple affected sibs have been described.

Prognosis and Treatment These patients may suffer from failure to thrive, skin infections due to eczema, and prolapse of the rectum from chronic diarrhea. Many patients have normal intelligence despite the microcephaly, however, mild mental retardation and behavioral problems consisting of hyperactivity, stubbornness, shyness, and short attention span have been noted. Surgery may be indicated for the various congenital anomalies. These children may require special schooling. The disorder probably does not affect life span.

REFERENCES

Dubowitz, V. Familial low birth weight dwarfism with an unusual facies and skin eruption. *J. Med. Genet.* 2: 12–17, 1965.

Opitz, J.M., Pfeiffer, R.A., Herrmann, J.P.R. et al. Studies of malformation syndromes of man XXIVB: the Dubowitz syndrome. Further observations. *Z. Kinderheilkd. 116:* 1–12, 1973.

Orrison, W.W., Schnitzler, E.R., and Chun, R.W.M. The Dubowitz syndrome: further observations. *Am. J. Med. Genet. 7:* 155–170, 1980.

M.R. [+ / few, mild]

- microcephaly / high sloping forehead
- facial asymmetry / blepharophimosis
- sparse hair / eyebrows
- low-set ears

Dubowitz Syndrome

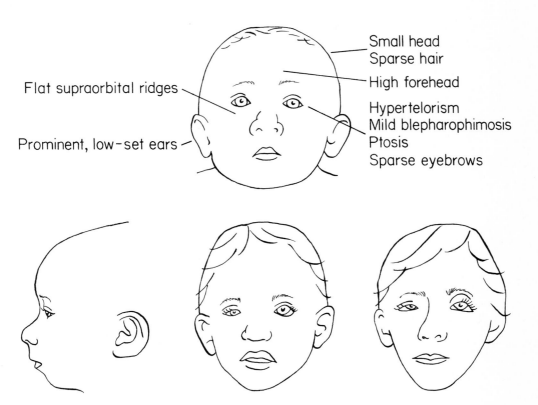

Flat supraorbital ridges

Prominent, low-set ears

Small head
Sparse hair

High forehead

Hypertelorism
Mild blepharophimosis
Ptosis
Sparse eyebrows

Note micrognathia, facial asymmetry, hypertelorism, blepharophimosis, ptosis and sparse eyebrows

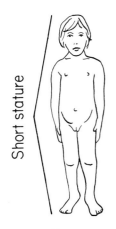

Short stature

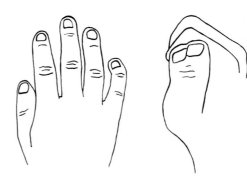

Clinodactyly and preaxial polydactyly may be present

117. ECTRODACTYLY-ECTODERMAL DYSPLASIA-CLEFTING SYNDROME

Clinical Features This syndrome can easily be recognized at birth by varying manifestations of lobster-claw deformity (ectrodactyly) of the hands and feet, nasolacrimal duct obstruction, cleft lip/palate, and various alterations in the skin and hair. More specifically, the cleft lip/palate is usually bilateral but may not be present in some patients. Other oral features include lack of permanent incisors, anodontia, oligodontia, enamel hypoplasia, deeply furrowed tongue, and dryness of the mouth. The absence of lacrimal punctas observed in most cases is associated with tearing, blepharitis, dacrocystitis, keratoconjunctivitis, and photophobia. A reduction in the number of Meibomian orifices also has been noted. The scalp hair, eyelashes, and eyebrows are usually sparse, while the nails may be hypoplastic and brittle. In some patients albinoid changes in the skin and hair have been observed as well as the presence of numerous pigmented nevi. The ectrodactyly usually involves all four extremities but exceptions are known. Cutaneous syndactyly may be present, especially of the toes. Other findings less commonly observed include microcephaly, mental retardation, prominent ears, flat tip of nose, conduction deafness, anomalies of the kidney and ureter, cryptorchidism, and inguinal hernia.

Specific Diagnosis The diagnosis of this syndrome is a clinical one based on the above features. In addition, a skin biopsy commonly shows an absence of sebaceous glands while dermatoglyphic studies may reveal dysplastic ridges with multiple irregular furrows and disorganized arrangement of sweat pores.

Differential Diagnosis Ectrodactyly (split hand or lobster-claw deformity) can occur by itself or in a number of syndromes such as *mandibulofacial dysostosis, perceptive deafness, congenital nystagmus, fundal changes* and *cataract syndrome, anonychia,* and the *acrorenal syndrome. Lacrimal duct obstruction* occurs in 1–6% of the general population and has an increased frequency in cleft lip/palate patients.

Prenatal Diagnosis Theoretically with improved ultrasound techniques this syndrome should be diagnosable in most pregnancies at risk by detecting the ectrodactyly.

Basic Defect, Genetics, and Other Considerations The basic defect in this disorder is not known. Although many cases are isolated examples, several families have been reported showing autosomal dominant inheritance with incomplete penetrance and variable expressivity. There is some evidence to suggest that genetic heterogeneity may be present in this syndrome.

Prognosis and Treatment Most patients are of normal intellect and do well after certain surgical procedures. Surgical repair of oral and skeletal malformations is usually indicated along with correction of the stenosed lacrimal duct orifices. If the latter are not corrected, chronic inflammation of the eyes may lead to blindness due to corneal damage. In early childhood a decrease in sweating may produce problems in regulating body temperature.

REFERENCES

Penchaszadeh, V.B. and De Negrotti, T.C. Ectrodactyly-ectodermal dysplasia clefting (EEC) syndrome: dominant inheritance and variable expression. *J. Med. Genet. 13:* 281–284, 1976.

Preus, M. and Fraser, F.C. The lobster claw defect, cleft lip-palate, tear duct anomaly and renal anomalies. *Clin. Genet. 4:* 369–375, 1973.

Rosenmann, A., Shapira, T., and Cohen, M.M. Ectrodactyly, ectodermal dysplasia and cleft palate (EEC syndrome): report of a family and review of the literature. *Clin. Genet. 9:* 347–353, 1976.

M.R. [+ / few]

- **cleft lip / palate**
- **sparse eyebrows / lashes**
- **scant scalp hair**
- **ectrodactyly**

Ectrodactyly-Ectodermal Dysplasia-Clefting Syndrome

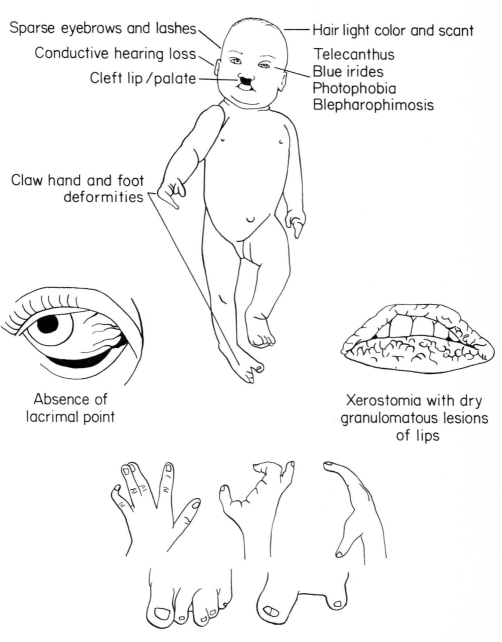

Sparse eyebrows and lashes

Conductive hearing loss

Cleft lip / palate

Hair light color and scant

Telecanthus
Blue irides
Photophobia
Blepharophimosis

Claw hand and foot deformities

Absence of lacrimal point

Xerostomia with dry granulomatous lesions of lips

Syndactyly, clinodactyly, ectrodactyly and nail dystrophy of hands and feet

118. FAMILIAL DYSAUTONOMIA

Clinical Features This disorder usually presents itself during infancy and is marked by feeding problems due to dysphagia, recurrent bouts of pneumonia, indifference to pain, hypotonia, and absent or decreased tearing. Growth retardation is usually evident by early childhood. Abnormalities in the autonomic, sensory, and central nervous systems become apparent during childhood and are reflected by the following: hypoactive corneal reflex, dysarthria, hypersalivation, excessive sweating, erratic temperature control, cyclic vomiting, difficulty in swallowing, vasomotor instability as manifested by blotching with excitement or eating, emotional lability, cold hands and feet, diarrhea and constipation, absence or hypoactivity of deep-tendon reflexes, ataxia, poor motor coordination, convulsions, and a relative indifference to pain. A pathognomonic feature is the complete absence or severe hypoplasia of the fungiform and circumvallate papillae of the tongue. A characteristic facial expression has been noted consisting of a sad, empty, and frightened look and a tendency to grimace. Patients also tend to have a thin face and transverse mouth. Facial asymmetry and hypertelorism may be present. Patients may appear pale and have a grayish complexion. Kyphoscoliosis is a common finding as these children begin to develop. Malocclusion and crowding of the teeth associated with comparatively small maxillary and mandibular arches have been noted frequently.

Specific Diagnosis This disease should be considered in any Ashkenazi Jewish infant who has feeding problems due to dysphagia and shows an indifference to pain and the absence of or diminution in tearing. The most striking feature is the absence of fungiform papillae. A number of functional abnormalities have been described in these patients and may be useful in making a diagnosis. They include: (1) diffuse pain and absence of a red flare after intradermal injection of 1:10,000 histamine; (2) hyperreactivity to administered methacholine; (3) inappropriate or prolonged hypoglycemic response to insulin; (4) pressor hyperreactivity to administered norepinephrine; (5) absence of cardiovascular autonomic reflexes; (6) decreased vanillylmandelic acid excretion in the urine; (7) decreased dopamine-betahydroxylase activity; and (8) abnormal release of renin with high plasma renin activity.

Differential Diagnosis No condition exactly mimics familial dysautonomia but many progressive sensory neuropathies such as *congenital indifference to pain, radicular sensory neuropathy, sensory neuropathy with anhidrosis,* and *congenital sensory neuropathy* have similar features. Absence of fungiform and circumvallate papillae is an important differential finding found in familial dysautonomia and not in the others.

Prenatal Diagnosis Not presently available for this disorder.

Basic Defect, Genetics, and Other Considerations The basic defect is not known. Postmortem studies have shown no consistent pathological changes in the CNS. It has been postulated that the primary defect may involve a developmental arrest in portions of the nervous system due to an insufficiency or alteration in some factor that controls differentiation, e.g. nerve growth factor. However, the role of nerve growth factor in familial dysautonomia is far from clear. Ninety-nine percent of all cases occur in children of Ashkenazi Jewish descent. The disorder has an autosomal recessive inheritance. The frequency of this condition in Ashkenazi Jews is between 1:10,000 and 1:20,000 live births. Accurate detection of the carrier state is not yet possible.

Prognosis and Treatment Death during infancy and childhood is usually due to aspiration or bronchopneumonia. With improved respiratory care patients live longer. Proper and early treatment must be given to such complications as corneal ulceration, vasomotor instability, vomiting, and excessive sweating. A Milwaukee brace and spinal fusion should be considered for treatment of the kyphoscoliosis. It is myth that these patients are impaired intellectually. Some individuals have married and have normal children. Patients frequently need help with their emotional problems.

REFERENCES

Axelrod, F.B., Nachtigal, R., and Dancis, J. Familial dysautonomia: Diagnosis, pathogenesis and management. *Adv. Pediatr. 21:* 75–96, 1974.

Brunt, P.W. and McKusick, V.A. Familial dysautonomia: a report of genetic and clinical studies with a review of the literature. *Medicine 49:* 343–374, 1970.

Schwartz, J.P. and Breakefield, X.O. Altered nerve growth factor in fibroblasts from patients with familial dysautonomia. *Proc. Natl. Acad. Sci. 77:* 1154–1158, 1980.

- **hypotonia**
- **indifference to pain / decrease tearing**
- **absent or hypoplastic fungiform papillae**
- **thin, sad face / transverse mouth**

Familial Dysautonomia

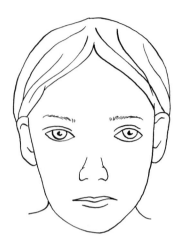

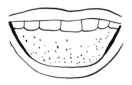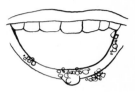

Normal tongue with fungiform papillae–tongue of a patient with absence of fungiform papillae, note drooling

Sad facial expression, slit–like shape to mouth, reduced or absent tears

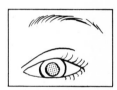

2.5% methacholine in right eye producing miosis–no effect on a normal pupil

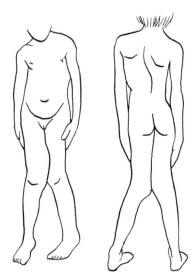

Genu valgum with Charcot joint–like changes, asymmetric thorax and kyphoscoliosis

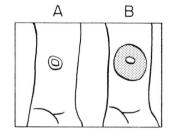

Histamine test in a patient (A), wheal but no large flare as in the normal (B)

119. FANCONI PANCYTOPENIA SYNDROME

Clinical Features This syndrome is characterized by the presence of multiple congenital anomalies, pancytopenia, and chromosome abnormalities. Many affected children have been noted to have low birth weights and decreased linear growth rates resulting in reduced stature. Abnormal skin pigmentation is a very common feature and usually consists of fine, generalized hypermelanosis with or without numerous cafe-au-lait spots. The most frequent congenital anomalies involve the thumb, radius, and urinary tract. Various deformities of the thumb may include: supernumerary, bifid, hypoplastic, or totally absent. The radius may also be hypoplastic or absent. Other skeletal anomalies include absent first metacarpal, reduced carpal bones, clinodactyly, syndactyly, absence of the forearm, hypoplasia of humerus, congenital hip dislocation, and various rib and vertebral malformations. Urinary tract anomalies consist of unilateral renal agenesis, duplication of renal pelvis and ureters, horseshoe kidney, kidney dystopia, hydronephrosis and hydroureter, and congenital renal cystic disease. Microphthalmia, strabismus, hypogenitalism with cryptorchidism in males, and facial asymmetry may also be observed in this disorder. Numerous other congenital malformations involving the heart, gastrointestinal tract, brain, eye, and skeletal systems have been reported. The pancytopenia is characterized by hypoplasia of erythropoietic, myeloid, and megakaryocytic marrow elements, which has its onset around the age of eight years. Bone marrow failure appears earlier in boys (7½ years) than in girls (8½ years).

Specific Diagnosis There is known to be a wide range in the clinical and hematologic manifestations of this syndrome, which at times presents a diagnostic problem. In addition to proper hematologic and roentgenographic studies for renal and skeletal anomalies, a chromosomal analysis should be done. An increased number of chromatid breaks, gaps, exchange figures, and endoreduplications are the main chromosomal aberrations observed. Mitomycin C and diepoxybutane stress tests appear to be the most reliable means for confirming the diagnosis.

Differential Diagnosis There are other syndromes involving upper limb anomalies associated with hematologic conditions. These include *thrombocytopenia associated with aplasia of the radius (TAR syndrome)* and *hypoplastic anemia–triphalangeal thumb syndrome (Aase syndrome)*. The hematologic and skeletal findings in Fanconi syndrome make for relative ease in differentiation. A few children have been reported with pancytopenia like that in the Fanconi syndrome with chromosome changes but without congenital malformations.

Prenatal Diagnosis Prenatal diagnosis has been done by showing an increase in chromosome breakage in cultured amniotic cells both before and after exposure to diepoxybutane. In a pregnancy at risk, ultrasound studies would also be helpful in trying to detect some of the more common skeletal and renal malformations.

Basic Defect, Genetics, and Other Considerations The basic defect is not known. A DNA repair defect and superoxide dismutase have been implicated. There may be failure of the cellular system to protect against exogenous toxicity. Most consider the disorder to be autosomal recessive in inheritance. Genetic heterogeneity has been demonstrated. At present it is not possible cytogenetically to determine the carrier state; however, there is evidence to show that male heterozygotes have a risk of malignant neoplasm three to four times that of the general population.

Prognosis and Treatment The prognosis is guarded as the patients frequently develop leukemias and other forms of cancer. The pancytopenia is usually progressive, however, it seems to be milder in those patients without associated congenital malformations. Renal anomalies and other malformations may also influence the prognosis. Mental retardation and deafness have been noted in a small number of patients. Splenectomy followed by use of androgen and steroid therapy have been reported useful in treating the pancytopenia. Surgical intervention should be considered when indicated for possible correction of the various congenital malformations.

REFERENCES

Auerbach, A.D., Adler, B., and Chaganti, R.S.K. Pre- and postnatal diagnosis and carrier detection of fanconi anemia by cytogenetic method. *Pediatrics 67:* 128–134, 1981.

Fanconi, G. Familial constitutional panmyelocytopa-thy, Fanconi's anemia (F.A.) I. Clinical aspects. *Sem. Hematol. 4:* 233–240, 1966.

Schroeder, T.M., Tilgen, D., Krüger, J. et al. Formal genetics of Fanconi's anemia. *Hum. Genet. 32:* 257–288, 1976.

M.R. [+ / few]

- thumb / radial anomalies
- skin hyperpigmentation / cafe-au-lait spots
- eye / renal anomalies
- anemia

Fanconi Pancytopenia Syndrome

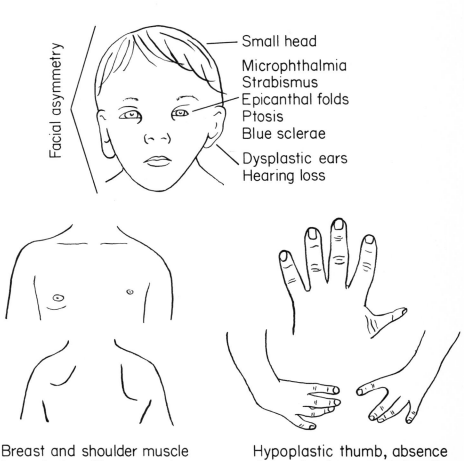

Facial asymmetry

Small head

Microphthalmia
Strabismus
Epicanthal folds
Ptosis
Blue sclerae

Dysplastic ears
Hearing loss

Breast and shoulder muscle
hypoplasia with asymmetry

Hypoplastic thumb, absence
of thumbs, forearm deformity

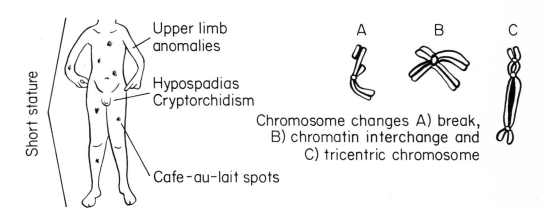

Short stature

Upper limb
anomalies

Hypospadias
Cryptorchidism

Cafe-au-lait spots

A   B   C

Chromosome changes A) break,
B) chromatin interchange and
C) tricentric chromosome

259

120. FETAL FACE SYNDROME
(Robinow syndrome)

Clinical Features This disorder derives its name from the fact that the facial features are similar to those seen in a fetus of approximately eight weeks. Facial findings include a disproportionately large neurocranium, bulging forehead, wide palpebral fissure with S-shaped lower lids, hypertelorism, short nose, anteverted nares, flat face, and triangular mouth with downturned angles. Dental malalignment, crowding, gingival hyperplasia, macroglossia, trapezoidal maxillary arch, cleft lip/palate, and minor clefting of the lower lip and tongue have all been reported. Short stature is a common feature due to vertebral and long bone involvement. Scoliosis, fused vertebrae, and hemivertebrae may be observed, while mesomelic brachymelia affects the upper extremities more than the lower. The hands may be short and stubby with hypoplastic nails, while the feet may show bulbous halluces. Clinodactyly with hypoplasia of the middle phalanx of the fifth finger may be present. Varying degrees of genital hypoplasia are seen in both males and females. Normal size penis, micropenis, and penile agenesis have been reported. Cryptorchidism has been noted. Hypoplasia of the clitoris and labia minora may be seen in females.

Specific Diagnosis The clinical features are distinct from birth and when these are combined with radiographic studies of the vertebral column and upper extremities, the diagnosis can easily be made. Radiographs show mesomelic brachymelia, malformed radial head, hypoplasia of middle phalanx of fifth fingers, dorsal hemivertebrae, segmentation anomalies of lower ribs, and short femora.

Differential Diagnosis This syndrome should be differentiated from the *Aarskog syndrome*. Saddle scrotum in the latter and genital hypoplasia in the former are important distinguishing features. Facial findings and stature in the fetal face syndrome can also be confused with those noted in *acrodysostosis*.

Prenatal Diagnosis Ultrasound studies with measurement of the fetal length of the radius and ulna may make possible the prenatal diagnosis of this syndrome in those pregnancies at risk.

Basic Defect, Genetics, and Other Considerations The basic defect is not known. Chromosome studies have been normal. In most instances this disorder is transmitted as an autosomal dominant condition. There is evidence for autosomal recessive inheritance in some families, which suggests genetic heterogeneity.

Prognosis and Treatment Life expectancy and general health are apparently not affected. In females the disorder does not interfere with reproduction; however, reproductive fitness in the male is less certain. Scoliosis is progressive and proper orthopedic measures should be instituted.

REFERENCES

Giedion, A. et al. The radiological diagnosis of the fetal-face (Robinow syndrome)—(mesomelic dwarfism and small genitalia). Report of 3 cases. *Helv. Pediatr. Acta 30:* 409–423, 1975.

Robinow, M., Silverman, F.N., and Smith, H.D. A newly recognized dwarfing syndrome. *Am. J. Dis. Child. 117:* 645–651, 1969.

Kelly, T.E. et al. The Robinow syndrome: an isolated case with a detailed study of the phenotype. *Am. J. Dis. Child. 129:* 383–386, 1975.

M.R. [+ / few,
   mild]

- **large head /
  bulging forehead**
- **S-shaped lower lids /
  hypertelorism**
- **short nose /
  anteverted nares**
- **flat face /
  triangular mouth**

Fetal Face Syndrome
[Robinow syndrome]

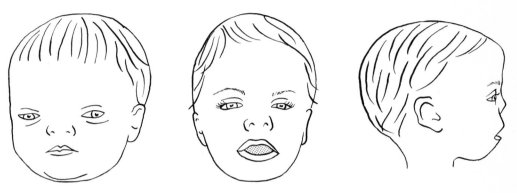

Large head, frontal bossing, hypertelorism,
S-shaped lower lids, short anteverted nose,
long philtrum and triangular mouth

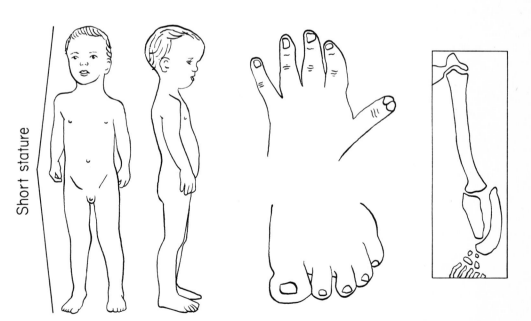

Short stature

Mesomelic brachymelia, hypoplastic genitalia, large head,
bifid thumb, hypoplastic nails, brachydactyly,
clinodactyly, bulbous hallux, short bent radius and ulna

261

121. FRONTONASAL DYSPLASIA
(median cleft face syndrome)

Clinical Features Frontonasal dysplasia is not a well-defined syndrome but rather a nonspecific developmental alteration in which the defect occurs with a variety of low-frequency anomalies. The facial malformation can be graded from mild to severe. Secondary telecanthus or narrowing of the palpebral fissures is observed in severe cases. Epibulbar dermoids are common. Anophthalmia, microphthalmia, upper eyelid colobomas, and congenital cataracts have been reported in rare instances. Nasal anomalies may vary from mild colobomas of the nostrils to flattening of the nose with widely spaced nares and a broad nasal root. Notching or clefting of the nasal alae is present in some patients. Nasal tags have been rarely observed. The anterior hairline may extend in a V-shape onto the center of the forehead (widow's peak configuration). Other findings include median cleft of the upper lip, rarely cleft palate, preauricular tags, absent tragus, low-set ears, conductive deafness, occasionally polydactyly, syndactyly, clinodactyly, umbilical hernia, cryptorchidism, and other anomalies.

Specific Diagnosis The diagnosis of this entity is a clinical one based on the above clinical features in conjunction with certain roentgenographic findings. These include mainly anterior cranium bifidum and hypoplastic frontal sinuses. Other reported observations have been coronal craniosynostosis, brachycephaly, anterior encephalocele, absence of the corpus callosum, and hydrocephalus.

Differential Diagnosis Certain physical findings such as epibulbar dermoids, upper eyelid colobomas, and preauricular tags are noted in the *oculoauriculovertebral dysplasia* syndrome. Bifid nose without ocular hypertelorism may be a distinct and separate disorder. Ocular hypertelorism is seen in numerous malformation syndromes.

Prenatal Diagnosis It is conceivable that ultrasonography and fetoscopy could detect the facial abnormalities in a severely affected fetus.

Basic Defect, Genetics, and Other Considerations The basic defect in this syndrome complex is not known. However, from an embryological viewpoint if the nasal capsule fails to develop properly, the primitive brain vesicle fills the space normally occupied by the capsule, thus producing anterior cranium bifidum occultum, a morphokinetic arrest in the positioning of the eyes, and lack of formation of the nasal tip. The widow's peak scalp-hair anomaly results from ocular hypertelorism, since the two periocular fields of hair growth suppression are also farther apart than usual. Most cases are sporadic. Autosomal dominant inheritance has been suggested in some families, while others have proposed multifactorial transmission, but at present it is not possible to assign a definite genetic mode of inheritance to this condition. For some unknown reason, instances of twinning are greater in families with frontonasal dysplasia than in the general population.

Prognosis and Treatment Mental retardation is present in some patients and seems to be directly related to the severity of the hypertelorism and extracephalic anomalies. Longevity is not compromised in this condition. Severe psychological problems are common when the facial features are markedly distorted, and psychiatric help should be given. Maxillofacial surgery should be considered in all patients where improvement is possible.

REFERENCES

De Myer, W. The median cleft face syndrome: differential diagnosis of cranium bifidum occultum, hypertelorism and median cleft nose, lip and palate. *Neurology 17:* 961–971, 1967.

Sedano, H.O., Cohen, M.M. Jr., Jirasek, J.E., et al. Frontonasal dysplasia. *J. Pediatr. 76:* 906–913, 1970.

Moreno Fuenmayor, H. The spectrum of frontonasal dysplasia in an inbred pedigree. *Clin. Genet. 17:* 137–142, 1980.

- **flat, broad nasal root**
- **hypertelorism**
- **split nares**
- **cleft lip / palate**

Frontonasal Dysplasia
[median cleft face syndrome]

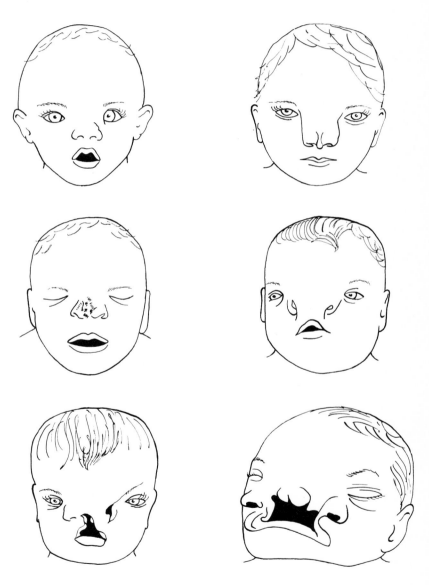

Varying degrees of facial alteration producing
severe hypertelorism, flattened nose, broad
nasal root, widely spaced to split nares
and clefting of lip and palate

122. G–SYNDROME
(hypertelorism with esophageal abnormality and hypospadias)

Clinical Features From birth, the facial appearance is characteristic and consists of hypertelorism, flat bridge of nose, prominence of parietal eminences and occiput with dolichocephaly and large anterior fontanel, slit-like palpebral fissures with mild mongoloid or antimongoloid slant, epicanthal folds with or without an accessory fold following the upper lid partly to the outer canthus, relative entropion of lower lid, strabismus, anteverted nares, flat and inapparent philtrum, micrognathia and dysplastic ears with some degree of posterior rotation. Oral features may include a broad or bifid uvula, ankyloglossia or a shortened lingual frenum and rarely, cleft lip/palate. The male genital and anal anomalies when severe are so unusual that they may be diagnostic. The degree of hypospadias varies from mild coronal to a scrotal type with an associated urethral groove. In markedly affected cases the scrotum is cleft and chordee may be so severe as to draw the tip of the glans to the anterior edge of the anus. The testes may be descended and of normal size. Occasionally an imperforate anus with rectourethral fistula has been reported. Bilateral ureteral reflex has been noted. Affected females have normal genitalia. Some infants have stridorous respiration with a hoarse cry. Various other findings have been reported which include patent foramen ovale and ductus arteriosus, anomalous venous return to the heart, midline position of the heart, unlobed lungs, absence of gallbladder, Meckel diverticulum, duodenal stricture, and bifid renal pelvis with double ureter.

Specific Diagnosis The combination of the previously described facial and genital anomalies with a hoarse or stridorous cry is diagnostic and studies should be done to rule out an esophageal functional defect. Cinefluoroscopic studies have shown apparent neuromuscular dysfunction of the swallowing mechanism with up to half of each bolus entering the tracheobronchial tree with gastroesophageal reflex. Achalasia may also be present.

Differential Diagnosis This syndrome is quite distinctive. Facial features may be confused with the *Aarskog syndrome,* but dysphagia and pulmonary difficulties are not part of the latter.

Prenatal Diagnosis This syndrome has not yet been diagnosed prenatally.

Basic Defect, Genetics, and Other Considerations The basic defect is not known, but midline organs and structures are primarily affected. There is good evidence to suggest that this condition is transmitted as an autosomal dominant trait with some male sex limitation. Most severely affected patients are male. X-linked inheritance is considered, as this could account for the greater heterogeneity of clinical features in females versus males.

Prognosis and Treatment In severe cases, although infants suck eagerly, they have difficulty in swallowing as manifested by choking, coughing, and cyanosis. This may be followed by respiratory distress, increase in stridor, aspiration pneumonia, patchy atelectasis, and emphysema. In chronic cases there is often bronchiectasis. After a swallowing defect has been demonstrated, a feeding jejunostomy should be done and if the patient survives, at approximately one year of age the esophagus can be reanastomosed. In successfully treated patients prognosis for life, growth, and reproduction is presumably normal, although some individuals may have mild mental retardation. Repair of the hypospadias is indicated in those patients who survive infancy.

REFERENCES

Arya, S., Viseskul, C., and Gilbert, E.F. The G-syndrome—additional observations. *Am. J. Med. Genet. 5:* 321–324, 1980.

Opitz, J.M., Frias, J.L., Gutenberger, J.E. et al. The G-syndrome of multiple congenital anomalies *Birth Defects 5 (2):* 95–110, 1969.

Van Biervliet, J. P. and van Hemmel, J.D. Familial occurrence of the G-syndrome. *Clin. Genet. 7:* 238–244, 1975.

M.R. [+ / some, mild]

- **asymmetric skull**
- **stridorous cry / dysphagia**
- **slit-like palpebral fissures / epicanthal folds**
- **hypospadias / genital / anal anomalies**

G-Syndrome
[hypertelorism with esophageal abnormality and hypospadias]

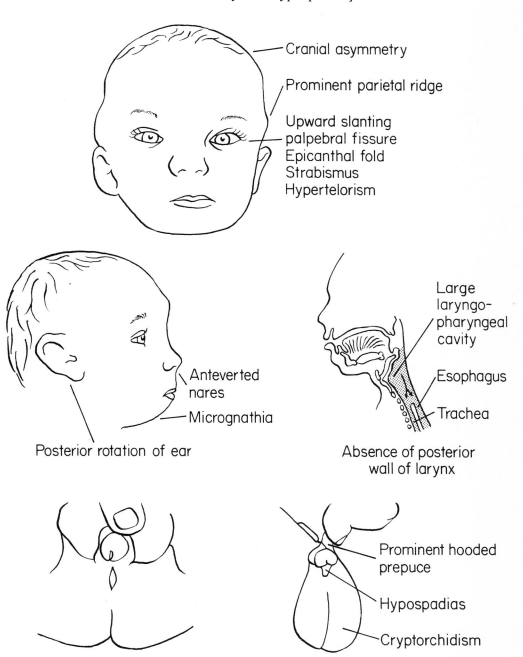

Cranial asymmetry

Prominent parietal ridge

Upward slanting palpebral fissure
Epicanthal fold
Strabismus
Hypertelorism

Anteverted nares

Micrognathia

Posterior rotation of ear

Large laryngo-pharyngeal cavity

Esophagus

Trachea

Absence of posterior wall of larynx

Prominent hooded prepuce

Hypospadias

Cryptorchidism

Cleft scrotum, hypospadias and cryptorchidism

265

123. INFANTILE CORTICAL HYPEROSTOSIS
(Caffey disease)

Clinical Features This disorder usually presents itself early in infancy, at age two to four months (average nine weeks). However, it has been diagnosed radiographically as early as five months prenatally and as late as twenty months after birth. The characteristic facial appearance consists of symmetric swelling of the face involving the body and ramus of the mandible. The soft tissue swelling may not only involve the face and orbits but also the thorax and extremities. It is firm, brawny, and frequently painful enough to produce pseudoparalysis of a limb. It is not associated with increased heat or redness. Pain, fever of a mild degree, and hyperirritability have been observed in approximately two-thirds of the patients. These signs usually precede the appearance of the swelling and bone involvement. Pallor is common. About 75% of all patients show mandibular involvement. The clavicle, tibia, ulna, scapula, femur, rib, humerus, maxilla, and fibula are less commonly involved, but usually several bones are affected at the same time.

Specific Diagnosis The diagnosis of this condition is a clinical one based on the above features plus roentgenographic changes. Initially the soft tissue swelling is all that is visible radiographically. Cortical hyperostoses may be present at the clinical onset indicating prior disease. With progression of the disorder there is variable external cortical thickening of the affected bones. In the mandible, massive thickening gives a structureless appearance of fibrous dysplasia, but serial subperiosteal layers of new bone may be identified in appropriate projections. Anemia, leukocytosis, and elevation of the sedimentation rate are found in more than half the patients. Elevation in the immunoglobins has been reported. Serum alkaline phosphatase level is raised in those patients with marked bone deposition.

Differential Diagnosis The facial and bone changes in this disease must be differentiated from *mumps, vaccinial* and *pyogenic osteomyelitis, rickets, congenital syphilis, scurvy, subperiosteal hematoma, parotid tumor,* and *vitamin A intoxication.*

Prenatal Diagnosis This disorder has been diagnosed prenatally using radiographic methods, however the majority of cases do not show prenatal bone changes.

Basic Defect, Genetics, and Other Considerations The basic defect is not known. A number of theories have been proposed regarding its etiology and which include some viral agent, milk allergy, collagen disorder, congenital anomaly of vessels supplying the periosteum and an altered gene. Both autosomal dominant and recessive inheritance have been suggested by several reports. Most cases have been sporadic. Despite the familial aggregation, this disorder seems to have an infectious rather than genetic origin. Perhaps its etiology is multifactorial or autosomal dominant with incomplete penetrance. A nongenetic phenocopy has also been suggested. It has been estimated that it occurs in 3 of every 1000 registered patients under six months of age.

Prognosis and Treatment Complete clinical resolution takes place within three to thirty months (average nine months). Rare deaths have been reported, but the relationship of the death to the disease is uncertain. A few chronic cases have been described. Treatment is symptomatic. Steroids produce a remission within three days but relapses after cessation of treatment for ten days are not uncommon.

REFERENCES

Caffey, J. Infantile cortical hyperostosis: a review of the clinical and radiographic features. *Proc. R. Soc. Med. 50:* 347–354, 1957.

Saul, R. A. Lee, W.H., and Stevenson, R. E. Caffey's disease revisited. *Am. J. Dis. Child. 136:* 56–60, 1982.

Van Buskirk, F.W., Tampas, J.P., and Peterson, O.S. Infantile cortical hyperostosis: an inquiry into its familial aspects. *Am. J. Roentgenol., 85:* 613–632, 1961.

- **symmetric swelling of face / mandible**
- **facial pallor**
- **soft tissue swelling thorax / extremities**

Infantile Cortical Hyperostosis
[Caffey disease]

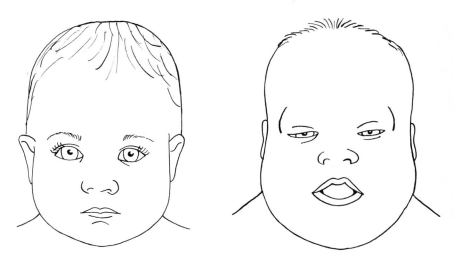

Infants with marked symmetrical facial
swelling over body and ramus of mandible

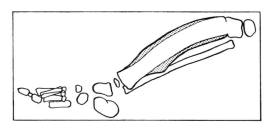

Forward bowing of tibia due to thickening
of periosteum and new bone formation

267

124. LENZ MICROPHTHALMIA SYNDROME

Clinical Features The disorder presents at birth with multiple anomalies involving mainly the eye, skeletal, and urogenital systems. Unilateral or bilateral eye defects range from microphthalmia to anophthalmia. Microcornea, strabismus, nystagmus, epicanthal folds, downward slanting palpebral fissures, and other eye defects have been described. The ears are frequently protuberant, asymmetric, and dysplastic. Micrognathia may be present. High-arched palate, crowded teeth, and agenesis of the permanent maxillary lateral incisors are the oral manifestations of this syndrome. Musculoskeletal features include short stature, cylindrical thorax with sloping shoulders, clavicular anomalies, low scapulas, cubitus valgus, limited extension in both hip joints, internally rotated knees, and prominent fibulas. Hand findings consist of camptodactyly of the fifth fingers, clinodactyly of the second, and duplication of the thumb. Foot anomalies include pes planus, calcaneovalgus and varus deformity, cutaneous syndactyly of the third and fourth toes, and a wide gap between the first and second toes. Urogenital features are unilateral renal agenesis, bilateral renal agenesis, renal dysgenesis, hydroureter, hypospadias, and cryptorchidism. Less common findings include congenital heart disease, atresia of the ileum, umbilical hernia, defective speech, and microcephaly.

Specific Diagnosis The diagnosis of this syndrome is mainly a clinical one based on the above features. Roentgenographic studies are indicated to detect possible renal anomalies. Various skeletal findings, as mentioned previously, may also be observed including notching of the vertebral bodies. Unusual dermatoglyphic changes have been reported.

Differential Diagnosis *Microphthalmia* and *anophthalmia* may occur in the same family as an autosomal dominant trait. *Isolated anophthalmia* is often inherited as an autosomal recessive condition or may be part of the findings associated with *trisomy 13 syndrome*. *Microphthalmia*, likewise, may be part of numerous syndromes or inherited as a dominant, recessive, or X-linked recessive trait.

Prenatal Diagnosis Has not yet been achieved, but theoretically ultrasound studies should be able to detect some of its renal features.

Basic Defect, Genetics, and Other Considerations The basic defect is not known. X-linked recessive inheritance seems likely. Minor anomalies have been noted in female heterozygous carriers. Female carriers have also been noted to have an increased abortion rate, suggesting that many cases may only appear to be sporadic. Linkage with G6PD has been excluded.

Prognosis and Treatment Mental retardation has been observed in some patients. Blindness or near blindness is common depending on the status of the eye anomalies. This syndrome may be life threatening due to the renal involvement. Treatment is supportive.

REFERENCES

Goldberg, M.F. and McKusick, V.A. X-linked colobomatous microphthalmos and other congenital anomalies. *Am. J. Ophthalmol. 71:* 1128–1138, 1971.

Herrmann, J. and Opitz, J.M. The Lenz microphthalmia syndrome. *Birth Defects 5(2):* 138–143, 1969.

Lenz, W. Recessiv-geschlechtsgebundene Mikrophthalmie mit multiplen Missbildungen. *Z. Kinderheilkd. 77:* 384–390, 1955.

- **microphthalmia / anophthalmia**
- **protruding dysplastic ears**
- **cylindrical thorax / sloping shoulders**
- **hand / foot anomalies**

Lenz Microphthalmia Syndrome

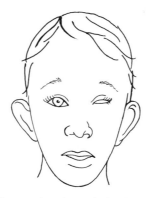

Unilateral microphthalmia with
large protruding dysplastic ears

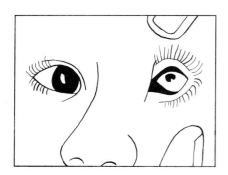

Strabismus, microcornea
and microphthalmia

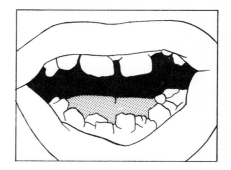

Crowding of the teeth

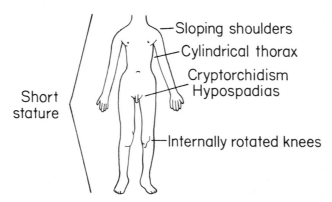

Short
stature

Sloping shoulders
Cylindrical thorax
Cryptorchidism
Hypospadias
Internally rotated knees

269

125. LEPRECHAUNISM
(Donohue syndrome)

Clinical Features Affected infants usually have low birth weight and rather striking physical features. Characteristic manifestations include grotesque elfin facies with a flat nasal bridge and flaring nostrils, thick lips, large, low-set ears, hirsutism, breast enlargement (also in males), prominent clitoris and labia minora in females and a large penis in males, deficiency of subcutaneous tissue with the presence of excessive folding of the skin especially involving the limbs, and motor and mental retardation. Other less common features are microcephaly, ocular hypertelorism, high or narrow-arched palate, cardiac malformation, umbilical and inguinal hernias, hypotonia, cryptorchidism, cholestatic jaundice, large hands and feet, and delayed skeletal maturation.

Specific Diagnosis No laboratory test as yet is known to be diagnostic for this disorder, however, the clinical features are so striking at birth that they readily suggest the diagnosis. A number of abnormal endocrine functions have been observed such as low fasting blood sugar, prolonged response to insulin, hyperinsulinemia, and growth hormone deficiency. Some affected infants also have hyperbilirubinemia, a low level of serum alkaline phosphatase, and nonspecific aminoaciduria.

Differential Diagnosis *Marasmic infants* may show similar facies. *Congenital total lipodystrophy (Seip-Lawrence syndrome)* shares many features with leprechaunism and there indeed may be a pathogenetic relationship between these two disorders.

Prenatal Diagnosis As yet prenatal diagnosis of this syndrome has not been made, but our studies suggest that such a diagnosis may be possible by demonstrating increased numbers of microfilaments as seen in electron microscopy from cultured fibroblasts obtained by amniocentesis (see below).

Basic Defect, Genetics, and Other Considerations The basic defect is not known. Based on our investigations we have proposed that it involves an alteration in insulin-receptor binding sites. Evidence for this hypothesis is the abundance of microfilamentous material observed under the electron microscope; this material is known to play a crucial role in the regulation of cell-surface receptors. No more than 30 well-documented cases of this syndrome have been reported in the literature. It is transmitted as an autosomal recessive condition and parental consanguinity and more than one affected sib have been noted.

Prognosis and Treatment Leprechaunism is invariably fatal and most infants die between the ages of six months and one year. All cases have shown severe motor-mental retardation and progressive marasmus.

REFERENCES

Bier, D.M., Schedewie, H., Larner, J. et al. Glucose kinetics in leprechaunism; accelerated fasting due to insulin resistance. *J. Clin. Endocrinol. Metab. 51:* 988–994, 1980.

Goodman, R.M. *Genetic Disorders Among the Jewish People,* Baltimore, Johns Hopkins University Press, 1979, pp. 255–259.

Rosenberg, A.M., Haworth, J.C., Degroot, G.W. et al. A case of leprechaunism with severe hyperinsulinemia. *Am. J. Dis. Child. 134:* 170–175, 1980.

- **grotesque facies / thick lips**
- **hirsutism**
- **emaciation**
- **enlarged external genitalia**

Leprechaunism
[Donohue syndrome]

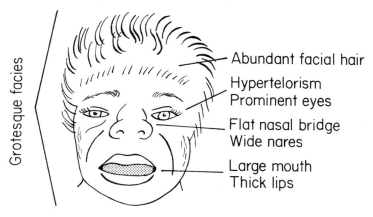

Grotesque facies

Abundant facial hair

Hypertelorism
Prominent eyes

Flat nasal bridge
Wide nares

Large mouth
Thick lips

Emaciated appearance

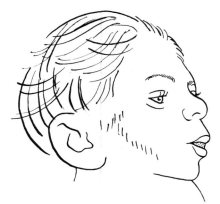

Large, low-set
ears, facial hair

Muscle wasting, large
hands and feet

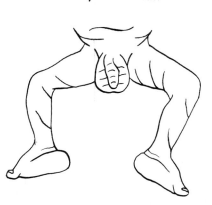

Enlarged external
genitalia – excess
wrinkling of skin

271

126. MANDIBULOFACIAL DYSOSTOSIS
(Treacher Collins syndrome)

Clinical Features This syndrome can be recognized at birth due to a typical facial appearance. The eyes may show several anomalies which include the following: antimongoloid obliquity of the palpebral fissures, coloboma of the outer third of the lower lid with a deficiency of cilia medial to the coloboma, iridial coloboma, absence of the lower lacrimal points, Meibomian glands, and intermarginal strip; and microphthalmia. The nose appears large due to a lack of malar development, while the nares are often narrow and the alar cartilages hypoplastic. The nasofrontal angle is commonly obliterated and the bridge of the nose raised. Choanal atresia has been noted. Micrognathia is almost always present; other oral manifestations include cleft palate (30%), high-arched palate, dental malocclusion, and unilateral or less often bilateral macrostomia. The external ear is frequently deformed, crumpled forward, or misplaced. Some patients have an absence of the external auditory canal or ossicle defects associated with conductive deafness. Anomalies of the ossicles include a fixed malleus, fusion of malformed malleus and incus, monopodal stapes, absence of stapes and oval window, and complete absence of the middle ear and epitympanic space. Extra ear tags and blind fistulas may be found anywhere between the tragus and angle of the mouth. Other anomalies occasionally mentioned are absence of the parotid gland, congenital heart disease, cervical vertebral malformations, congenital defects of the extremities, cryptorchidism, and renal anomalies.

Specific Diagnosis The diagnosis of this syndrome is a clinical one based on the above features. Radiographic studies may show a wide variety of findings involving the skull such as poorly developed supraorbital ridges, increased digital markings, hypoplastic malar bones with nonfusion of the zygomatic arches, sclerotic and nonpneumatized mastoids, sclerosis of the middle ear (and rarely the inner ear) with poor delineation of their structures, hypoplasia of the mandible, and flat or aplastic coronoid and condyloid processes. The undersurface of the body of the mandible is markedly concave.

Differential Diagnosis This syndrome must be differentiated from *acrofacial dysostosis (Nager syndrome)* which may have multifactorial inheritance and involves not only the face but also the upper extremities with absent or hypoplastic thumbs, radioulnar synostosis, absence or hypoplasia of the radius and/or one or more metacarpals. Many have confused mandibulofacial dysostosis with *oculoauriculovertebral dysplasia* which usually has multifactorial inheritance and is associated with hemifacial microsomia and various vertebral anomalies. Other isolated and rare syndromes may exhibit some of the facial features seen in mandibulofacial dysostosis, but the two mentioned here are the more common ones.

Prenatal Diagnosis In pregnancies at risk for this syndrome the use of fetoscopy and sonography may be helpful in making a prenatal diagnosis, but because the phenotypic range of expression is so variable it would not be easy to detect a minimally affected fetus.

Basic Defect, Genetics, and Other Considerations The basic defect is not known, although various theories have been postulated. Most involved structures derive from the first branchial arch, groove, and pouch. This syndrome is inherited as an autosomal dominant trait with high penetrance and marked variability in expressivity. More than half the cases arise as new mutations, but before a patient is considered to represent a new mutation, careful examination of family members must be done, looking for minimal signs of the syndrome. The gene may have a lethal effect since miscarriage or early postnatal death is common.

Prognosis and Treatment Mental retardation has been noted in some patients, but this may be due to a severe hearing deficit. Life span is not affected unless there is severe cardiac or renal malformation. Treatment for the conductive hearing loss may involve the use of hearing aids or surgical intervention. Plastic surgery can improve facial features, and orthodontic treatment and speech therapy must be considered.

REFERENCES

Caldarelli, D.D., Hutchinson, J.G. Jr., Pruzansky, S. et al. A comparison of microtia and temporal bone anomalies in hemifacial microsomia and mandibulofacial dysostosis. *Cleft Palate J. 17:* 103–110, 1980.

Franceschetti, A. and Klein, D. Mandibulo-facial dysostosis: a new hereditary syndrome. *Acta Ophthal. 24:* 143–224, 1949.

Herring, S.W., Rowlatt, U.F., and Pruzansky, S. Anatomical abnormalities in mandibulofacial dysostosis. *Am. J. Med. Genet. 3:* 225–229, 1979.

- **downward slant palpebral fissures / lower eyelid coloboma**
- **micrognathia**
- **dysplastic ears / hearing loss**
- **ear tags / fistulas**

Mandibular Dysostosis
[Treacher Collins syndrome]

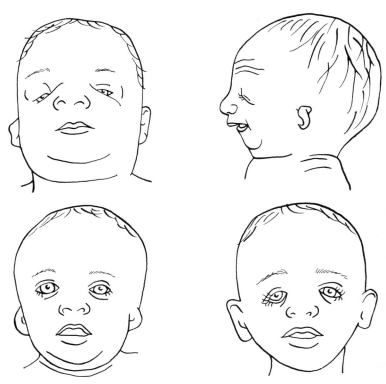

Degrees of lateral downward slant of palpebral fissures, coloboma of outer portion lower lids, deformed ears and facial asymmetry

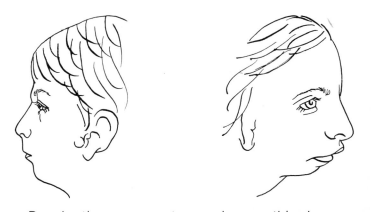

Dysplastic ears, ear tags, micrognathia, large appearing nose with narrow nares

273

127. MECKEL SYNDROME

Clinical Features. The key features of this syndrome consist of microcephaly with occipital encephalocele, cleft palate, polydactyly, polycystic kidneys, and external genital ambiguity in males. Microcephaly (30%) with associated holoprosencephaly, hydrocephaly with and without Arnold-Chiari malformation (15%), and occipital encephalocele (80%) are common CNS anomalies. Anencephaly (10%) and agenesis, hypoplasia, or dysplasia of the cerebellum and also agenesis of olfactory lobes, optic tract, corpus callosum, and septum pellucidum have occasionally been observed. Some brain anomaly is found in nearly all cases. Facial findings include sloping forehead, various eye anomalies (35%) (anophthalmia, microphthalmia, coloboma), cleft lip and/or cleft palate (30%), micrognathia, and dysplastic ears. Malformations of the tongue and larynx have been recorded. Cystic dysplasia of the kidney is seen in all cases, while cysts and/or fibrosis of the liver and/or pancreas are less common (about 40%). Genital anomalies (30%) in the male include hypoplastic penis and cryptorchidism, while females tend to have imperforate vagina and hypoplastic or bicornuate uterus. The urinary bladder may also be hypoplastic (10%). Postaxial polydactyly, noted in about 75%, when present always involves the hands, less often the feet. Congenital heart anomalies (40%) include VSD, ASD, aortic coarctation, complex rotational anomalies, and a host of other developmental abnormalities. Talipes equinovarus is seen in about 25% but probably results from oligohydramnios. Less common findings include hypoplastic adrenals (10%), imperforate anus, missing or accessory spleen (20%), intestinal malrotation, and various other anomalies.

Specific Diagnosis The anomalies present at birth in this syndrome are usually quite prominent and severe, enabling one to easily suspect this condition. The characteristic features have been noted above.

Differential Diagnosis This disorder must be differentiated mainly from *trisomy 13;* when in doubt, chromosomal studies are helpful. Clinically the polydactyly is usually more extreme in the Meckel syndrome and polycystic kidneys, cysts of the liver and pancreas, and occipital encephalocele are not usually a part of trisomy 13. The genital anomalies may cause confusion with the *Smith-Lemli-Opitz syndrome*. The face may appear somewhat similar to that in *holoprosencephaly*.

Prenatal Diagnosis It is possible to diagnose the syndrome early in fetal development by sonography or fetoscopy. Increased α-fetoprotein level is common in this disorder.

Basic Defect, Genetics, and Other Considerations The basic defect is not known. Numerous examples of affected sibs, concordance in presumably monozygotic twins, roughly equal occurrence in males and females, and parental consanguinity in some families establishes autosomal recessive inheritance. Among Jews, this syndrome is more common in the Oriental communities originating from Yemen and Iraq. Its prevalence among Jews in Israel is estimated to be 1:50,000. This syndrome has also been noted to occur among the Hutterites. There is some clinical evidence to suggest that there may be genetic heterogeneity in this disorder.

Prognosis and Treatment Patients are either stillborn or die shortly after birth.

REFERENCES

Fraser, F.C. and Lytwyn, A. Spectrum of anomalies in the Meckel syndrome: or, 'Maybe there is a malformation syndrome with at least one constant anomaly.' *Am. J. Med. Genet. 9:* 67–73, 1981.

Nevin, N.C., Thompson, W., Davison, G. et al. Prenatal diagnosis of the Meckel syndrome. *Clin. Genet. 15:* 1–4, 1979.

Opitz, J.M. and Howe, J.J. The Meckel syndrome (dysencephalia splanchnocystica, the Gruber syndrome). *Birth Defects 5(2):* 167–179, 1969.

- **microcephaly / occipital encephalocele**
- **cleft palate**
- **polydactyly**
- **protruding abdomen / polycystic kidneys**

Meckel Syndrome

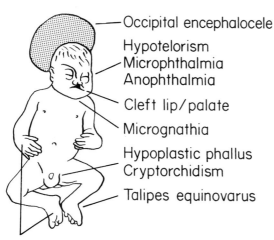

Occipital encephalocele

Hypotelorism
Microphthalmia
Anophthalmia

Cleft lip/palate

Micrognathia

Hypoplastic phallus
Cryptorchidism

Talipes equinovarus

Postaxial polydactyly
hands and feet

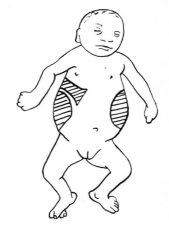

Microcephalic infant with
polycystic kidneys and liver

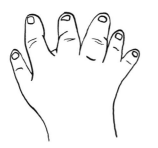

Postaxial polydactyly of hand and foot,
syndactyly, short hallux and talipes

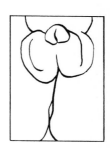

Hypoplastic phallus,
hypospadias and
cryptorchidism

128. MULTIPLE ENDOCRINE ADENOMATOSIS
(multiple mucosal neuromas; MEA, type III)

Clinical Features This syndrome is characterized by multiple mucosal neuromas, pheochromocytoma, medullary carcinoma of the thyroid, and asthenic build with muscle wasting of the extremities. Neuromas involving the oral and labial mucosa are the first component of the syndrome to appear usually before the eighth year of life. They have also been described in early infancy. The mucosal neuromas involve mainly the lips and tongue but buccal, gingival, palatal, pharyngeal, nasal, conjunctival, and other mucosal surfaces may also be affected. Both lips are extensively enlarged and nodular. The tongue lesions appear primarily on the anterior dorsal surface as pink pedunculated nodules. The eyelid margins are thickened and often everted. White medullated nerve fibers appear on the cornea and can be seen under slit-lamp examination. These fibers extend into the pupillary area where they anastomose. Mucosal neuromas may be found throughout the gastrointestinal tract, bronchi, bladder, and spinal nerve roots. Persistent diarrhea, megacolon, and diverticulosis are common intestinal problems. Cafe-au-lait spots and/or diffuse freckling have been reported. Most patients have an asthenic Marfanoid habitus with severe muscular wasting of the extremities. Lordosis, kyphoscoliosis, pes cavus, joint hypermobility, and prognathism have been described. Pheochromocytoma is present in about half of all cases during the second to third decades of life. Medullary carcinoma of the thyroid has been diagnosed in over 85% of these patients between the ages of 18 to 25 years. Parathyroid hyperplasia is quite rare.

Specific Diagnosis The facies and body physiognomy are frequently striking and diagnostic. Catecholamine assays and plasma calcitonin levels are useful in detecting pheochromocytoma and medullary thyroid carcinoma, respectively. Microscopically the mucosal nodules are plexiform neuromas, i.e. unencapsulated masses of convoluted myelinated and unmyelinated nerves which may also elaborate calcitonin.

Differential Diagnosis Both *pheochromocytoma* and *medullary carcinoma of the thyroid* may occur as an isolated tumor or in combination. When in binary combination it is called the *Sipple syndrome* or MEA, type II and also inherited as an autosomal dominant disorder. Five percent of cases of *neurofibromatosis* are associated with pheochromocytoma.

Prenatal Diagnosis This is not yet possible.

Basic Defect, Genetics, and Other Considerations The basic defect in this syndrome is not known, but its clinical features can be explained by hyperplasia and/or neoplasia of neural crest derivatives. The condition is transmitted as an autosomal dominant with variable expressivity. Penetrance is thought to be high.

Prognosis and Treatment Prognosis must be guarded depending on tumor type and the stage at which it is detected. Some surgeons recommend prophylactic thyroidectomy if the facies is typical and certainly if the plasma calcitonin level is elevated. Periodic tests should be done for the possible presence of pheochromocytoma.

REFERENCES

Gorlin, R.J. and Mirkin, B.L. Multiple mucosal neuromas, pheochromocytoma, medullary carcinoma of the thyroid and Marfanoid body build with muscle wasting. Syndrome of hyperplasia and neoplasia of neural crest derivatives. A unitarian concept. *Z. Kinderheilkd. 113:* 313–321, 1972.

Miller, R.L., Burzynski, N.J., and Giammara, B.L. The ultrastructure of oral neuromas in multiple mucosal neuromas, pheochromocytoma, medullary thyroid carcinoma syndrome. *J. Oral. Pathol. 6:* 253–263, 1977.

Moyes, C.D. and Alexander, F.W. Mucosal neuroma syndrome presenting in a neonate. *Develop. Med. Child Neurol. 19:* 518–521, 1977.

- **oral neuromas / large nodular lips**
- **everted thick eyelids**
- **asthenic habitus**
- **muscular wasting**

Multiple Endocrine Adenomatosis
[multiple mucosal neuromas; MEA, type III]

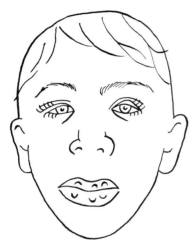 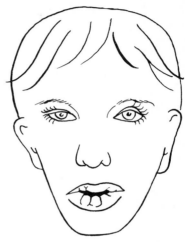

Coarse, thin facial features, large nodular
lips and everted upper eyelids

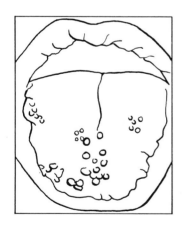 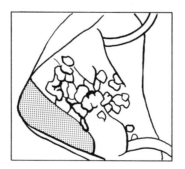

Mucosal neuromas of lips,
tongue and buccal mucosa

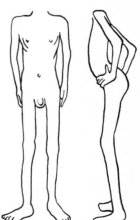

White nerve fibers
in pupillary area

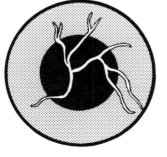

Asthenic body build
with muscle wasting
and lumbar lordosis

277

129. MYOTONIC DYSTROPHY
(Steinert disease)

Clinical Features Polyhydramnios and reduced fetal movements are common in pregnancies where the fetus is affected. Hypotonia during infancy has been occasionally recorded. Although the average age of detection is in the second decade, it is potentially recognizable during infancy and early childhood. Presenting symptoms are usually weakness of the hands and difficulty in walking with a tendency to fall. Myotonia or muscular stiffness may have been present prior to the above complaints. The facies is characteristically expressionless due to weakness of the facial muscles. Ptosis is common with symmetric impairment of ocular movement and difficulty in closing the eyes. The mouth shows retraction at the corners and pursing of the lips with drooping of the lower lip. Oral findings may include a high-arched palate, malocclusion, micrognathia, prognathism, high rate of dental caries, and retention of saliva in the oral cavity. Wasting of the masseter, temporal, and sternocleidomastoid muscles produces a haggard appearance. Dysarthria is common. As the disease progresses, mature cataracts occur in over 85% of patients. A variety of eye defects have been reported including microphthalmia, choroidal coloboma, and optic atrophy. Partial alopecia in the frontal and parietal areas may be seen in male patients. Small testes due to testicular atrophy and cryptorchidism are common in males while amenorrhea, dysmenorrhea, and ovarian cysts may be noted in females. Cardiac involvement is frequent as manifested by conduction defects with arrhythmias. Respiratory distress, pulmonary infections, and chronic pulmonary disease result from weak chest muscles and inability of the esophagus to empty adequately. The myotonia is often clinically limited to the tongue, forearm, and hand muscles but at times may be generalized. The deep tendon reflexes are reduced in the affected muscles. Weakness and wasting of the limbs affect mainly the muscles of the forearm and anterior tibial group, and to lesser extent the calves and peronei. Abdominal wall muscular weakness is invariable.

Specific Diagnosis Infants with neonatal myotonic dystrophy have thin ribs. Myotonia may be detected using electromyographic studies before the clinical signs and features are apparent. Also the use of slit-lamp examination for "myotonic dust," decreased IgG and IgM levels, along with insulin secretion studies showing an excessive insulin response to glucose, may be helpful in the early detection of this disorder.

Differential Diagnosis Myotonia may be seen in other conditions such as *myotonia congenita* (*Thomsen syndrome*), *paramyotonia congenita, generalized myotonia, Schwartz-Jampel syndrome,* and *Gamstorp-Wohlfahrt syndrome.*

Prenatal Diagnosis Prenatal diagnosis is possible as the gene for this condition is closely linked to the secretor locus. However, only 5–10% of the matings can be used for this type of detection. The secretor status of the fetus can be determined by examination of the amniotic fluid.

Basic Defect, Genetics, and Other Considerations The basic defect is not known but evidence suggests a generalized defect of cell membranes. The disorder has autosomal dominant inheritance with complete penetrance and variable expressivity. One-third of the cases may be due to a new mutation. Stillbirth and infant mortality rates are high. Genetic heterogeneity is suggested by three possible types based on times of onset; (1) during infancy, (2) early childhood to 20 years, and (3) 20–60 years.

Prognosis and Treatment In general this is a slowly progressive condition leading to incapacitation and death before the sixth decade. Mental deterioration may occur with progression of the disease. These patients are particularly at risk during anesthesia. Prednisone may be useful for short-term therapy. Orthopedic measures along with physical therapy should be used for muscle weakness. Correction of ptosis and removal of cataracts may be indicated.

REFERENCES

Brumback, R.A. et al. Myotonic dystrophy as a disease of abnormal membrane receptors: an hypothesis of pathophysiology and a new approach to treatment. *Med. Hypotheses 7(8):* 1059–1066, 1981.

Harper, P.S. Congenital myotonic dystrophy in Britain. I. Clinical aspects. *Arch. Dis. Childh. 50:* 505–521, 1975.

Schrott, H.G., Karp, L., and Omenn, G.S. Prenatal prediction in myotonic dystrophy: guidelines for genetic counseling. *Clin. Genet. 4:* 38–45, 1973.

M.R. [mental
deterioration
in some]

- **difficulty in walking /
  weakness in hands**
- **expressionless face /
  ptosis**
- **myotonia / cataracts**
- **frontal / parietal
  alopecia**

Myotonic Dystrophy
[Steinert disease]

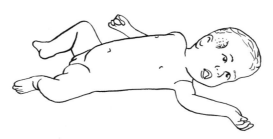

Marked hypotonia, open mouth, poor suck reflex and temporal atrophy

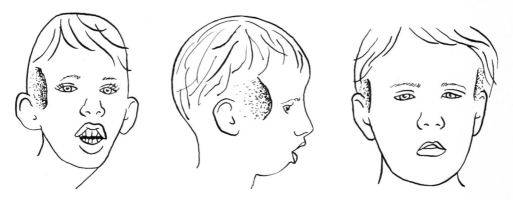

Thin expressionless facies, ptosis of eyelids,
drooping lower lip and temporal atrophy

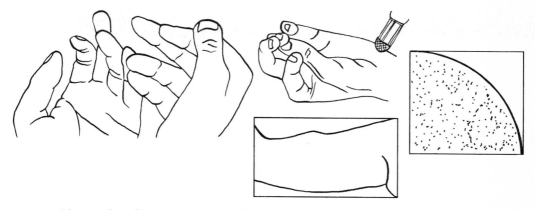

Myotonia of hands, myotonic response to blow to thenar and
biceps muscle, cataract (myotonic dust) seen from slit lamp

279

130. NAGER SYNDROME
(acrofacial dysostosis)

Clinical Features The disorder is most often mistaken for mandibulofacial dysostosis (Treacher Collins syndrome). The mandible is quite small, often resulting in respiratory distress and feeding difficulties. There is usually antimongoloid obliquity of the palpebral fissures. Often there is absence of lashes on the medial portion of the lower eyelids. The pinnae and the external ear canals are narrow or atretic. Preauricular tags may be present. The thumbs are hypoplastic or absent. The radius and ulna may be fused and there may be absence or hypoplasia of the radius and one or more metacarpals. In some cases the humerus may be short and radial-ulnar synostosis has been reported. Often there is reduction in full elbow extension due to posterior dislocation of the head of the radius. Pronation and supination of the arms are thereby impaired.

Specific Diagnosis Patients almost always exhibit growth retardation. Diagnosis is predicated upon recognition of the phenotype, that is, a patient who has what appears to be mandibulofacial dysostosis but who has absent or hypoplastic thumbs and/or radii. The frequency of cleft palate may be as high or even higher than in Treacher Collins syndrome. The mild mental retardation which has been reported in several cases is probably not valid but is based on severe conductive hearing loss.

Differential Diagnosis The only condition that one would consider in differential diagnosis would be *mandibulofacial dysostosis (Treacher Collins syndrome)*. In contrast to the latter, in Nager syndrome the zygomata are less hypoplastic and hence there is less antimongoloid obliquity of the palpebral fissures. Lower lid colobomas are less common than in mandibulofacial dysostosis, but the mandibular hypoplasia is far more severe. The main differentiating point, however, is hypoplasia of the thumb and/or radius in Nager syndrome, while there is a lack of any extracephalic anomalies in mandibulofacial dysostosis.

Prenatal Diagnosis The absence or severe hypoplasia of the thumb (rarely radius) theoretically may be noted by fetoscopy or ultrasonography, but we are not aware of this having been done.

Basic Defect, Genetics, and Other Considerations In spite of the occurrence of this disorder in one pair of siblings, all other cases have been isolated. There has been one report of the parents being first cousins, but we do not believe that this disorder has single gene inheritance. Approximately 25 cases have been reported. The sex ratio of affected infants does not seem to be altered.

Prognosis and Treatment Severe cases require immediate tracheostomy. Maxillofacial correction of the small mandible and zygomatic hypoplasia has been carried out successfully. Pollicization is also possible, but we are not aware of it being attempted in any case of Nager syndrome.

REFERENCES

Bowen, T. and Harley, F. Mandibulofacial dysostosis with limb malformations (Nager's acrofacial dysostosis). *Birth Defects 10(5):* 109–115, 1974.

Halal, F., Herrmann, J., Pallister, P.D. et al Differential diagnosis of Nager acrofacial dysostosis syndrome: report of four patients with Nager syndrome and discussion of other related syndromes. *Am. J. Med. Genet. 14:* 209–224, 1983.

Meyerson, M.D., Jensen, K.M., Meyers, J.M. et al. Nager acrofacial dysostosis. Early intrauterine and longterm planning. *Cleft Palate J. 14:* 35–40, 1977.

- **small mandible**
- **hypoplastic or absent thumbs**
- **upper limb anomalies**
- **downward slant palpebral fissures**

Nager Syndrome
[acrofacial dysostosis]

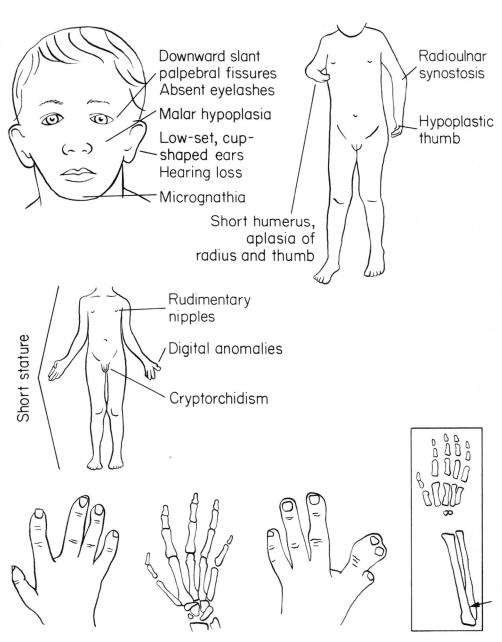

Downward slant palpebral fissures
Absent eyelashes

Malar hypoplasia

Low-set, cup-shaped ears
Hearing loss

Micrognathia

Short humerus, aplasia of radius and thumb

Radioulnar synostosis

Hypoplastic thumb

Rudimentary nipples

Digital anomalies

Cryptorchidism

Short stature

Hypoplastic thumb, preaxial attachment to thumb and index finger mass, radioulnar synostosis (arrow)

131. NOONAN SYNDROME

Clinical Features The key features in this syndrome are facial anomalies, congenital heart disease, skeletal abnormalities with short stature, genital malformations, and mild mental retardation. At birth the facies may exhibit a broad forehead, micrognathia, unilateral or bilateral ptosis of the eyelids, epicanthal folds, mild antimongoloid obliquity of palpebral fissures, hypertelorism, strabismus, saddle nose, and low-set fleshy ears with folding of the upper transverse portion of the helix. In approximately half the patients there is pterygium colli with a low posterior hairline. Oral findings include a high-arched palate, malocclusion, bifid uvula, and rarely cleft palate. Half of the patients have cardiovascular anomalies with the right side of the heart most frequently involved with valvular pulmonic stenosis, patent ductus arteriosus, and aortic stenosis. Coarctation of the aorta and the Ebstein anomaly of the tricuspid valve occasionally have been reported. Multiple cardiac anomalies may also be present. Lymphedema of the lower extremities is seen in about 15% of the patients and intestinal lymphangiectasis is less frequent. Cryptorchidism with a normal or a large penis is common. Hypospadias and renal duplication have been described. Gonadal differentiation and function may vary from normal function and fertility to complete absence. Hypoplastic, inverted, and accessory nipples have been described. Skeletal features commonly include retarded bone age, osteoporosis, proximal pectus carinatum, distal pectus excavatum, cubitus valgus, and clinodactyly, and occasionally there is polydactyly, scoliosis, kyphosis, lordosis, spina bifida occulta, and the Klippel-Feil anomaly. Hypoplastic nails, curly hair, hirsutism, and hemangiomas may be noted. Other findings are sensorineural deafness, hydrocephaly, seizures, autoimmune thyroiditis, hypoparathyroidism, hypotonia, inguinal and umbilical hernia, plus a variety of miscellaneous anomalies.

Specific Diagnosis The diagnosis of this syndrome is a clinical one based on the above features. Recently a comprehensive scoring system of clinical features was devised for aid in diagnosis. Chromosomal studies are normal. Dermatoglyphic findings are not specific but simian creases are common and a distally placed axial triradius has been noted in some patients.

Differential Diagnosis This syndrome in phenotypic females must be differentiated from the *Turner syndrome* in which gonadal dysgenesis is invariably present and mental deficiency is extremely rare. Chromosomal studies will make possible this differentiation plus individuals mosaic for *XO/XY*. Other syndromes that may share some of the clinical features of the Noonan syndrome are *multiple pterygium, Aarskog, leopard, fetal alcohol,* and *18p- syndromes*.

Prenatal Diagnosis In a pregnancy considered to be at risk for this syndrome the early prenatal detection of a cardiovascular anomaly by sonography may indicate an affected fetus.

Basic Defect, Genetics, and Other Considerations The basic defect is not known. Most cases are sporadic, however, there are several affected families reported, compatible with autosomal dominant inheritance. It has been described in multiple sibs of apparently unaffected but consanguineous parents, suggesting autosomal recessive transmission. Genetic heterogeneity is certainly possible in this syndrome. Prevalence is not known but it may be as high as 1 in 1000. There is no apparent racial or ethnic predilection.

Prognosis and Treatment Mental deficiency is present in more than half the patients, ranging from mild to an IQ below 50. Short stature is common with adult males and females averaging 165 and 152 cm, respectively. Patients may or may not reproduce, depending on their gonadal status. Life span may be normal or shortened depending on the severity of the cardiac defect. Therapy may include surgical correction of a cardiovascular anomaly or cryptorchidism. Hormonal substitution therapy may also be indicated.

REFERENCES

Char, F., Rodriquez-Fernandez, H.L., Scott, C.I. Jr. et al. The Noonan syndrome—a clinical study of forty-five cases. *Birth Defects 8(5):* 110–118, 1972.

Duncan, W.J., Fowler, R.S., Farkas, L.G. et al. A comprehensive scoring system for evaluation of Noonan syndrome. *Am. J. Med. Genet. 10:* 37–50, 1981.

Wilroy, R.S., Summitt, R.L., Tipton, R.E. et al. Phenotypic heterogeneity in the Noonan syndrome. *Birth Defects 15*(5B): 305–311, 1979.

- **broad forehead**
- **ptosis / eye anomalies**
- **low-set, thick ears**
- **pterygium colli /
  low posterior hairline**

Noonan Syndrome

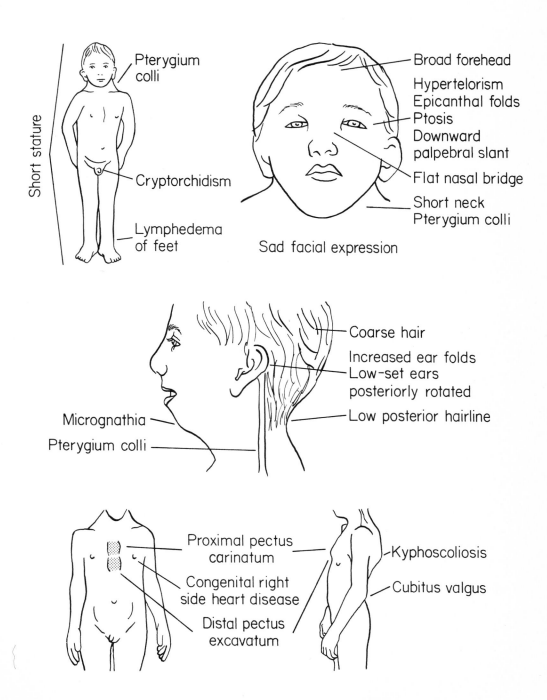

Short stature

Pterygium colli

Cryptorchidism

Lymphedema of feet

Broad forehead
Hypertelorism
Epicanthal folds
Ptosis
Downward palpebral slant
Flat nasal bridge
Short neck
Pterygium colli

Sad facial expression

Coarse hair
Increased ear folds
Low-set ears posteriorly rotated
Low posterior hairline

Micrognathia
Pterygium colli

Proximal pectus carinatum
Congenital right side heart disease
Distal pectus excavatum

Kyphoscoliosis
Cubitus valgus

132. OCULOAURICULOVERTEBRAL DYSPLASIA
(Goldenhar syndrome)

Clinical features The facial and ear anomalies may be so striking that recognition is readily made at birth. Facial asymmetry is common, partly due to hypoplasia and/or displacement of the pinna. The maxillary, temporal, and malar bones on the involved side are reduced in size and flattened. The ipsilateral eye may be set lower than that on the opposite side. Frontal bossing is common. Though the disorder is usually more severe on one side (the right), bilateral involvement is present in approximately 10% of patients. Malformation of the external ear may vary from complete aplasia to a crumpled, distorted pinna displaced anteriorly and inferiorly. Supernumerary ear tags may occur anywhere from the tragus to the angle of the mouth. When epibulbar dermoids are present, ear tags tend to be bilateral. Blind-ended fistulas are common in the same area but are not always bilateral. Conduction hearing loss due to middle ear abnormalities and/or absence or deficiency of the external auditory meatus is found in approximately 40%. Epibulbar dermoid and/or lipodermoid is a variable finding. It is white to yellow in color, flattened, ellipsoidal, and solid. The dermoid is usually located at the limbus or corneal margin in the lower outer quadrant; in contrast, the lipodermoid is usually in the upper outer quadrant. Some patients have both lesions in the same eye. Unilateral coloboma of the superior lid is common in those patients with epibulbar dermoids. Choroidal or iridial coloboma and congenital cystic eye may be observed in this disorder. Mental retardation is more common when unilateral microphthalmia or anophthalmia is present. Vertebral anomalies found in about half the patients include: occipitalization of the atlas, cuneiform vertebra, complete or partial synostosis of two or more vertebrae, supernumerary vertebrae, hemivertebrae, and spina bifida. Anomalous ribs, talipes equinovarus, and other skeletal defects have been reported. Hypoplasia of muscles such as the masseter, temporalis, pterygoideus, and those of facial expression on the involved side has been observed. The palatal and tongue muscles may be hypoplastic and/or paralyzed. Within the mouth there is decreased palatal width from the midline palatal raphe to the lingual surface of the teeth on the affected side. Agenesis of the mandibular ramus is found in conjunction with macrostomia, i.e. lateral facial cleft of a mild degree. It is nearly always unilateral and on the side of the more affected ear. Various dental malocclusions are present. Cleft lip/palate may be seen in some patients. Other anomalies include: occipital encephalocele, congenital heart disease, homolateral pulmonary agenesis or hypoplasia, various renal abnormalities (absent kidney, double ureter, anomalous blood supply to the kidney, etc.), and agenesis of the ipsilateral parotid gland.

Specific Diagnosis The diagnosis of this disorder is a clinical one based on the above clinical features. Radiographic study of the vertebral column may be a useful diagnostic aid.

Differential Diagnosis This disorder should be differentiated from the *Robin anomaly, Moebius syndrome,* and *mandibulofacial dysostosis.* Epibulbar dermoids may be observed in *frontonasal dysplasia.*

Prenatal Diagnosis In families in which autosomal dominant inheritance has been shown, the use of ultrasound and fetoscopy may be of value.

Basic Defect, Genetics, and Other Considerations The basic defect in this syndrome is not known. Although most cases are sporadic and of unknown etiology there is good evidence for genetic heterogeneity. The occurrence of the disorder in two or more generations and in sibs has been reported, but multifactorial transmission has been postulated by most authors. The frequency of the condition is about 1 in 3000 live births. Recurrence risk in the isolated case is about 1%.

Prognosis and Treatment This condition is usually compatible with normal life span and intellect. In those patients with conductive deafness, hearing aids should be utilized from early infancy. Correction of the malocclusion is frequently necessary. Plastic and/or maxillofacial surgery are often required.

REFERENCES

Baum, J.L. and Feingold, M. Ocular aspects of Goldenhar's syndrome. *Am. J. Ophthalmol. 75:* 250–257, 1973.

Poswillo, D. Otomandibular deformity: pathogenesis as a guide to reconstruction. *J. Maxillofac. Surg. 2:* 64–72, 1974.

Regenbogen, L., Godel, V., Goya, V. et al. Further evidence for an autosomal dominant form of oculoauriculovertebral dysplasia. *Clin. Genet. 21:* 161–167, 1982.

- **facial asymmetry**
- **dysplastic ears / ear tags / hearing loss**
- **eye anomalies / epibulbar dermoid**
- **prominent forehead**

Oculoauriculovertebral Dysplasia
[Goldenhar syndrome]

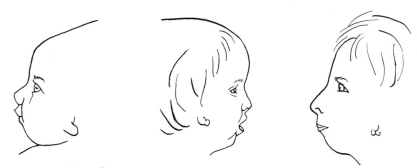

Mandibular hypoplasia, prominent forehead
and varying types of malformed displaced pinnae

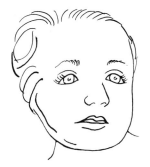

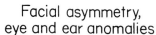

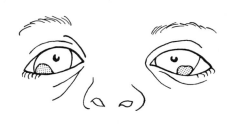

Facial asymmetry,
eye and ear anomalies

Bilateral epibulbar dermoids
with downward slant to palpebral fissures

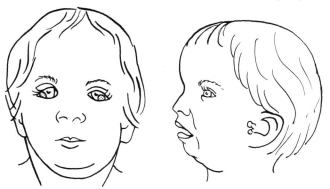

Note epibulbar dermoids, facial asymmetry,
frontal bossing, mandibular hypoplasia
and preauricular appendages

133. OCULOCEREBRORENAL SYNDROME
(Lowe syndrome)

Clinical Features The syndrome can be recognized at birth by the presence of congenital glaucoma, hypotonia, mental retardation, and various abnormalities in renal function. A high, prominent forehead is common with thin, sparse hair along with cataracts which are white and opaque. These cataracts may be nuclear or located on the anterior or posterior surface of the lens. Glaucoma develops in the first few months of life and its cause is not known. Other eye features include miotic pupils unresponsive to mydriatics, pigmentary degeneration in the area of the macula, and posterior synechiae between the lens and iris. Cryptorchidism is common. The hypotonia which is present at birth tends to remain throughout infancy. Deep tendon reflexes are usually absent but may be present in older children. Many patients have protruding ears. Some patients are hyperexcitable and scream for no apparent reason.

Specific Diagnosis The diagnosis of this syndrome is based on the above clinical features in conjunction with various laboratory findings. A generalized aminoaciduria develops in the first few weeks after birth, but the amount excreted shows wide daily fluctuation. Proteinuria, intermittent glucosuria, and deficient renal ammonia production have been noted. More recently, it has been shown that these patients have excess excretion of bound sialic acid and of undersulfated chondroitin sulfate A. The jejunal mucosa in some patients shows defective transport of lysine and arginine. Electroencephalographic studies show diffuse abnormalities.

Differential Diagnosis This syndrome shares many features (hypotonia, glaucoma or cataracts, high, broad forehead, and proteinuria) with that of the *cerebrohepatorenal syndrome,* but in the latter the presence of stippled epiphyses, joint contractures, renal cortical cysts, elevated serum iron, and autosomal recessive inheritance make differentiation relatively easy. *Marked hypotonia* as well as *congenital cataracts* and *glaucoma* are features of a number of syndromes which can present in infancy, but each must be differentiated by various physical findings and genetic and laboratory studies.

Prenatal Diagnosis To the best of our knowledge this syndrome has not yet been diagnosed prenatally.

Basic Defect, Genetics, and Other Considerations The basic defect in this disorder is not known. The reported pathologic changes are nonspecific and variable. No specific eye pathology has been described, but some have reported congenital anomalies of the canal of Schlemm. This syndrome is transmitted as an X-linked recessive condition and the female carrier state can be detected in some individuals. The presence of lens opacities and aminoaciduria after ornithine loading is an indication of the heterozygous state. Some have reported a high incidence of maternal cataract. Genetic heterogeneity is probable in this syndrome.

Prognosis and Treatment All reported patients have been mentally retarded, usually to a severe degree. During infancy and childhood, height is usually below the 3rd percentile. Most infants fail to thrive and the main cause of death in infancy is chronic renal insufficiency. Patients with metabolic acidosis and rickets respond to treatment with alkali supplement and vitamin D. Some patients have survived to adulthood and one developed an acute arthritis involving the joints of the extremities. The average life expectancy is not known.

REFERENCES

Abbassi, V., Lowe, C.U., and Calcagno, P.L. Oculocerebro-renal syndrome. A review. *Am. J. Dis. Child. 115:* 145–168, 1968.

Akasaki, M. et al. Urinary excretion of a large amount of bound sialic acid and of undersulfated chondroitin sulfate A by patients with the Lowe syndrome. *Clin. Chim. Acta 89:* 119–125, 1978.

Delleman, J.W., Bleeker-Wagemakers, E.M., and van Veelen, A.W. Opacities of the lens indicating carrier status in the oculo-cerebro-renal (Lowe) syndrome. *J. Pediatr. Ophthalmol. 14:* 205–212, 1977.

- **prominent forehead**
- **thin, sparse hair**
- **congenital glaucoma / cataracts**
- **protruding ears**

Oculocerebrorenal Syndrome
[Lowe syndrome]

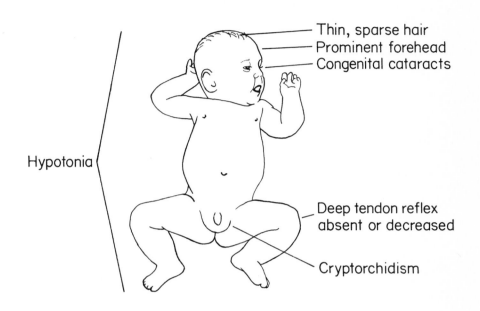

Thin, sparse hair
Prominent forehead
Congenital cataracts

Hypotonia

Deep tendon reflex absent or decreased

Cryptorchidism

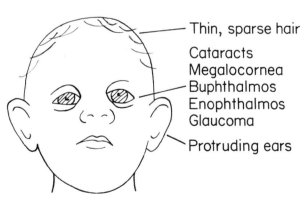

Thin, sparse hair

Cataracts
Megalocornea
Buphthalmos
Enophthalmos
Glaucoma

Protruding ears

Older child with list
of eye findings

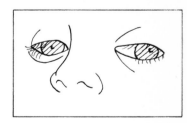

Congenital white opaque
cataracts at birth

134. OCULODENTOOSSEOUS DYSPLASIA

Clinical Features The syndrome is characterized in part by a distinct facial appearance that is present at birth and consists of ocular hypotelorism, sunken eyes, epicanthal folds, and a thin nose with absent alar flare. Eye anomalies include iris defects (fine, porous spongy tissue), microcornea, and in some, small palpebral apertures and secondary glaucoma. Other ophthalmologic findings sometimes present are microphthalmia with small orbits, eccentric pupils, and narrowed visual fields. The external ears are frequently dysplastic and conduction deafness has been noted in a few patients. Head circumference may be reduced. Dry, lusterless hair, which fails to grow to normal length has been noted in some patients. Amelogenesis imperfecta is common. In addition, cleft lip/palate, high-arched palate, and a wider than normal alveolar ridge of the mandible have been described in some cases. The most common finding involving the extremities is camptodactyly of the fifth or less often of the fourth and fifth fingers. Bilateral soft tissue syndactyly of the fourth and fifth fingers with ulnar clinodactyly and syndactyly of the third and fourth toes are usually present. Other skeletal features may include cubitus valgus, congenital hip dislocation, poor posture, and increased bone density.

Specific Diagnosis The diagnosis of this syndrome is a clinical one based on the above clinical features and radiographic findings which include bony orbital hypotelorism, enamel hypoplasia of the teeth, cube-shaped middle phalanx of the hand, hypoplasia or aplasia of the middle phalanx of one or more toes, and lack of modeling of the metaphyseal area of the long bones. Recently intracranial calcification of the basal ganglia has been observed in two patients along with low levels of serum inorganic phosphate and other nonspecific endocrine abnormalities.

Differential Diagnosis Some of the eye anomalies seen in this syndrome may be found in the *Rieger syndrome* but microcornea and enamel hypoplasia are not in the latter. The nasal appearance in oculodentoosseous dysplasia somewhat resembles that seen in the *trichorhinophalangeal syndrome* but the latter disorder is not associated with the eye, tooth, and skeletal anomalies seen in the former.

Prenatal Diagnosis Theoretically, prenatal diagnosis may be possible in a fetus at risk by observing syndactyly of the fourth and fifth fingers using fetoscopy or sonography.

Basic Defects, Genetics, and Other Considerations The basic defect is not known. Autosomal dominant inheritance with variable expressivity has been well established. A paternal age effect has been observed in new mutations for this condition.

Prognosis and Treatment This is not considered to be a life-threatening disorder. Intellect is normal. Eye anomalies with the development of secondary glaucoma may result in blindness. Treatment is directed toward the eye pathology, correction of the syndactyly, and crowning of the teeth.

REFERENCES

Barnard, A., Hamersma, H., De Villiers, J.C. et al. Intracranial calcification in oculodentoosseous dysplasia. *S. Afr. Med. J. 59 (21):* 758–762, 1981.

Judisch, G.F., Martin-Casals, A., Hanson, J.W. et al. Oculodentodigital dysplasia. Four new reports and a literature review. *Arch. Ophthalmol. 97:* 878–884, 1979.

Reisner, S.H., Kott, E., Bornstein, B. et al. Oculodentodigital dysplasia. *Am. J. Dis. Child. 118:* 600–607, 1969.

- **microphthalmia /
  hypertelorism**
- **thin nose /
  absent alar flare**
- **amelogenesis
  imperfecta**
- **digital anomalies /
  4–5 syndactyly fingers**

Oculodentoosseous
Dysplasia

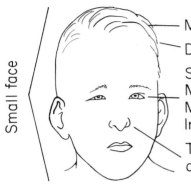

Small face

Mild microcephaly

Dry hair

Sunken eyes
Microphthalmia
Microcornea
Iris anomalies

Thin nose without
alar flare

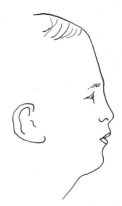

Small face – nose
without alar flare

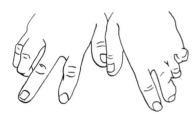

Bilateral camptodactyly
of 4th–5th fingers

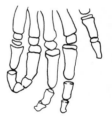

Bony fusion of terminal
phalanges of 4th–5th fingers

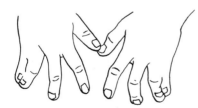

Bilateral syndactyly 4th–5th
fingers with ulnar deviation

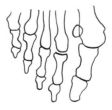

Absence of middle
phalanges of toes

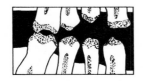

Small teeth with
marked enamel hypoplasia

135. OCULOMANDIBULOFACIAL SYNDROME
(Hallermann-Streiff syndrome)

Clinical Features The syndrome is characterized by distinct craniofacial features along with proportionate dwarfism, hypotrichosis, and congenital cataracts. The face is small, with a small mouth, and a long beak-like nose with a tendency to septal deviation; micrognathia accompanied by a double cutaneous chin (with a central cleft or dimple) and brachycephaly with frontal and parietal bossing make up the other distinguishing features. Mild microcephaly, malar bone hypoplasia, gaping of the longitudinal and lambdoidal sutures, as well as delayed closure of the fontanels have been described. Oral findings include a high and narrow palate, absence of teeth, persistence of deciduous teeth, malocclusion, malformed teeth, and severe and premature caries. Supernumerary as well as natal teeth have been reported. Microphthalmia of variable severity and bilateral congenital cataracts are constant features. Other eye findings include blue sclerae in 15–25% of patients, posterior synechiae, aphakia, prepupillary membrane, nystagmus, strabismus, and secondary glaucoma. Hypotrichosis involving the scalp, brows, and cilia is a frequent feature. Sparse axillary and pubic hair may also be present. Alopecia is prominent about the frontal and occipital areas. The scalp skin is thin and taut with prominent scalp veins. Similar skin changes can be noted on the nose. Skeletal anomalies are infrequent, but syndactyly, spina bifida, lordosis, scoliosis, osteoporosis, and winging of the scapulae have been described. Hypogenitalism and cryptorchidism are relatively common. All patients have proportionally diminished height of 2–5 standard deviations below the mean. Adult height for females is approximately 152 cm with males 2.5–5.0 cm taller.

Specific Diagnosis The craniofacial features in this syndrome are present at birth and their distinctness aids in the recognition of the disorder. Radiographic examination of the temporomandibular joints shows a characteristic change. The joint is displaced approximately 2 cm forward. Normally the joint is located just in front of the external auditory meatus.

Differential Diagnosis The facial features in this syndrome should be differentiated from those in *progeria* and *mandibulofacial dysostosis*. Brachycephaly with persistently open fontanels and wide sutures, high palatal vault, and malar bone flattening are seen in *cleidocranial dysplasia* and *pyknodysostosis*.

Prenatal Diagnosis Not yet possible for this syndrome.

Basic Defect, Genetics, and Other Considerations The basic defect is not known. Most cases have been sporadic with no sex predilection. It has been described both as concordant and discordant in identical twins. An affected female has had two normal children. Although the syndrome has been reported in a father and daughter there is doubt regarding the accuracy of the diagnosis. Over 70 cases of this condition have been reported in the literature.

Prognosis and Treatment During early infancy feeding difficulties and respiratory problems present the greatest challenge and may be fatal. The congenital cataracts may resorb spontaneously, but visual acuity may decrease to the point of total blindness. Mental retardation has been noted in about 15% of the patients. Reproductive fitness is greatly reduced. Treatment consists of possible surgical intervention to improve oral and eye defects.

REFERENCES

Chandra, R.K., Joglekar, S., and Antonio, Z. Deficiency of humoral immunity and hypoparathyroidism associated with Hallermann-Streiff syndrome. *J. Pediatr. 93:* 892–893, 1978.

Crevits, L., Thiery, E., and van der Eecken, H. Oculomandibular dyscephaly associated with epilepsy. *J. Neurol. 215:* 225–230, 1977.

Ronen, S., Rozenmann, Y., Isaacson, M. et al. The early management of a baby with Hallermann-Streiff-François syndrome. *J. Pediatr. Ophthalmol. Strabismus 16:* 119–121, 1979.

M.R. [+ / few]

- frontal / parietal bossing
- small face / mouth / pinched nose
- microphthalmia / congenital cataracts
- micrognathia / double chin

Oculomandibulofacial Syndrome
[Hallermann-Streiff syndrome]

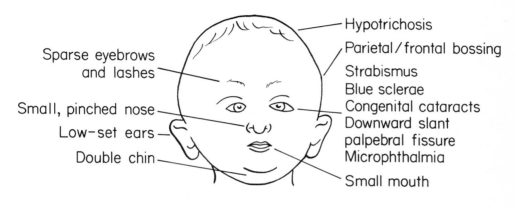

Hypotrichosis
Parietal / frontal bossing
Strabismus
Blue sclerae
Congenital cataracts
Downward slant palpebral fissure
Microphthalmia
Small mouth

Sparse eyebrows and lashes
Small, pinched nose
Low-set ears
Double chin

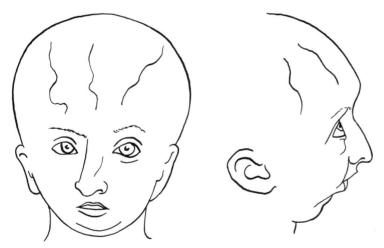

Beaking and deviation of nose, prominent scalp veins, frontal/parietal bossing, small mouth, micrognathia, double chin

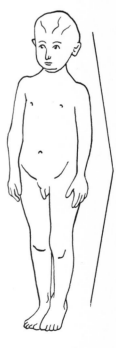

Proportionally short stature

Sparse body hair

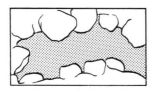

Hypodontia and malformed teeth

291

136. ORAL-FACIAL-DIGITAL SYNDROME I

Clinical Features The syndrome can be recognized at birth by its distinct oral, facial, and digital findings. The eyes commonly show euryopia and frequently there is lateral displacement of the inner canthi. The nose appears thin with lack of nasal alar flare due in part to hypoplasia of the alar cartilage. The nasal root is broad. One nostril may be smaller than the other and there may be flattening of the nasal tip. The midfacial region is flat in the majority of patients. Oral manifestations are many and include a short upper lip with a small midline cleft extending through the vermilion border, thick frenula, and clefting of the palate such that the maxilla is divided into an anterior segment containing the canine teeth and two posterior segments. The soft palate is completely and asymmetrically cleft in most patients. Numerous thick, fibrous bands traverse the lower mucobuccal fold frequently clefting the tongue into two or more lobes; small white, hamartomatous masses may be on the dorsal or ventral surfaces of the tongue or between the lobes. Ankyloglossia is present in a third of the cases. Malposition of the maxillary canine teeth, supernumerary maxillary deciduous canines and premolars, aplasia of the mandibular lateral incisors, infraocclusion, and hypoplasia of the mandible with a short ramus account for the more common oral anomalies. Malformations of the hands in decreasing order of frequency are clinodactyly, syndactyly, and brachydactyly. Alterations involving the feet are less common and include unilateral hallucal polysyndactyly and brachydactyly. The hallux is often inclined laterally with brachydactyly and hypoplasia of the second to fifth toes. The skin of affected infants frequently shows transient milia of the face and ears which usually disappear before the third year. More than half of the patients have dryness of the skin and alopecia of the scalp. Various anomalies of the CNS have been reported which include hydrocephaly, porencephaly, hydranencephaly, and partial agenesis of the corpus callosum. Polycystic kidneys have been reported in a few cases.

Specific Diagnosis The diagnosis of the syndrome is clinical. Radiographs of the hands and feet show irregularly short and thick tubular bones. Areas of osteoporosis may be seen in the metacarpals and phalanges. Cone-shaped epiphyses of the digits have been reported in some patients. Dermatoglyphic findings suggest a preponderance of whorls.

Differential Diagnosis This syndrome must be differentiated from the *Oral-facial-digital syndrome II (Mohr syndrome)* which has autosomal recessive inheritance. In *OFD II* there are no hyperplastic frenula, skin and hair are normal, the lower central incisors may be absent, and frequently there is a hearing defect. Central upper lip cleft in OFD I may be seen in the *Ellis-van Creveld syndrome,* while lateral displacement of the inner canthi and hypoplasia of the alar cartilage is common to the *Waardenburg syndrome.*

Prenatal Diagnosis It is conceivable in those pregnancies at risk that prenatal diagnosis could be made by fetoscopy or ultrasonography in those affected fetuses having polydactyly.

Basic Defect, Genetics, and Other Considerations The basic defect is not known. This condition is inherited as an X-linked dominant disorder limited to females and lethal in males. A patient with XXY was reported with this disorder which supports that inheritance pattern. The incidence of this syndrome is probably 0.0225 per 1000 live births.

Prognosis and Treatment Approximately a third of the patients die in early infancy. Mild mental retardation has been noted in over half the patients with the IQ ranging from 70–90. Polycystic renal disease may be a delayed manifestation of the syndrome. Treatment is directed toward surgical correction of the oral clefts and dental care.

REFERENCES

Gorlin, R.J. The oral-facial-digital (OFD) syndrome. *Cutis 4:* 1345–1349, 1968.

Jacquemart, C.J. et al. The oral-facial-digital syndromes reviewed: the role of computerized axial tomography in management. *Ariz. Med. 37:* 261–264, 1980.

Melnick, M. and Shields, E.D. Orofaciodigital syndrome, type I: a phenotypic and genetic analysis. *Oral Surg. 40:* 599–610, 1975.

M.R. [+ / most, mild]

- **thin nose / lack of alar flare / broad nasal root**
- **flat midface**
- **short upper lip / midline cleft**
- **digital anomalies**

Oral-Facial Digital Syndrome I

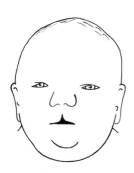
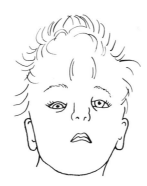
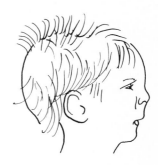

Note pseudocleft midline of upper lip, broad nasal root, small nares, down–turned mouth, dystopia canthorum and patchy alopecia

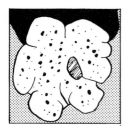
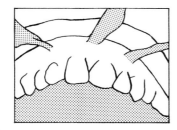
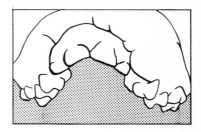

Cleft tongue with hamartoma

Multiple hyperplastic frenula

Maxilla divided into anterior segment and two posterior segments

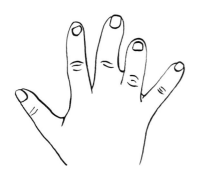
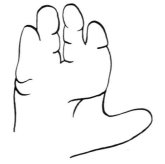
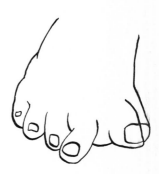

Brachydactyly/syndactyly of fingers – preaxial polysyndactyly of hallux

137. ORAL-FACIAL-DIGITAL SYNDROME II
(Mohr syndrome)

Clinical Features This syndrome can be recognized at birth and is characterized by the presence of cleft tongue, polydactyly of the hand, and bilateral polysyndactyly of the halluces. Facial features include low nasal bridge with a broad nasal tip which at times is slightly bifid. Frequently there is lateral displacement of the inner canthi and a midline cleft of the upper lip. Other facial features may be altered due to hypoplasia of the zygomatic arch, maxilla, and body of the mandible. A rather constant oral finding is a cleft tongue generally associated with a general ankyloglossia. Cleft palate and a bifid uvula have been reported in a few cases. Multiple frenula, missing central incisors, and fatty hamartomas have been reported in some patients. The skeletal changes generally are limited to the hands and feet, and consist of bilateral manual ulnar hexadactyly and bilateral polysyndactyly of the halluces. At times there may be one or more postminimus digits. Bimanual hexadactyly is not always present. There may be five fingers with ulnar deviation of the fifth, syndactyly of three and four with extra bones in the web, or hexadactyly of just one hand. Wormian cranial bones, scoliosis, and pectus excavatum have been occasionally described. Various CNS alterations have been noted which include internal hydrocephaly, microcephaly, porencephaly, conduction deafness due to a malformed incus, choroid coloboma, and muscular hypotonia with poor coordination. Cryptorchidism and inguinal hernia have been reported.

Specific Diagnosis The diagnosis of this syndrome is a clinical one based on the above features.

Radiographs of the feet show short, broad naviculars and first metatarsals, while the medial cuneiform bones may be broad or duplicated. Audiograms may reveal bilateral conductive hearing deficit.

Differential Diagnosis This syndrome can easily be differentiated from *OFD I* by the presence of bilateral polysyndactyly of the halluces, normal skin and hair, broad bifid tip of nose, and autosomal recessive inheritance. A true median cleft, bifid nose, and ocular hypertelorism may be seen in *frontonasal dysplasia*.

Prenatal Diagnosis In pregnancies at risk for this disorder sonography and fetoscopy could detect the hand and feet anomalies, thus making possible a prenatal diagnosis.

Basic Defect, Genetics, and Other Considerations The basic defect is not known. There are several families with affected sibs and parental consanguinity, supporting autosomal recessive inheritance.

Prognosis and Treatment There appears to be an increased susceptibility to respiratory infection which has resulted in death during infancy. Tachypnea has also been reported. Mental retardation has been observed in several patients. Stature tends to be moderately short. Treatment is symptomatic, consisting of proper treatment of respiratory infections, surgical treatment of ossicular defect, use of a hearing aid, removal of lingual hamartomas, and possible use of speech therapy.

REFERENCES

Gustavson, K.H., Krueger, A., and Petersson, P.O. Syndrome characterized by lingual malformation, polydactyly, tachypnea and psychomotor retardation. (Mohr syndrome). *Clin. Genet. 2:* 261–266, 1971.

Levy, E.P., Fletcher, B.D., and Fraser, F.C. Mohr syndrome with subclinical expression of bifid great toe. *Am. J. Dis. Child. 128:* 531–540, 1974.

Rimoin, D.L. and Edgerton, M.T. Genetic and clinical heterogeneity in the oral-facial-digital syndrome. *J. Pediatr. 71:* 94–102, 1967.

- cleft tongue
- low nasal bridge / broad nasal tip
- polydactyly of hands
- polysyndactyly of halluces

Oral-Facial-Digital Syndrome II
[Mohr syndrome]

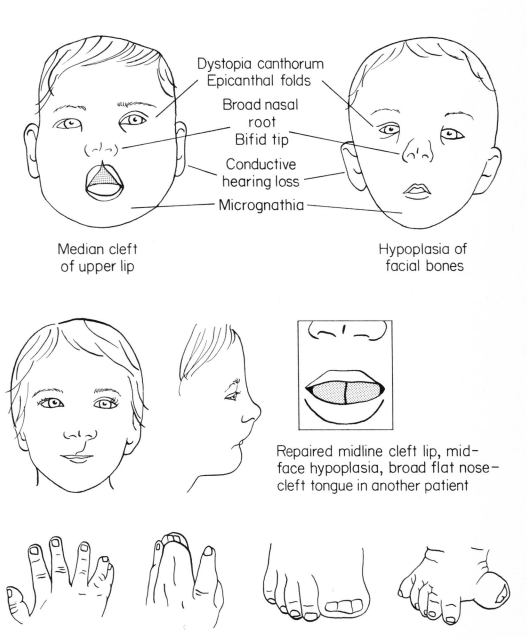

Dystopia canthorum
Epicanthal folds
Broad nasal root
Bifid tip
Conductive hearing loss
Micrognathia

Median cleft of upper lip

Hypoplasia of facial bones

Repaired midline cleft lip, mid-face hypoplasia, broad flat nose-cleft tongue in another patient

Digital anomalies of brachydactyly, syndactyly and polydactyly

295

138. OTOPALATODIGITAL SYNDROME

Clinical Features Affected males tend to have characteristic facies due to overhanging brows, prominent supraorbital ridges, low-set slanted ears with poorly modelled pinnae, broad nasal root, low vertical nasal bridge, hypertelorism, antimongoloid slant of palpebral fissures, increased mandibular angle, small mouth with downturned corners, and a flat midface. Cleft palate is common. Otologic studies have shown abnormalities of the ossicles with conduction deafness in some patients. Skeletal growth is retarded and all patients are below the 10th percentile. Pectus excavatum is common and the trunk is small. The occiput is prominent. The appearance of the hands and feet is quite characteristic. The thumb and hallux are spatulate and abbreviated. The clefting between the hallux and the rest of the toes is exaggerated. The toes and fingers are irregular in form and in direction of curvature. Limited elbow extension and wrist supination have been noted in several patients and some have shown subluxation of the radial heads. Females exhibit some features similar to, but usually much milder and more variable than, those of affected males.

Specific Diagnosis The above clinical features in conjunction with certain radiographic findings make for ease in diagnosis. The changes in the hands and feet, in combination with an altered relationship between the clivus and cervical vertebrae on skull roentgenograms appear to be pathognomonic for this syndrome in patients over five years of age. The hand findings include shortening of the radial side of the middle phalanx of the fifth finger, clinodactyly, short distal phalanx of the thumb which in develop-ment has a cone-shaped epiphysis, accessory ossification center of second metacarpal, tear-drop lesser multangular and transverse capitate. Female carriers have a higher frequency than normal of great multangular-navicular fusion.

Differential Diagnosis This disorder should be differentiated from the *Larsen syndrome* which also has joint dislocation and cleft palate. Unusual radiographic changes in the *Larsen syndrome* include the presence of multiple small carpal bones and juxtacalcaneal bone or bifid calcaneus. Dislocation of the radial heads may be seen in many disorders: *nail-patella syndrome, de Lange syndrome, Ehlers-Danlos syndromes, arthrogryposis,* etc.

Prenatal Diagnosis Has not yet been achieved for this syndrome.

Basic Defect, Genetics, and Other Considerations The basic defect is unknown. The condition is an X-linked recessive trait with some female carriers manifesting minimal features. More specifically, the carrier female may show mild skeletal alterations, hypertelorism, and lateral frontal prominence with lateral extension of eyebrows.

Prognosis and Treatment Male patients usually are mildly retarded. Speech development may be slow and this may be related to the conductive hearing loss. Chronic serous otitis media has been observed in several patients. None of the anomalies is life-threatening. Surgical intervention may be indicated to repair the cleft palate and improve the hearing.

REFERENCES

Gall, J.C. Jr., Stern, A.M., Poznanski, A.K. et al. Oto-palato-digital syndrome: comparison of clinical and radiologic manifestations in males and females. *Am. J. Hum. Genet. 24:* 24–36, 1972.

Gorlin, R.J., Poznanski, A.K., and Hendon, I. The oto-palato-digital (OPD) syndrome in females. *Oral Surg. 35:* 218–224, 1973.

Salinas, C.F., Jorgenson, R.J., and Lorenzo, R.L. Variable expression in otopalato-digital syndrome; cleft palate in females. *Birth Defects 15(5B):* 329–345, 1979.

- **prominent occiput**
- **overhanging brows**
- **flat midface / small mouth**
- **spatulate thumbs-hallux / irregular digits**

Otopalatodigital Syndrome

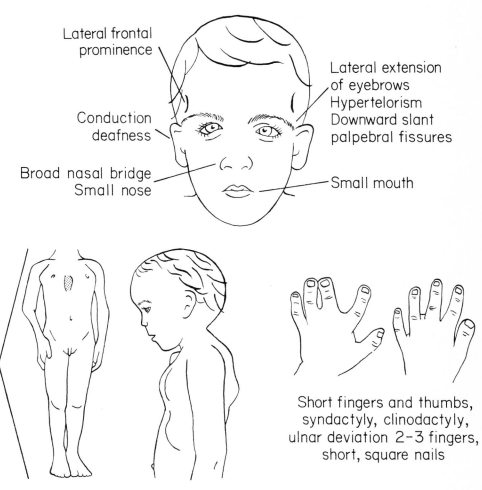

Lateral frontal prominence

Lateral extension of eyebrows
Hypertelorism
Downward slant palpebral fissures

Conduction deafness

Broad nasal bridge
Small nose

Small mouth

Short stature

Short fingers and thumbs, syndactyly, clinodactyly, ulnar deviation 2–3 fingers, short, square nails

Elbow deformity, pectus excavatum, small nose and occipital bossing

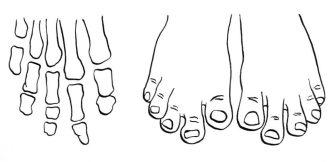

Short, broad hallux, toes irregular in form and curvature

139. PFEIFFER SYNDROME

Clinical Features The disorder can be recognized at birth and consists of craniosynostosis resulting in turribrachycephaly, broad thumbs and great toes, and variable partial cutaneous soft tissue syndactyly of the hands and feet. Additional craniofacial features include depressed nasal bridge, hypertelorism, antimongoloid slant to the palpebral fissures, proptosis, strabismus, maxillary hypoplasia with relative mandibular prognathism, facial asymmetry in some patients, low-set ears, and occasionally a cloverleaf skull deformity. Reported oral manifestations are high-arched palate, malocclusion and crowding of the teeth and, rarely, bifid uvula. The thumbs and great toes are broad and usually show varus deformity. In some patients the great toes may be shortened but without varus deformity. Cutaneous syndactyly is usually present, involving digits two and three and at times three and four of both hands and feet. Clinodactyly and symphalangism of both hands and feet have been reported. Other features occasionally seen are pyloric stenosis, bicuspid aortic valve, hypoplasia of the gallbladder, single umbilical artery, umbilical hernia, preauricular tags, hearing loss, choanal atresia, various CNS anomalies when the cloverleaf skull deformity is present, and a variety of other malformations.

Specific Diagnosis The diagnosis of this disorder is a clinical one based on the above features plus certain skeletal radiographic findings which include the following: craniosynostosis (especially coronal), increased digital markings with age, maxillary hypoplasia, shallow orbits, brachymesophalangy of hands and feet, absence of middle phalanges in some cases, usually a trapezoidal shape to the proximal phalanges of the thumbs and great toes with varus deformity of the big toes. Other radiographic findings may involve fusion of numerous bones such as carpals, tarsals, proximal ends of metacarpals and metatarsals, fused vertebrae, and radiohumeral and radioulnar synostoses.

Differential Diagnosis The Pfeiffer syndrome must be differentiated from other *craniosynostosis syndromes,* mainly the *Apert* and *Saethre-Chotzen* syndromes. Facially it is similar to the *Apert syndrome* but in the latter the degree of syndactyly involving the digits is extreme and characteristic. The facial findings of asymmetry, low hairline, and beaking of the nose in the *Saethre-Chotzen syndrome* are not typical of the Pfeiffer syndrome. In *Crouzon syndrome* the hands are normal. Other syndromes have large thumbs and toes but their facial features are much different from those in the Pfeiffer syndrome.

Prenatal Diagnosis To the best of our knowledge this disorder has not yet been diagnosed prenatally, but the digital findings when severe could possibly be recognized using fetoscopy and sonography.

Basic Defect, Genetics, and Other Considerations The basic defect is not known. This relatively rare syndrome is transmitted as an autosomal dominant with complete penetrance and variable expressivity. Sporadic cases have been reported but no increased paternal age effect has been noted. More information is needed on the variability in the phenotypic expression of this condition.

Prognosis and Treatment Intellect is usually normal but mental retardation has been described in some patients. Depending on the severity of craniosynostosis, the facial appearance tends to improve with age. Surgical correction of the cutaneous syndactyly is possible in more severe cases.

REFERENCES

Baraitser, M., Bowen-Bravery, M., and Saldana-Garcia, P. Pitfalls of genetic counselling in Pfeiffer's syndrome. *J. Med. Genet. 17:* 250–256, 1980.

Martsolf, J.T., Cracco, J.B., Carpenter, G.G. et al. Pfeiffer syndrome: an unusual type of acrocephalo-syndactyly with broad thumbs and great toes. *Am. J. Dis. Child. 121:* 257–262, 1971.

Naveh, Y. and Friedman, A. Pfeiffer syndrome: a report of the family and review of the literature. *J. Med. Genet. 13:* 277–280, 1976.

- **turribrachycephaly**
- **broad thumbs / halluces / syndactyly**
- **proptosis / strabismus**
- **midface hypoplasia / prognathism**

Pfeiffer Syndrome

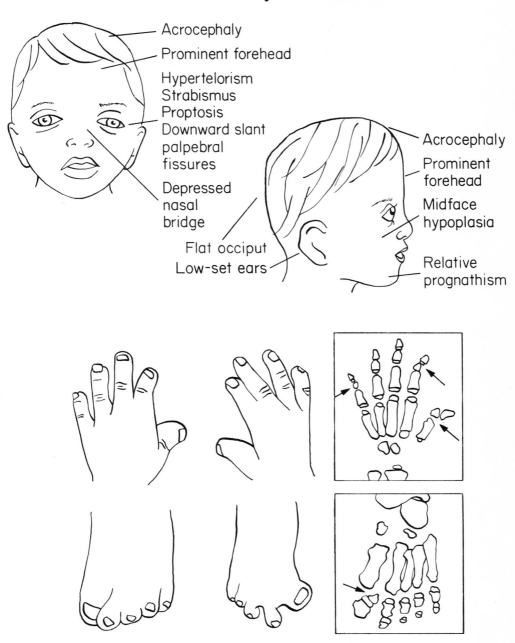

Acrocephaly
Prominent forehead
Hypertelorism
Strabismus
Proptosis
Downward slant palpebral fissures
Depressed nasal bridge
Flat occiput
Low-set ears

Acrocephaly
Prominent forehead
Midface hypoplasia
Relative prognathism

Broad distal phalanges of thumb and hallux with medial deviation, partial syndactyly fingers 2–3, toes 2–4, small middle phalanges of fingers (arrows), and delta proximal phalanx of thumb and hallux (arrows)

140. PROGRESSIVE HEMIFACIAL ATROPHY
(Parry-Romberg syndrome)

Clinical Features Facial changes usually appear during the first decade of life and tend to involve the paramedian part of the face. The condition slowly progresses and spreads so that atrophy of the underlying muscle, bone, and cartilage soon becomes apparent. From the initial site of the temporal or buccinator muscles, the process extends to the brow, angle of the mouth, neck, and may even involve half the body. The left side of the face tends to be more involved than the right. Frequently the overlying skin becomes darkly pigmented. Atrophy of half of the upper lip and tongue is common. The maxillary teeth on the involved side are exposed. Loss of periorbital fat produces enophthalmos. Resolution of bone may cause the outer canthus to be displaced downward. Muscular paralysis, ptosis of the eyelid, and inability to shut the eyes completely have been described. The Horner syndrome, heterochromia iridis, and dilated and fixed pupil have also been noted. The affected side may exhibit circumscribed but complete alopecia limited to the paramedian scalp area, eyelashes, and median portion of the eyebrow. Blanching of the hair has been observed in some patients. Such neurologic findings as trigeminal neuralgia and/or facial paresthesia may appear early and precede the rest of the changes. Migraine is a common finding. Epilepsy of the sensory Jacksonian type often appears later in the disease process.

Specific Diagnosis The diagnosis of this disorder is a clinical one based on the above features.

Radiographic studies of the jaw have shown that the body and ramus of the mandible are shorter on the involved side and that there is a delay in development. The teeth on the involved side may be retarded in eruption or may have atrophic roots.

Differential Diagnosis *Congenital facial hypoplasia* can be differentiated from this disorder by its presence at birth and diminution in the size of teeth on the involved side. Other conditions to be considered include the *oculoauriculovertebral syndrome, fat necrosis,* and *scleroderma.*

Prenatal Diagnosis Prenatal diagnosis is not possible as the initial findings occur during childhood.

Basic Defect, Genetics, and Other Considerations The basic defect is not known. Some patients give a history of prior trauma. Most emphasis has been placed on alterations in the peripheral trophic sympathetic system. The majority of cases have been sporadic but a few familial instances have been reported.

Prognosis and Treatment In general the condition slowly progresses for several years and then becomes stationary for the rest of life. The average progress of the disease lasts about three years. Hemografts from the abdomen and other parts of the body have been helpful in improving the facial appearance.

REFERENCES

Muchnick, R.S., Aston, S.J., and Rees, T.D. Ocular manifestations and treatment of hemifacial atrophy. *Am. J. Ophthalmol. 88:* 889–897, 1979.

Rees, T.D., Facial atrophy. *Clin. Plast. Surg. 3:* 637–646, 1976.

Wells, J.H. and Edgerton, M.T. Correction of severe hemifacial atrophy with a free dermis flap from the lower abdomen. *Plast. Reconstr. Surg. 59:* 223–230, 1977.

- unilateral facial atrophy
- left side more affected
- hyperpigmentation of overlying skin
- upper lip / tongue involvement

Progressive Hemifacial Atrophy
[Parry-Romberg syndrome]

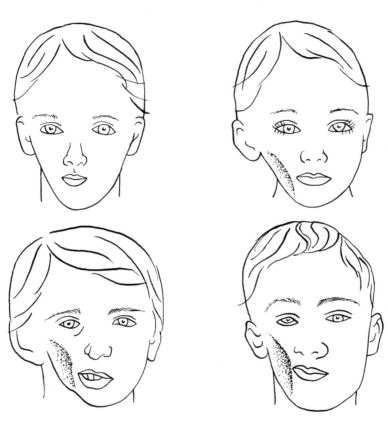

Increased severity of disorder in patients

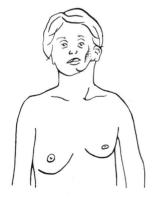

Half of body involved

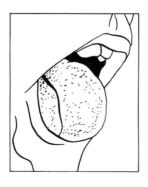

Atrophy of half of tongue

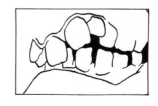

Severe dental malocclusion

301

141. RIEGER SYNDROME

Clinical Features The disorder is characterized mainly by a reduction in the number of teeth, associated with anomalies involving the anterior chamber of the eye. The eye findings consist of hypoplasia of the iris and anterior synechiae running from the iris to the cornea across the anterior chamber. In most instances these patients have slit-like pupils due to the traction of the synechiae. Posterior embryotoxon, which is an unusual prominence and forward displacement of the Schwalbe line appearing like an encircling glass rod inside the limbus, is a constant feature. Other eye findings may include microcornea, megalocornea, corneal opacity, iris coloboma, blue sclerae, aniridia, glaucoma, and strabismus. Mild telecanthus with or without hypertelorism is present in approximately half the patients. As these individuals develop, they tend to show certain common facial features. A broad, flat nasal root, prominent supraorbital ridges, and relative prognathism with a protruding lower lip due to underdevelopment of the maxilla or to loss of vertical height because of the oligodontia have been described. The maxillary incisors, less often mandibular incisors, are commonly missing. Peg-shaped crowns of the lower incisors and canines are frequently observed. Microdontia occurs in about 80%. Anal stenosis has been noted in some cases. Meckel's diverticulum has recently been described in this syndrome. Failure of the periumbilical skin to involute properly is seen in at least 75% of the patients.

Specific Diagnosis The diagnosis of this syndrome is a clinical one based on the above features.

Differential Diagnosis A distinct *autosomal recessive syndrome* has been described with the eye anomalies of the Rieger syndrome in conjunction with severe growth retardation, inguinal hernia, joint hypermobility, deep-set eyes, and delayed teething. Absence of teeth and conical crown formation can be noted in several disorders including *hypohidrotic ectodermal dysplasia, chondroectodermal dysplasia,* and *incontinentia pigmenti.*

Prenatal Diagnosis This disorder has not yet been diagnosed prenatally.

Basic Defect, Genetics, and Other Considerations The basic defect is not known but is thought to be a developmental aberration of the mesodermal and possibly ectodermal germ layers of the anterior ocular segment. The condition is rare and its frequency has been estimated to be 1 per 200,000 population. Mode of inheritance is autosomal dominant with almost complete penetrance and extreme variability in expression.

Prognosis and Treatment These patients have normal intelligence and their life span is not impaired. Vision may be poor and proper evaluation of the eye defects with possible surgical intervention is often indicated. Specific eye problems include control of glaucoma, cataract extraction, and possible corneal transplant and enucleation to relieve pain.

REFERENCES

Feingold, M., Shiere, F., Fogels, H.R. et al. Rieger's syndrome. *Pediatr. 44:* 564–569, 1969.

Jorgenson, R.L., Levin, L.S., Cross, H.E. et al. The Rieger syndrome. *Am. J. Med. Genet. 2:* 307–318, 1978.

Langdon, J.D. Rieger's syndrome. *Oral Surg., 30:* 788–795, 1970.

- **anterior chamber eye anomalies**
- **midface hypoplasia / prognathism**
- **short philtrum**
- **hypodontia**

Rieger Syndrome

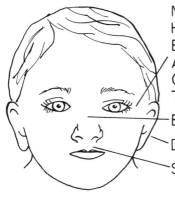

Microcornea
Hypoplasia of iris
Blue sclerae
Aniridia
Glaucoma
Telecanthus
Broad nasal root
Dysplastic ears
Short philtrum

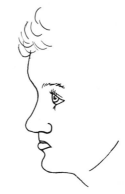

Midfacial hypoplasia with prognathism, protruding lower lip, short philtrum

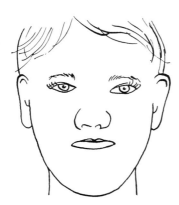

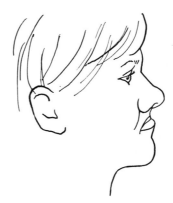

Older patient with more advanced changes

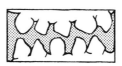

Hypodontia with cone-shaped teeth

142. ROBERTS SYNDROME

Clinical Features The main features of the syndrome recognizable at birth include bilateral cleft lip/palate, tetraphocomelia with reduced number of digits, ocular proptosis with hypertelorism, and growth deficiency. Bilateral cleft lip with or without cleft palate is present in almost all patients. Additional findings may include colobomas of the eyelids, shallow orbits, bluish sclerae, cataracts, and corneal opacity. The external ears tend to be dysplastic and rudimentary. Other common craniofacial features are microbrachycephaly, midfacial capillary hemangioma, thin nares, and sparse, silvery-blond scalp hair. Limb malformations are almost all symmetric aplasias or hypoplasias of all the bones resulting in shortening of the limbs and sometimes phocomelia. Most commonly absent are the radius alone, radius and ulna, fibula, and marginal digits. In nearly all cases, the number of digits has been reduced more frequently in the hands than in the feet. Malposition of the thumb is a frequent finding. Cutaneous syndactyly is seen in approximately 70% of patients. Low birth weight (less than 2200 g) and growth deficiency are common. Although an enlarged phallus has been described, it is possible that the marked growth deficiency in this disorder may account for making a normal-sized phallus appear enlarged. Cryptorchidism is found in most affected males. In females a vaginal septum, enlarged clitoris, and cleft labia minora have been reported. Occasional anomalies include frontal encephalocele, hydrocephalus, spina bifida, short neck, atrial septal defect, patent ductus arteriosus, bicornuate uterus, polycystic kidneys, and horseshoe-shaped kidney.

Specific Diagnosis The diagnosis of this syndrome is a clinical one. Based on a review of the literature, about 75% of all reported cases showed (1) tetraphocomelia, (2) cleft lip (bilateral) and palate, (3) ectrodactyly and malposition of the thumb, (4) syndactyly, (5) ocular hypertelorism with exophthalmus at birth, (6) prominent clitoris or penis at birth, (7) cryptorchidism, (8) low birth weight, and (9) failure to thrive either in utero or after delivery.

Differential Diagnosis This syndrome must be differentiated from the *pseudothalidomide syndrome*. Some think these two disorders are the same, while others (we) consider them as separate entities. Cleft lip/palate, ocular proptosis, hypertelorism, genital abnormalities, and a higher frequency of renal anomalies seen in the Roberts syndrome help to differentiate it from the pseudothalidomide syndrome. In *thalidomide embryopathy* the limbs are usually asymmetrically malformed. Hypoplastic limbs may be seen in the *TAR syndrome (thromocytopenia-aplasia of radius)* but cleft palate is not a feature.

Prenatal Diagnosis Possible in this syndrome, but the accuracy of using sonography or fetoscopy will depend on the severity of the limb anomalies. The chromosome changes described below can also serve to diagnosis this condition prenatally and this method has been used in some families at risk.

Basic Defect, Genetics, and Other Considerations The basic defect is not known. Prophase and metaphase chromosomes in this disorder have shown premature sister-chromatid separation and interphase nuclei have exhibited a striking distortion in their contours. These findings have been interpreted as evidence for the presence of a genetically determined disturbance affecting the normal mechanism for pairing and disjoining of sister chromatids. Although most cases have been sporadic, there is good evidence for autosomal recessive inheritance, as families with multiple affected sibs and close parental consanguinity have been reported.

Prognosis and Treatment Most cases are stillborn or die in early infancy. Those who survive show marked growth deficiency and many are mentally retarded. When indicated, surgical intervention should be considered for repair of the various anomalies.

REFERENCES

Freeman, M.V.R., Williams, D.W., Schimke, R.N. et al. The Roberts syndrome. *Clin. Genet. 5:* 1–16, 1974.

German, J. Roberts' syndrome. I. Cytological evidence for a disturbance in chromatid pairing. *Clin. Genet. 16:* 441–447, 1979.

Herrmann, J. and Opitz, J.M. The SC phocomelia and the Roberts syndrome: nosologic aspects. *Europ. J. Pediatr. 125:* 117–134, 1977.

M.R. [+ / most]

- **tetraphocomelia**
- **cleft lip [bilateral] / palate**
- **ectrodactyly / mal-position of thumbs**
- **hypertelorism / exophthalmos**

Roberts Syndrome

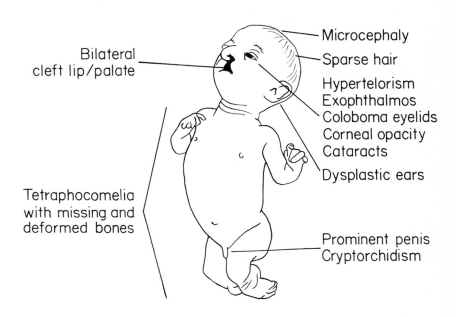

Bilateral cleft lip/palate

Microcephaly

Sparse hair

Hypertelorism
Exophthalmos
Coloboma eyelids
Corneal opacity
Cataracts

Dysplastic ears

Tetraphocomelia with missing and deformed bones

Prominent penis
Cryptorchidism

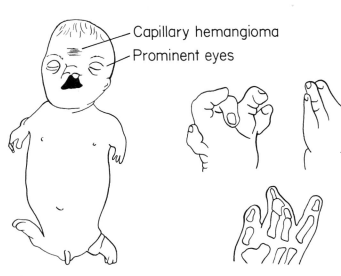

Capillary hemangioma
Prominent eyes

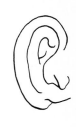

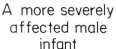

A more severely affected male infant

Malformed hands with hypoplastic or absent thumbs, ectrodactyly and syndactyly

Malformed ear with hypoplastic lobule

143. RUBINSTEIN-TAYBI SYNDROME

Clinical Features The syndrome is recognizable at birth and is characterized by the presence of distinct facies, mental retardation, and broad thumbs and toes. The unusual facial appearance is characterized by microcephaly, prominent forehead, antimongoloid obliquity of the palpebral fissures, epicanthal folds, strabismus, broad nasal bridge, beaked nose with the nasal septum extending below the alae, and mild micrognathia. Other findings may include heavy eyebrows; long eyelashes; ptosis of eyelids; hypertelorism; nasolacrimal duct obstruction; refractive error; minor abnormalities in the shape, position, and degree of rotation of the ears; and nevus flammeus about the forehead. Grimacing or an unusual smile frequently is observed. A high-arched palate and dental malocclusion are frequent, while bifid uvula and tongue, macroglossia, short lingual frenum, and thin upper lip are only rarely observed. Characteristically broad thumbs and halluces are present. In most instances the terminal phalanges of the fingers are also broad. Angulation deformities of the thumbs and halluces together with abnormally shaped proximal phalanges are common. Clinodactyly of the fifth finger and overlapping of the toes are present in more than 50% of the patients. Hexadactyly of the feet, partial cutaneous syndactyly of the toes, and absence of the distal phalanx of the hallux have been reported occasionally. Skeletal anomalies include short stature, pectus excavatum, kyphoscoliosis, and lordosis. Although the gait may be stiff, patients tend to be hypotonic with lax ligaments and hyperextensible joints. Numerous other findings have been reported some of which include congenital heart disease, supernumerary nipples, absence of the corpus callosum, hyperactive deep-tendon reflexes, hirsutism, cryptorchidism, hypospadias, angulation of penis, and various anomalies of the urinary tract such as duplication of the kidney and ureter and renal agenesis.

Specific Diagnosis The diagnosis of this syndrome is a clinical one based on the above features and certain radiographic and dermatoglyphic findings. Radiographs show broad and enlarged digits, frequently enlarged anterior fontanel with delayed closure, foramen magnum and parietal foramina; vertebral, sternal and rib anomalies, flat acetabular angles, flared ilia, and delayed bone age. Significant dermatoglyphic findings include an increased frequency of thenar, interdigital, and hypothenar patterns. Simian creases have been observed in many patients.

Differential Diagnosis In the newborn period this disorder may be confused with the *de Lange syndrome* and *trisomy 13*. Broad thumbs may be seen in the *Apert* and *Pfeiffer syndromes*. When the classical features of the syndrome are not present, it is best not to consider such individuals as having an "incomplete form" of the syndrome.

Prenatal Diagnosis Although distinct clinical features of this syndrome are present at birth, it is not known whether such findings would be recognizable, using current diagnostic means, early in fetal development.

Basic Defect, Genetics, and Other Considerations The basic defect is not known. Almost all cases have been sporadic. Affected sibs, identical twins, and consanguinity have rarely been noted. Normal karyotypes are the rule, although inconsistent chromosomal variations have been reported occasionally. The frequency in the mentally retarded population has been variously estimated between 1 : 267 and 1 : 720. The frequency in the general population is unknown. Parental age does not seem to be a factor. The syndrome has been reported from many parts of the world.

Prognosis and Treatment All patients show mental, motor, language, and social retardation. In the majority of cases the IQ is below 50. During infancy feeding problems and upper respiratory infections are common. Life span is shortened in these patients, but to what extent is not accurately known. Treatment is supportive.

REFERENCES

Atasu, M.J. Dermatoglyphic findings in Rubinstein-Taybi syndrome. *J. Ment. Defic. Res. 23:* 111–121, 1979.

Padfield, C.J., Partington, M.W., and Simpson, N.E. The Rubinstein-Taybi syndrome. *Arch. Dis. Child. 43:* 94–101, 1968.

Rubinstein, J.H.: The broad thumbs syndrome—progress report, 1968. *Birth Defects,* 5(2): 25–41, 1969.

- microcephaly
- long eyelashes / heavy eyebrows
- beaked nose
- broad thumbs / halluces

Rubinstein-Taybi Syndrome

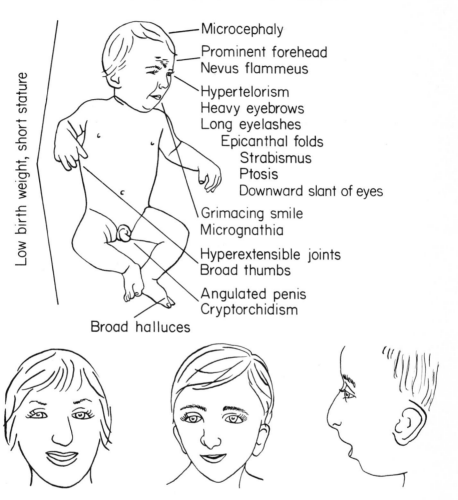

Low birth weight, short stature

Microcephaly
Prominent forehead
Nevus flammeus

Hypertelorism
Heavy eyebrows
Long eyelashes
Epicanthal folds
Strabismus
Ptosis
Downward slant of eyes

Grimacing smile
Micrognathia

Hyperextensible joints
Broad thumbs

Angulated penis
Cryptorchidism

Broad halluces

Note heavy eyebrows, long eyelashes, beaking nose, low-set ears, micrognathia and grimacing smile

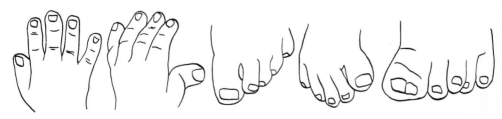

Broad thumbs, halluces with angulation, brachydactyly, clinodactyly and polydactyly

144. RUSSELL-SILVER SYNDROME

Clinical Features At birth affected infants are unusually small for gestational age. Their pattern of growth usually parallels the normal growth curve but remains below the 3rd percentile. One of the main features of this syndrome is asymmetry which is present at birth but can be quite variable in extent and degree. In some, one entire side of the body may be significantly larger than the other, while in others the asymmetry may be limited and involve only the skull, spine, or all or part of a limb. The heads of these children are disproportionately large for the small facial mass which tapers to a narrow jaw, producing the characteristic triangular-shaped face. On facial profile patients tend to show frontal bossing and mandibular hypoplasia. Other facial features include prominent eyes, long eye lashes, and thin lips with the corners of the mouth turned down. The palate is high and narrow and the teeth are crowded. Variation in sexual development has been found in approximately 30% of patients. There is usually normal puberty and rarely cryptorchidism, enlarged clitoris, or hypospadias. Other findings include clinodactyly of the fifth fingers, syndactyly between second and third toes, poor muscular development, delay in early gross motor performance, cafe-au-lait spots, hyperhidrosis, renal, ureteral, and cardiac anomalies, and rarely mild mental retardation.

Specific Diagnosis Basically this is a clinical diagnosis determined by the above findings. Those infants who display many of the above features but have no asymmetry have been termed the "Russell variant" of the Russell-Silver syndrome. Various radiographic alterations may be noted which include the following: delayed closure of the anterior fontanel, retarded bone age in relation to sexual development and chronologic age, hip or bone dislocation, shortened humerus, clinodactyly with hypoplasia of the middle phalanges of the fifth fingers and pseudoepiphyses at the base of the second metacarpals. Urinary gonadotropin levels have been elevated in about 10% of patients. Hypo-glycemia following short periods of fasting has been reported in some individuals.

Differential Diagnosis Clinically the syndrome must be differentiated from a multitude of conditions associated with short stature and precocious sexual development. There is similarity in phenotype to those with autosomal recessive *mulibrey nanism* (short stature, mild hypotonia, pericardial constriction, and hypoplastic choroid). Cafe-au-lait spots may be seen with *neurofibromatosis, hemihypertrophy, McCune-Albright syndrome* and the *Klippel-Trenaunay-Weber* syndrome.

Prenatal Diagnosis Not yet possible in this disorder.

Basic Defect, Genetics, and Other Considerations The basic defect in this syndrome is not known. The finding of elevated levels of growth hormone in a few cases suggests that short stature may be due to an unresponsiveness to this hormone, however, there has been a normal response to the administration of this hormone. Almost all of the 100 or more cases reported have been sporadic. A few familial instances have been recorded, suggesting autosomal dominant inheritance, while the great majority of cases probably represent a fresh gene mutation in the affected individual. Monozygotic twins concordant for the syndrome have been reported. Genetic heterogeneity may be present in terms of the "Russell variant" without asymmetry. This syndrome has been reported in association with various chromosomal disorders such as 45X/46XY mosaicism, XXY, 18 trisomy mosaicism, and 18 short-arm deletion.

Prognosis and Treatment Adult height ranges from 147 to 153 cm. Approximately one-third of the patients have some degree of mental retardation. Functional impairment depends on the degree of asymmetry, but most patients have no functional disturbance. Treatment is symptomatic. Periodic examination is indicated to rule out the presence of a tumor of the kidney or adrenal.

REFERENCES

Escobar, V., Gleiser, S., and Weaver, D.D. Phenotypic and genetic analysis of the Silver-Russell syndrome. *Clin. Genet. 13:* 278–288, 1978.

Gareis, F.J., Smith, D.W., and Summitt, R.C. The Russell-Silver syndrome without asymmetry. *J. Pediatr. 79:* 775–781, 1971.

Tanner, J.M., Lejarraga, H., and Cameron, N. The natural history of the Silver-Russell syndrome: a longitudinal study of thirty-nine cases. *Pediatr. Res. 9:* 611–623, 1975.

M.R. [+ / few,
    mild]

• **asymmetry body /
  limb / face**
• **triangular face /
  long eyelashes**
• **frontal bossing**
• **micrognathia**

Russell-Silver Syndrome

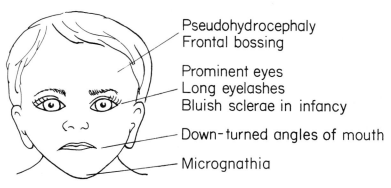

Pseudohydrocephaly
Frontal bossing

Prominent eyes
Long eyelashes
Bluish sclerae in infancy

Down-turned angles of mouth

Micrognathia

Small triangular face with facial asymmetry

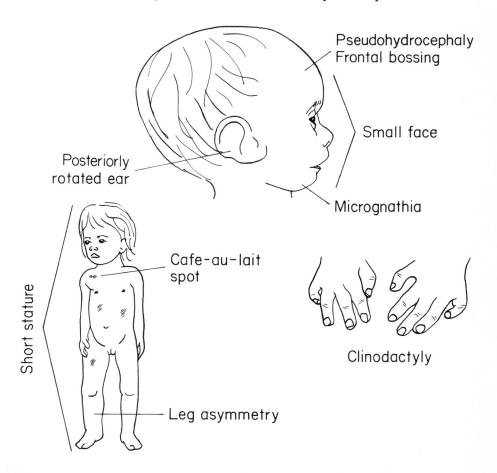

Pseudohydrocephaly
Frontal bossing

Small face

Posteriorly
rotated ear

Micrognathia

Cafe-au-lait
spot

Short stature

Clinodactyly

Leg asymmetry

145. SAETHRE-CHOTZEN SYNDROME

Clinical Features Although the time of onset and degree of craniosynostosis usually involving the coronal sutures are variable, altered facial features may be present at birth. Asymmetrical involvement producing plagiocephaly and facial asymmetry is common, with a tendency for the left side to be more frequently affected. Acrocephaly is more commonly noted, but scaphocephaly has been observed in some instances. Frontal and parietal bossing and flattened occiput also have been described. Head circumference is reduced and often there is a low frontal hairline. Eye findings consist of strabismus, myopia, and hyperopia, eyelid ptosis, hypertelorism, optic atrophy, and occasionally lacrimal duct abnormalities. Oral features include peg-shaped or missing maxillary lateral incisors in half the patients. High arched or narrow palate, cleft palate, mandibular prognathism and enamel hypoplasia have been described in some cases. The ears may be dysplastic with folded helices, prominent antihelices, small, posteriorly rotated, and even low-set. A minor degree of hearing loss is common. The nose tends to be beaked with deviation of the nasal septum. The nasofrontal angle is flattened in some patients. Partial cutaneous syndactyly can be observed frequently between the second and third fingers and occasionally extending to the fourth finger. Similar changes can also involve the toes along with hallux valgus. Brachydactyly, including short fourth metacarpals, bifid terminal hallucal phalanx, radioulnar synostosis, and fifth finger clinodactyly have been reported. Other findings include short stature, cryptorchidism, renal anomalies, and congenital heart disease in a few cases.

Specific Diagnosis The diagnosis of this syndrome is a clinical one based on the above features in combination with abnormal roentgenographic and dermatoglyphic findings. Skeletal alterations usually show coronal synostosis, reduced length of posterior cranial base, low position of sella turcica, reduced facial depth, steep mandibular plane angle, and absence or reduced size of cranial sinuses. Dermatoglyphic changes include simian creases, distally placed axial triradii, increased frequency of thenar and hypothenar patterns, and low total ridge count.

Differential Diagnosis Since syndactyly is not a consistent finding in this disorder, an isolated case without this feature may be confused with the *Crouzon, Apert, Pfeiffer,* or *Weiss* syndromes or even *simple craniosynostosis.*

Prenatal Diagnosis To the best of our knowledge this disorder has not been diagnosed early in prenatal development. It is conceivable that in a pregnancy at risk, where the fetus was markedly affected, sonography may be able to detect some of the abnormal cranial features, but such a postulation awaits confirmation.

Basic Defect, Genetics, and Other Considerations The basic defect is not known. This relatively common form of craniosynostosis is transmitted as an autosomal dominant trait with complete penetrance and variable expressivity. In instances of a new mutation, advanced paternal age may be a factor.

Prognosis and Treatment Intelligence is usually normal, but mild to moderate mental retardation has been noted. It is not known whether this is secondary to the craniosynostosis. With growth during childhood the facial appearance tends to improve. At times surgical intervention may be necessary for correction of the premature sutural fusion, to improve the facial appearance. Plastic surgery can be helpful for the ptosis and tear duct anomalies. Glasses are indicated for correcting the refractive errors.

REFERENCES

Friedman, J.M., Hanson, J.W., Graham, C.B. et al. Saethre-Chotzen syndrome: a broad and variable pattern of skeletal malformations. *J. Pediatr. 91:* 929–932, 1977.

Kopysc, Z., Stanska, M., Ryzko, J. et al. The Saethre-Chotzen syndrome: partial bifidity of the distal phalanges of the great toes. *Hum. Genet. 56:* 195–204, 1980.

Pantke, O.A., Cohen, M.M. Jr., Witkop, C.J. Jr. et al. The Saethre-Chotzen syndrome. *Birth Defects 11(2):* 190–225, 1975.

M.R. [+ / few]

- **craniosynostosis / frontal-parietal bossing**
- **strabismus / hyper-telorism / ptosis**
- **dysplastic ears**
- **beaked nose / deviation of septum**

Saethre-Chotzen Syndrome

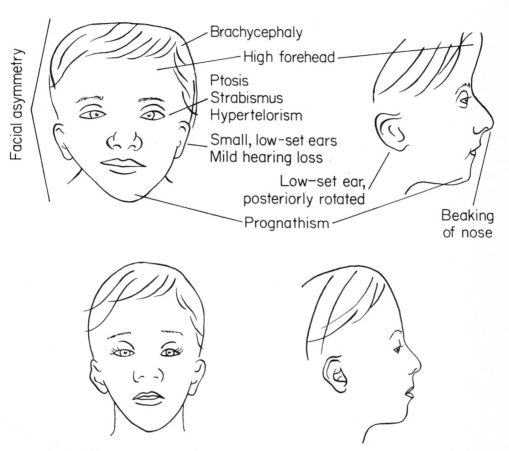

Facial asymmetry

Brachycephaly
High forehead
Ptosis
Strabismus
Hypertelorism
Small, low-set ears
Mild hearing loss
Low-set ear, posteriorly rotated
Prognathism
Beaking of nose

Older child with similar craniofacial features as noted above

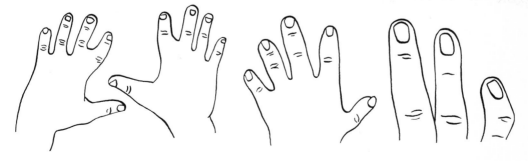

Cutaneous syndactyly between 2nd and 3rd fingers, brachydactyly with short 4th metacarpal and clinodactyly

311

146. SCHWARTZ-JAMPEL SYNDROME

Clinical Features An infant with this disorder may appear normal at birth but by the end of the first year or during the second year distinct physical findings become apparent. Because of tonic contraction of facial muscles, the facies develops a pinched, immobile mask-like appearance with puckered lips and narrow palpebral fissures due to medial displacement of the outer canthi. Other eye anomalies include increased distance between the inner angles of the eyes, intermittent unilateral ptosis, microcornea, microphthalmus, bilateral pseudoptosis, severe myopia, juvenile cataract, and eyelashes inserted in two or several rows instead of the normal single row. Skeletal deformities include short neck, pectus carinatum, kyphoscoliosis, hip dysplasia, and joint contractures. Limitation of motion at the hips is usually evident within the first six months of life. The gait becomes waddling and progressively difficult because of stiff hips and knees. Height is 2 standard deviations below the mean for age in children. Average adult height is 150 cm. The skeletal muscles tend to be small, show increased consistency, and display generalized hypertrophy. Repetitive contractures decrease the myotonia. Other associated anomalies may include transient lactosuria, umbilical and/or inguinal hernia, small testicles, patency of anal sphincter, high pitched voice, and high-arched palate.

Specific Diagnosis At present the diagnosis of this syndrome is a clinical one. The presence of muscle disease with myotonia is one of the essential features of the syndrome but is easily overlooked because the skeletal and oculofacial abnormalities are so predominant. Electromyography should be done to show the presence of myotonia. Ultrastructural studies of muscle have shown increased glycogen and electron-dense lamellar bodies along with vacuolization of muscle fibers.

Differential Diagnosis The facies in this syndrome shows a resemblance to that seen in *craniocarpotarsal dysplasia* and in the *Marden-Walker syndrome* but when viewed in its entirety the Schwartz-Jampel syndrome can be easily differentiated from these conditions. Growth retardation, platyspondyly, and hip dysplasia are seen in the *Morquio syndrome,* but again this disorder can be excluded based on other clinical and radiographic grounds. *Familial myotonia* may be seen in a number of conditions.

Prenatal Diagnosis At present this condition has not been diagnosed prenatally.

Basic Defect, Genetics, and Other Considerations The basic defect in this syndrome is not known although the main tissues involved are of mesodermal origin. It is thought that there is a generalized defect of enchondral ossification accounting for the retarded growth rate and anomalies of the face and skeleton. This is considered to be a rare syndrome inherited as an autosomal recessive trait. Parental consanguinity has been noted.

Prognosis and Treatment Patients have normal intelligence. There is no evidence that life expectancy is altered, although choking on cold liquids has been described during early childhood. Surgical intervention may be indicated to improve the ocular and skeletal abnormalities. Indistinct speech and drooling may persist beyond the age of two years. Spontaneous improvement in the myotonia during childhood has been noted in several cases.

REFERENCES

Aberfeld, D.C., Hinterbuchner, L.P., and Schneider, M. Myotonia, dwarfism, diffuse bone disease and unusual ocular and facial abnormalities (a new syndrome). *Brain 88:* 313–322, 1965.

Beighton, P. The Schwartz syndrome in southern Africa. *Clin. Genet. 4:* 548–555, 1973.

Fowler, W.M. Jr., Layzer, R.B., Taylor, R.G. et al. The Schwartz-Jampel syndrome: its clinical, physiological and histological expressions. *J. Neurol. Sci. 22:* 127–146, 1974.

- **pinched facies / puckered lips**
- **blepharophimosis / eye anomalies**
- **joint contractures / kyphoscoliosis**
- **pectus carinatum**

Schwartz-Jampel Syndrome

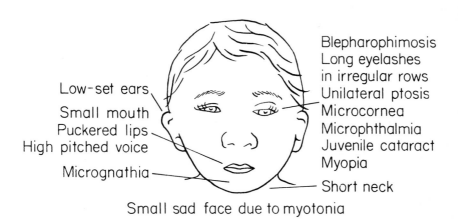

Low-set ears
Small mouth
Puckered lips
High pitched voice
Micrognathia

Blepharophimosis
Long eyelashes
in irregular rows
Unilateral ptosis
Microcornea
Microphthalmia
Juvenile cataract
Myopia
Short neck

Small sad face due to myotonia

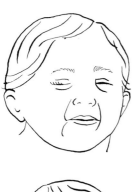

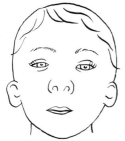

Small mouth, puckered lips
and blepharophimosis

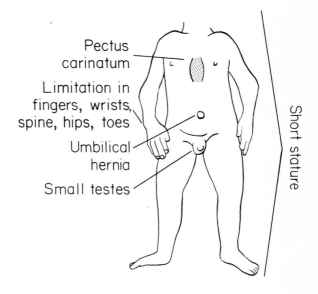

Pectus carinatum
Limitation in fingers, wrists, spine, hips, toes
Umbilical hernia
Small testes

Short stature

Joint contractures and
generalized muscular hypertrophy

313

147. SMITH-LEMLI-OPITZ SYNDROME

Clinical Features The disorder is recognizable at birth by the following characteristic features: ptosis of eyelids, slanted low-set ears, broad nasal tip with anteverted nares, micrognathia, broad maxillary alveolar ridges, cutaneous syndactyly of the second and third toes, and hypospadias and cryptorchidism. Prior to birth, fetal movements have been noted to be decreased. Breech presentation is common and birth weight may be less than 2500 g. The facies may be quite distinct exhibiting microcephaly, eyelid ptosis, strabismus, epicanthal folds, increased nasolabial distances, upturned nares, broad nasal tip, micrognathia, low-set and/or slanted ears, and short neck. Occasional findings may include congenital cataracts, hypertelorism, mild antimongoloid slant, minor ear anomalies, and plagiocephaly. The maxillary alveolar ridges are broad and the palate may be highly arched. Cleft palate or bifid uvula has been reported in some cases. The hands commonly show a simian crease while camptodactyly, rudimentary postaxial polydactyly, short fingers, clinodactyly, and proximally placed thumbs also have been noted. The feet usually display cutaneous syndactyly between the second and third toes; clinodactyly, hallucal hammer toes, metatarsus adductus, pes equinovarus, and other anomalies are seen in some patients. In males the genitalia can range from normal-appearing with small descended testes to severe perineoscrotal hypospadias with perineal urethral opening, cleft scrotum, and bilateral cryptorchidism. A variety of other anomalies have been reported which include partial agenesis of the cerebellar vermis and/or corpus callosum, hypoplasia of the frontal lobes, ventricular dilation, patent ductus arteriosus, ventricular septal defect, tetralogy of Fallot, aberrant right subclavian artery, pyloric stenosis, hypoplasia of thymus, renal anomalies, sacral dimple, deep cutaneous pit anterior to the anus, congenital hip dislocation, coxa valga, cubitus valgus, premature fusion of sternal ossification centers, short terminal phalanges secondary to stippled epiphyses, clenched hand with index fingers overlying third, acrocyanosis, widely spaced nipples, and inguinal hernia.

Specific Diagnosis The diagnosis of this syndrome is a clinical one based on the main clinical features mentioned above. In addition to simian creases, dermatoglyphic findings may show an increased number of digital whorls and also increased arches when there is severe camptodactyly. The axial triradius may be distally placed. EEG may be abnormal. Roentgenograms may show dysplasia epiphysialis punctata.

Differential Diagnosis This syndrome may be confused with *trisomy 13* and the *Meckel syndrome*. The presence of stippled epiphyses may also be seen in *chondrodysplasia punctata* and the *cerebrohepatorenal syndrome*.

Prenatal Diagnosis Not yet possible for this syndrome.

Basic Defect, Genetics, and Other Considerations The basic defect is not known. This disorder shows autosomal recessive inheritance and there are numerous reports of affected sibs. Parental consanguinity has only been noted in a few families, suggesting that the gene for this condition may be relatively common in the general population. Males have been reported far more frequently than females but this may be due to ascertainment bias of the more obvious genital anomalies in the male. Few adults have been described with this syndrome.

Prognosis and Treatment During the neonatal period vomiting, irritable behavior with shrill screaming, and increased susceptibility to infection pose problems for survival. Approximately half of all reported cases have died by the age of 18 months, usually from pneumonia. Moderate to severe mental retardation has been observed in all patients. Treatment is symptomatic.

REFERENCES

Cherstvoj, E.D., Lazjuk, G.I., Lurie, I.W. et al. The pathological anatomy of the Smith-Lemli-Opitz syndrome. *Clin. Genet 7:* 382–387, 1975.

Johnson, V.P. Smith-Lemli-Opitz syndrome: review and report of two affected siblings. *Z. Kinderheilkd 119:* 221–234, 1975.

Lowry, R.B. and Yong, S.L. Borderline normal intelligence with Smith-Lemli-Opitz (RSH) syndrome. *Am. J. Med. Genet. 5:* 137–143, 1980.

Smith-Lemli-Opitz Syndrome

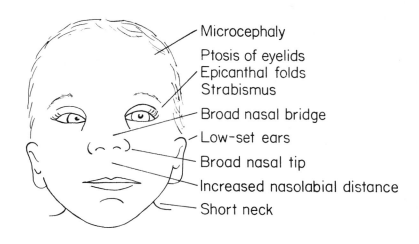

Microcephaly

Ptosis of eyelids
Epicanthal folds
Strabismus

Broad nasal bridge

Low-set ears

Broad nasal tip

Increased nasolabial distance

Short neck

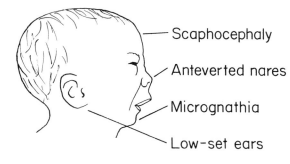

Scaphocephaly

Anteverted nares

Micrognathia

Low-set ears

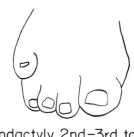

Syndactyly 2nd–3rd toes, short 5th with clinodactyly

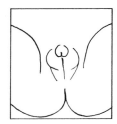

Small penis, hypospadias and cryptorchidism

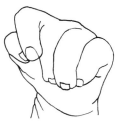

Clenched hand

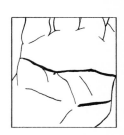

Dark lines show a simian crease and distal palmar axial triradius

148. TRICHORHINOPHALANGEAL SYNDROMES

Clinical Features The characteristic abnormalities in this syndrome involve the face, hair, and joints of the fingers. The hair and facial findings are present at time of birth. The scalp hair is sparse especially in the frontotemporal areas. Its texture is fine, brittle, and growth is slow. The eyebrows tend to broaden medially and narrow laterally. Eyelashes are sparse. Later on, the hair in other regions of the body is usually scant and the nails are thin. The distinct facial appearance is due to a bulbous nose, tented alae, and a prominent and elongated philtrum. The cartilaginous framework of the nose tends to be flabby. The upper lip is thin, and midfacial hypoplasia and mild micrognathia have been described. The ears may be large and protruding. A horizontal groove is often present on the chin. The fingers become progressively deformed during midchildhood, plateauing at puberty. There is swelling of the proximal interphalangeal joints resulting in ulnar deviation and clinobrachydactyly. The distal phalanges of the thumbs and halluces are usually short. Toes as well as fingers may be involved. Pes planus is common. Approximately 40% of the adults are below the 3rd percentile in height. Bone age is often several years behind chronologic age. Other infrequent findings include small teeth, dental malocclusion, high arched palate, kyphoscoliosis, pectus carinatum, winging of scapulae, gynecomastia, congenital heart disease, koilonychia and leukonychia. More recently such new findings as trigonocephaly, short frenum of tongue, and anomalies of the lower extremities (absence of patellae, hypoplasia and/or absence of fibula) have been reported.

Specific Diagnosis The clinical features described above in conjunction with certain radiographic findings allow for a specific diagnosis. There are cone-shaped epiphyses involving the middle phalanges of the second to the fourth fingers. The fourth and fifth metacarpals usually are shortened. Multiple cone-shaped epiphyses may also be seen in the toes. No specific abnormal laboratory findings have been described.

Differential Diagnosis The syndrome shares many features with those of the *Langer-Giedion* syndrome but multiple exostoses which are seen in the latter help distinguish the two disorders.

Prenatal Diagnosis Has not yet been achieved in this condition.

Basic Defect, Genetics, and Other Considerations The basic defect is not known. The combination of bone and hair hypoplasia with the proneness to upper respiratory tract infections raise the possibility of some immunologic alteration. Genetic heterogeneity is known to exist in this disorder since both autosomal dominant and recessive forms have been described. It is not possible to distinguish between these two types either clinically or radiographically. Most cases are of autosomal dominant inheritance.

Prognosis and Treatment During infancy and early childhood these patients have an increased susceptibility to upper respiratory tract infections. Progressive arthritic symptoms of the spine, elbows, and fingers may occur in midlife. A wig may be helpful if thin hair is of concern to the patient. Life expectancy is normal. Treatment is symptomatic.

REFERENCES

Felman. A.H. and Frias, J.L. The trichorhinophalangeal syndrome: study of 16 patients in one family. *Am. J. Roentgenol. 129:* 631–638, 1977.

Goodman, R.M., Trilling, R., Hertz, M. et al. New clinical observations in the trichorhinophalangeal syndrome. *J. Craniofacial Genet. Dev. Biol. 1:* 15–29, 1981.

Weaver, D.D., Cohen, M.M., and Smith, D.W. The tricho-rhino-phalangeal syndrome. *J. Med. Genet. 11:* 312–314, 1974.

- fine, sparse, brittle hair
- bulbous nose / tented alae / long philtrum
- thin upper lip
- horizontal groove on chin

Trichorhinophalangeal Syndromes

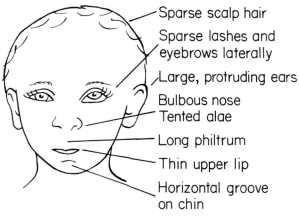

Sparse scalp hair

Sparse lashes and eyebrows laterally

Large, protruding ears

Bulbous nose
Tented alae

Long philtrum

Thin upper lip

Horizontal groove on chin

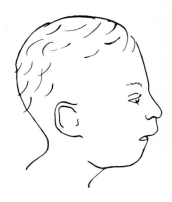

High forehead, micrognathia, long philtrum and tented alae

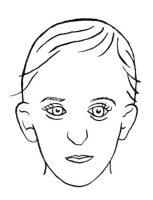 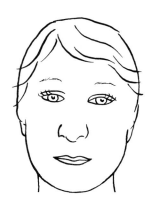 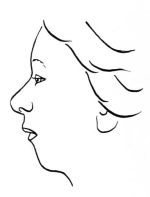

Similar facial features in older children

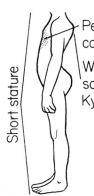

Short stature

Pectus carinatum

Winging of scapulae
Kyphoscoliosis

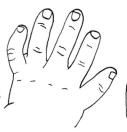 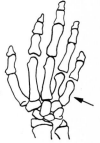

Clinobrachydactyly, later deviation of fingers at proximal interphalangeal joints, cone−shaped epiphyses and brachydactyly (arrow)

317

149. WILLIAMS SYNDROME

Clinical Features Affected infants present with distinct facial features which become more striking with age. The constellation of facial findings includes a depressed nasal bridge, anteverted nares, flat midface with full and dependent cheeks, long philtrum, thick lips with later drooping of lower lip, wide intercommissural distance, and open mouth. Common eye findings include short palpebral fissures, hypotelorism, epicanthal folds, medial eyebrow flare, strabismus, periorbital fullness, and blue eyes with a stellate iris pattern. Less commonly there may be corneal and/or lenticular opacities. There may be prominence of the ears and thyroid cartilage with age. Various oral anomalies have been described such as hypodontia, microdontia, hypoplasia of the mandible, dental malocclusion, bud-shaped deciduous molars, thickening of the buccal mucous membranes, and prominent and accessory labial frenula. Frequently the voice is hoarse. Numerous cardiovascular findings have been reported which include supravalvular aortic stenosis, valvular aortic stenosis, aortic hypoplasia, coarctation of the aorta, pulmonary artery stenosis, atrial and ventricular septal defect, anomalous pulmonary venous return, arteriovenous fistula of the lung, interruption of the aortic arch, aplasia of the portal vein, and peripheral artery stenosis. Other features may include craniosynostosis secondary to microcephaly, pectus excavatum, hallux valgus, clinodactyly, hypoplastic deep-set nails, multiple bladder diverticula, small penis, and inguinal and umbilical hernia.

Specific Diagnosis The diagnosis of this syndrome is mainly a clinical one based on the above features. Hypercalcemia is not observed in most cases, but when present it usually disappears during the second year of life. Radiographs may show increased calcification of the skull base, around the orbits, vertebral plates, and metaphyseal regions of the long bones. Angiographic studies are helpful in demonstrating the extent and types of vascular lesions.

Differential Diagnosis Isolated *supravalvular aortic stenosis* can be transmitted as an autosomal dominant trait, but usually occurs as a sporadic anomaly. *Idiopathic hypercalcemia* may have a familial occurrence. It has been shown that hypercalcemia with and without mental retardation and supravalvular aortic stenosis with and without mental retardation are the same entities.

Prenatal Diagnosis This is not yet possible.

Basic Defect, Genetics, and Other Considerations The basic defect in this disorder is not known. Some have shown an impaired ability of normocalcemic children with this syndrome to handle large intravenous calcium loads efficiently, thus suggesting a deficiency of calcitonin. There is no evidence at present to state that this condition is genetically determined since most cases have been sporadic.

Prognosis and Treatment Mild to moderate growth deficiency of prenatal onset with more striking growth deficiency during the postnatal period is found in most cases. Mental retardation (IQ from 40–80) with a mild neurologic dysfunction is a common feature. During childhood patients have been noted to be extremely friendly and loquacious. The prognosis is variable. If hypercalcemia is present treatment should be instituted to prevent nephrocalcinosis and deafness due to calcification of the labyrinth. Surgical correction of the vascular lesions should be done when indicated.

REFERENCES

Beuren, A.J. Supravalvular aortic stenosis: a complex syndrome with and without mental retardation. *Birth Defects 8 (5)*: 45–56, 1972.

Cortada, X., Taysi, K., and Hartmann, A.F. Familial Williams syndrome. *Clin. Genet. 18*: 173–176, 1980.

Jones, K.L. and Smith, D.W. The Williams elfin facies syndrome: A new prospective. *J. Pediatr. 86*: 718–723, 1975.

- **full, dependent cheeks**
- **open mouth / thick lips**
- **long philtrum**
- **heart murmur**

Williams Syndrome

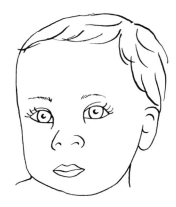
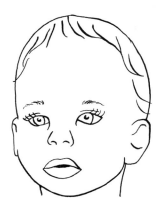

Full cheeks in the young, broad forehead, anteverted nares, depressed nasal bridge, long philtrum, strabismus, epicanthal folds, wide mouth and prominent lips

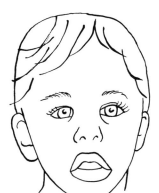
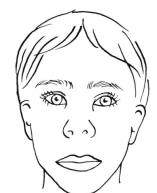

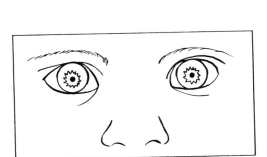

Stellate iris pattern

Pectus excavatum

Supravalvular aortic stenosis

Umbilical hernia

Small penis

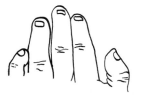
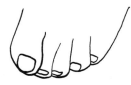

Hypoplastic nails, clinodactyly, hallux valgus

319

C. Genetic Syndromes
e. Skeletal Dysplasia

150. ACHONDROGENESIS SYNDROMES

Clinical Features Achondrogenesis is a lethal form of chondrodysplasia characterized by disproportionately large head and severe shortening of limbs and trunk. The condition is easily recognized at birth and most affected infants are either born dead or survive only a few days. Frequently there is a prenatal history of polyhydramnios. The enlarged head may exceed 40% of body length. There is a broad forehead and the face and scalp are swollen. The nose and nasal bridge are extremely flattened. The mouth is small and the ears are low set and blunted in shape. The neck is hidden by skin folds and thus the head appears attached directly to the trunk. The thorax is markedly shortened and dwarfed by a rotund abdomen. The extremities are exceedingly abbreviated and bowed ("flipper-like" appendages), in most cases rarely exceeding 20 cm in length. Hands and feet are broad with extremely short digits. Total body length at term seldom is greater than 36 cm. Other features include inguinal hernia, congenital heart defects (patent ductus arteriosus), and a hypoplastic respiratory system, mainly involving the tracheobronchial system.

Specific Diagnosis The radiographic findings allow for the distinction between Types I and II. Radiographically in Type I there is complete lack of ossification of the vertebral bodies, although the pedicles in the lumbar area ossify. The pelvis ossifies poorly, while skull ossification is variable. The ribs are very short with expanded costochondral junctions. The long tubular bones are extremely short and bowed, and spurs project at the borders of the expanded metaphyses. Type II exhibits normal ossification of calvaria, smooth ribs, diaphyseal constriction of long bones, and better ossified iliac bones. On histologic examination the chondrocytes are retarded and disturbed in proliferation as they approach the epiphyseal plate—in Type II there is degeneration of physeal and epiphyseal cartilage.

Differential Diagnosis This disorder should be differentiated from *thanatophoric dysplasia* and *Grebe disease*. The latter unfortunately has been called achondrogenesis of the Brazilian type, but there is no similarity other than name.

Prenatal Diagnosis Early prenatal diagnosis of both types using ultrasound and radiographs is possible based on the extremely abnormal skeletal findings.

Basic Defect, Genetics, and Other Considerations The basic defect is not known, however, in Type I it is postulated there is a fault in the normal maturation of cartilage, and in Type II there is an alteration in degeneration of cartilage. Both forms are considered to be rare and inherited in an autosomal recessive manner. Parental consanguinity and affected sibs have been reported. Probably there is genetic heterogeneity in achondrogenesis, as infants with this condition have been described with only mild abbreviation of the extremities.

Prognosis and Treatment Prematurity, fetal hydrops, and death either in utero or shortly thereafter characterize both forms.

REFERENCES

Saldino, R.M. Lethal short-limbed dwarfism: achondrogenesis and thanatophoric dwarfism. *Am. J. Roentgenol. 112:* 185–197, 1971.

Smith, W.L., Breitweiser, T.D., and Dinno, N. In utero diagnosis of achondrogenesis, type I. *Clin. Genet. 19:* 51–54, 1981.

Yang, S.S., Brough, A.J., Garewal, G.S., et al. Two types of heritable lethal achondrogenesis. *J. Pediatr.,85:* 796–801, 1974.

- large head
- severe shortening of limbs / trunk
- broad forehead and face
- small mouth

Achondrogenesis Syndromes

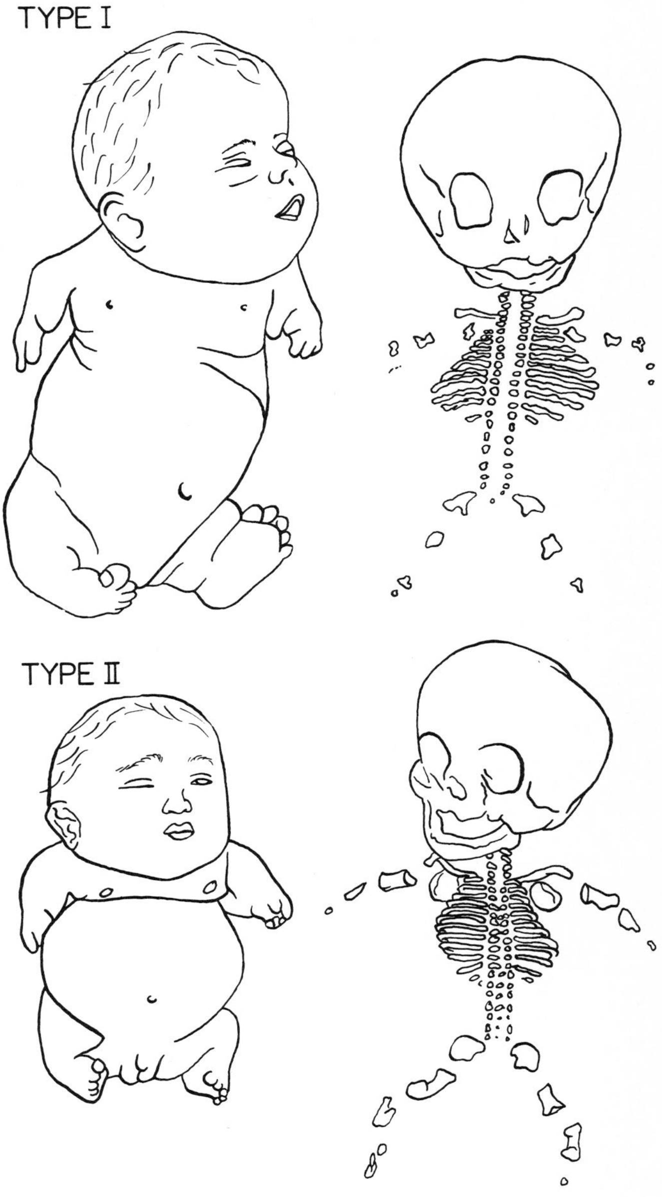

TYPE I

BOTH TYPES SHOW

Very short limbs

Large head

Short, hidden neck

Edematous facies

Broad forehead

Flat nose

Small mouth

Low-set, blunted ears

Protuberant abdomen

TYPE II

Type I – irregularly shaped ribs, poor ossification of
skull, vertebral bodies and pelvic bones
Type II – smooth ribs and better ossification of bones

151. ACHONDROPLASIA

Clinical Features At birth, the head is enlarged with frontal bossing and depression of the nasal bridge. Brachycephaly, relative mandibular prognathism, and mild midfacial hypoplasia with narrow nasal passages are other craniofacial alterations associated with this condition. Oral features include malocclusion with anterior crowding, anterior overjet, and various crossbites. The limb bones are shortened in a rhizomelic pattern, i.e. more pronounced in the upper extremities. Incomplete extension is observed at the elbows. The metacarpals and phalanges, although shortened, are disproportionately large in relation to the humerus, radius, and ulna. The fibula is excessively long at the ankle, producing in some cases a varus foot deformity. Lumbar lordosis with mild thoracolumbar kyphosis is seen in almost all cases. The hand has a characteristic shape being short, stubby, and typically trident. The three parts of the trident are: (a) the thumb, (b) fingers 2 and 3, and (c) fingers 4 and 5. A triangular cleft separates fingers 3 and 4. A trident hand may be absent in 5% of patients with achondroplasia. Mean birth length for males is 47.7 cm and 47.2 cm for females, while mean birth weight is 3500 g for boys and 3150 g for girls.

Specific Diagnosis The craniofacial, hand, and limb anomalies in this disorder are easily recognizable at birth. Radiographic findings include an enlarged calvaria with shortening of the cranial base and basilar kyphosis, small foramen magnum, hypoplastic maxilla, prominent frontal and occipital bones. There is partial occipitalization of the first cervical vertebra, progressive narrowing of the interpediculate distances from upper to lower spine, shortened pedicles in the anteroposterior diameter, concave vertebral bodies in the posterior aspect, and decreased bony spinal canal diameters especially in the lumbar region. The sacrum is narrow and horizontally oriented. The pelvis is broad and short. The superior acetabular margins are oriented horizontally and the sacrosciatic notch is acute. The legs are frequently bowed due to lax knee ligaments.

Differential Diagnosis This disorder should be distinguished from *thanatophoric dysplasia, achondrogenesis, metatropic dysplasia, diastrophic dysplasia, asphyxiating thoracic dysplasia, hypochondroplasia, Ellis-van Creveld syndrome,* and other forms of short-limbed dwarfism.

Prenatal Diagnosis The offspring of an achondroplastic patient who is at 50% risk for having the disorder can be accurately diagnosed during the second trimester using ultrasonographic methods to measure fetal femoral length.

Basic Defect, Genetics, and Other Considerations The basic defect is not known but histopathologic studies suggest that achondroplasia may be associated with a quantitative decrease in endochondral ossification and a normal rate of membranous ossification resulting in short, squat bones with cupped ends. Although this disorder is transmitted as an autosomal dominant, most cases (80%) represent sporadic new mutations associated with increased paternal age at time of conception. Achondroplasia is the most common form of short-limbed dwarfism. The homozygous state resembles thanatophoric dysplasia in many respects and is lethal during infancy.

Prognosis and Treatment Early motor progress is usually slow with poor head control until 3–4 months and delayed walking until 24–36 months, but eventually motor development is normal. Mentality is normal in most instances, however, internal hydrocephalus may impair intellect in a small number of patients. The narrow spinal canal predisposes to neurologic complications with age and almost 50% of all patients have some spinal complications and need close orthopedic-neurologic follow-up. Final height is approximately 130 cm for males and 123 cm for females. Mean adult weights are 55 kg for men and 46 kg for women. Since there is a tendency to obesity, dietary restrictions may be necessary.

REFERENCES

Cohen, M.E., Rosenthal, A.D., and Matson, D.D. Neurological abnormalities in achondroplastic children. *J. Pediatr. 71:* 367–376, 1967.

Filly, R.A., Golbus, M.S., Carey, J.C. et al. Short-limbed dwarfism: ultrasonographic diagnosis by mensuration of fetal femoral length. *Ultrasound 138:* 653–656, 1981.

Murdock, J.L., Walker, B.A., Hall, J.G. et al. Achondroplasia—a genetic and statistical survey. *Ann. Hum. Genet. 33:* 227–244, 1970.

M.R. [+ / few, secondary]

- **large head / frontal bossing**
- **depressed nasal bridge**
- **short extremities / rhizomelia**
- **short, stubby trident hand**

Achondroplasia

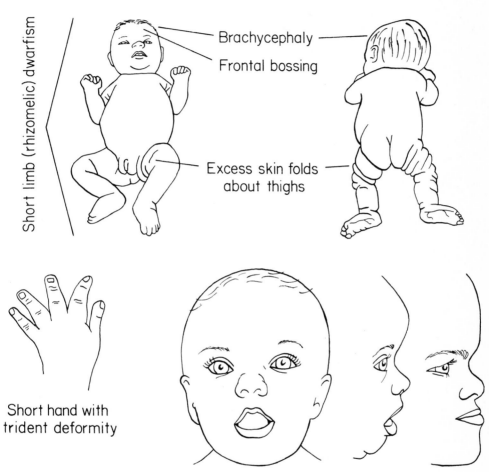

Short limb (rhizomelic) dwarfism

Brachycephaly

Frontal bossing

Excess skin folds about thighs

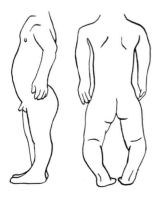

Short hand with trident deformity

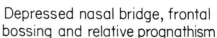

Depressed nasal bridge, frontal bossing and relative prognathism

Lumbar lordosis, protuberant abdomen, short extremities and genu varum

152. ACRODYSOSTOSIS

Clinical Features The characteristic features are present at birth and include peripheral dysostosis, nasal and midfacial hypoplasia, mental retardation, and growth failure. The nose tends to be markedly hypoplastic with a low nasal bridge and appears flat and short with a broad and often dimpled tip and anteverted nares. The center of the nasal tip is more severely reduced than the sides so that the alae extend below the columella. The philtrum is usually long. In some patients the nose is not especially short but the nasal bridge is depressed. Epicanthal folds and an apparent hypertelorism due to the low nasal bridge also have been described. Maxillary hypoplasia is common, producing a peculiar flattening of the cheeks. Open bite is frequent and relative mandibular prognathism may be conspicuous. Tooth formation may be delayed but the teeth are normal. The fingers and toes are characteristically short and stubby. This feature may be present at birth or not become obvious until months later. The nails are broad and very short. With age the skin and subcutaneous tissues outgrow the skeleton, forming bulges and excess folds over the dorsal surface of the hands and feet. Mesomelic brachymelia of the upper extremities is present but less conspicuous. Forearm shortening seems to become more severe with age. In the upright position the hands of affected adults barely reach the trochanters. In addition, the range of motion is usually limited in the elbows and may be considerably restricted in the spine. Some children start to walk late. Intrauterine growth retardation and short stature are almost constant findings. Birth weight at full term ranges from 1800 to 3000 g and birth length from 44 to 48 cm. Growth failure is progressive. Other findings occasionally observed include internal hydrocephalus, optic atrophy, choreoathetosis, seizures, hearing loss, strabismus, numerous pigmented nevi, and delayed puberty.

Specific Diagnosis Diagnosis is clinical based on the above findings in conjunction with certain radiographic features. The most striking roentgenographic anomalies are found in the hands and feet with severe shortening of metacarpals and phalanges. The growth disturbance is most severe in the metacarpals where the epiphyses are deformed and fuse prematurely. The phalanges have cone-shaped epiphyses which also fuse prematurely. Continued remodeling broadens and deforms the bones into more grotesque shapes. The distal radius and ulna are frequently malformed. A hypoplastic ulna with a poorly developed or absent styloid process is common. Foot changes are similar but less striking than those observed in the hands. Brachycephaly and occasionally mild microcephaly are present. Nasal bones are commonly hypoplastic or even missing.

Differential Diagnosis *Peripheral dysostosis* which refers to shortening of tubular bones associated with cone-shaped epiphyses may be seen as an isolated finding or found in various other bone disorders such as *pseudohypoparathyroidism* and the *trichorhinophalangeal syndrome*. It also plays a key role in an *autosomal recessive form of severe dwarfism* where the nose and facial features tend to be normal. The facial features in acrodysostosis share some common findings with those in the *fetal face syndrome*, but the latter shows macrocephaly with frontal bossing, and the hands and feet are not as severely affected as in the former.

Prenatal Diagnosis This has not yet been done.

Basic Defect, Genetics, and Other Considerations The basic defect is not known. Almost all cases have been sporadic with the exception of possible autosomal dominant inheritance in one family. Older paternal age (35 years) has been recorded in several cases, suggesting that all cases represent new autosomal dominant mutations.

Prognosis and Treatment Most patients have reduced intelligence with IQs ranging from 35 to 85. With age, arthritic changes are common; these involve the hands and feet and may even be generalized. Treatment is symptomatic.

REFERENCES

Reiter, S. Acrodysostosis: a case of peripheral dysostosis, nasal hypoplasia, mental retardation and impaired hearing. *Pediatr. Radiol. 7:* 53–55, 1978.

Robinow, M., Pfeiffer, R.A., Gorlin, R.J., et al. Acrodysostosis. A syndrome of peripheral dysostosis, nasal hypoplasia and mental retardation. *Am. J. Dis. Child. 121:* 195–203, 1971.

Singleton, E.B., Daeschner, C.W. and Teng, C.T. Peripheral dysostosis. *Am. J. Roentgenol. 84:* 499–505, 1960.

M.R. [+ / most]

Acrodysostosis

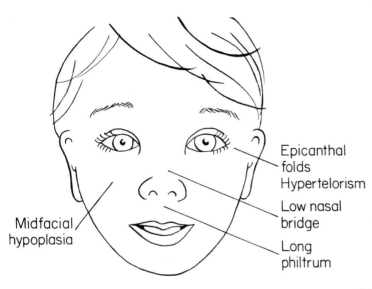

Midfacial hypoplasia

Epicanthal folds
Hypertelorism

Low nasal bridge

Long philtrum

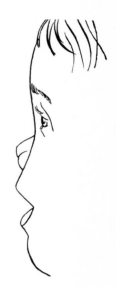

Marked hypoplasia of nose, anteverted nares

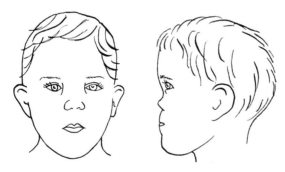

Similar features in older child plus relative prognathism

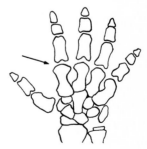

Brachydactyly hands and feet, short broad nails and cone-shaped epiphyses (arrow)

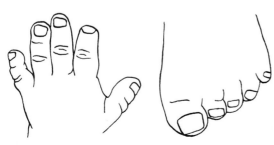

327

153. ALBRIGHT HEREDITARY OSTEODYSTROPHY
(pseudo and pseudopseudohypoparathyroidism)

Clinical Features Affected infants may present at birth with brachycephaly, round face, low nasal bridge, and rarely ptosis of the upper eyelid. A characteristic and striking finding is shortening of one or more fingers or toes due to shortening of corresponding metacarpals or metatarsals. The fourth and fifth metacarpals are nearly always involved, less often the first, third, and second. Shortened metacarpals are manifested when the patient makes a fist. The fourth and less frequently the third metatarsals are shortened. Short stature and obesity are common. Peripheral lenticular opacities develop in about a quarter of the patients. Tetany, muscle cramps, convulsions, delayed dental eruption, enamel hypoplasia with extensive dental caries, and ectopic calcification are findings related to the abnormal mineral metabolism. Other occasional features include short ulna, epiphyseal dysplasia, genu valgum, hypothyroidism, and hypogonadism with or without gonadal dysgenesis.

Specific Diagnosis In addition to the above clinical features, there are specific biochemical alterations associated with PHP which include hypocalcemia, hyperphosphatemia, diminished renal excretion of phosphate, and virtual lack of renal response to exogenous parathormone, i.e. failure to exhibit phosphorus diuresis. Patients with PHP also show a decreased urinary excretion of cyclic 3',5'-AMP following infusion of parathyroid hormone. Presumably the biochemical differences between PHP and pseudo-PHP depend on the ability of patients with the latter to compensate for the tubular phosphate reabsorption, perhaps through some degree of secondary hyperparathyroidism. Radiographs show calcification of soft tissues of the scalp and along the extremities, especially in periarticular areas of the hands and feet and the basal ganglia. There is thickening of the calvaria and shortening of metacarpals and metatarsals with cone-shaped epiphyses. An electrocardiogram may show prolonged Q-T interval. Dermatoglyphics are abnormal in some patients, showing distal palmar axial triradii.

Differential Diagnosis *Type E brachydactyly* resembles this disorder in respect to short stature,

hand anomaly, and round face, but mental retardation, ectopic calcification, and cataract are not present. Shortened metacarpals can also be noted in *Turner syndrome, peripheral dysostosis, acrodysostosis,* and *nevoid basal cell carcinoma syndrome.*

Prenatal Diagnosis This is not yet possible for this disorder.

Basic Defect, Genetics, and Other Considerations The basic defect is not entirely understood; there appears to be normal secretion of parathyroid hormone, however, a defect in receptor tissues produces little or no response to the hormone. It has been suggested that the basic alteration may be a deficient amount or function of parathormone-sensitive adenylcyclase in bone and kidney. Genetic heterogeneity is present in this syndrome as there are two different phenotypes of pseudohypoparathyroidism, Type 1 (PHP-1) and Type 2 (PHP-2). PHP-1 also has a normocalcemic and phosphophatemic form known as pseudopseudohypoparathyroidism (pseudo-PHP-1, which includes latent PHP-1). These phenotypes can be subdivided into an unexplained and variable somatotype, and events related to abnormal mineral metabolism. PHP-1 and pseudo-PHP-1 are thought to be transmitted as X-linked dominant traits due to the fact that females are more often affected (1M:2F) than males and there is a relative absence of male-to-male transmission. Sex-influenced autosomal dominant inheritance has also been postulated, as X-linked dominant transmission does not explain the fact that females are usually more severely affected than males. PHP-2 may be inherited as an autosomal recessive disorder.

Prognosis and Treatment Mental retardation (average IQ 60) is seen in more than half of the patients with PHP-1 but in fewer than 10% of those with pseudo-PHP-1. Seizures, tetany, and laryngospasm in childhood are due to the hypocalcemia. Treatment involves calcium supplements and high doses of vitamin D. Therapy should be reevaluated periodically since hypocalcemia may spontaneously correct itself. In general, patients can have a normal life span.

REFERENCES

Farfel, Z., Brickman, A. S., Kaslow, H.R. et al. Defect of receptor-cyclase coupling protein in pseudohypoparathyroidism, *N. Engl. J. Med. 303:* 237–242, 1980.

Kinard, R.E., Walton, J. E., and Buckwalter, J. A. Pseudohypoparathyroidism: report on a family

with four affected sisters. *Arch. Intern. Med. 139:* 204–207, 1979.

Steinbach, H.L. and Young D.A. The roentgen appearance of pseudohypoparathyroidism (PH) and pseudopseudohypoparathyroidism (PPH). *Am. J. Roentgenol. 97:* 49–66, 1966.

Albright Hereditary Osteodystrophy

[pseudo and pseudopseudohypoparathyroidism]

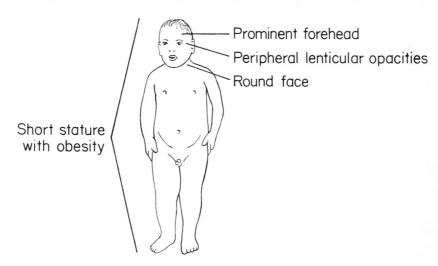

Prominent forehead

Peripheral lenticular opacities

Round face

Short stature with obesity

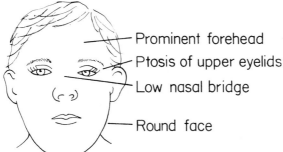

Prominent forehead

Ptosis of upper eyelids

Low nasal bridge

Round face

Features in an older child

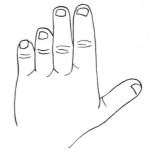

Short 4th and 5th digits with short broad nails

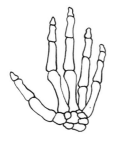

Short 4th digit due to brachydactyly of 4th metacarpal

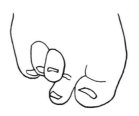

Shortening of toes due to brachydactyly of metatarsals also broad nails

154. ASPHYXIATING THORACIC DYSPLASIA
(Jeune syndrome)

Clinical Features This disorder is recognizable at birth by the presence of a narrow thorax which contrasts with the shortness of the limbs. The narrowness and immobility of the thorax lead to tachypnea and cyanosis. Respiration is diaphragmatic. Polydactyly of the hands and feet may be present, and the nails may be mildly dystrophic. The craniofacial morphology is normal except for poor dentition with dental anomalies.

Specific Diagnosis The above clinical features in conjunction with certain roentgenographic findings make for an easy diagnosis. The thoracic roentgenogram shows a high position of the clavicles; narrowing of the thoracic cage; and horizontal, short, and stubby ribs with the anterior portion widened. The pelvis also has distinct features consisting of square iliac wings, horizontal roof of the acetabulum with its medial portion deformed by a rounded protuberance limited on each side by a spur-shaped projection. The long bones may be short and stubby and the metaphyseal ends irregular. A small spine may be seen on the distal metaphysis of the humerus or on the proximal end of the tibia. Cone-shaped epiphyses and polydactyly may be observed involving the bones of the hands and feet. Abnormal concentrations of lipid have been noted in costochondral biopsies from affected individuals. Hypoplastic lungs with a marked reduction in the number of alveoli have been reported.

Differential Diagnosis This disorder shares many physical findings with that of *chondroectodermal dysplasia (Ellis-van Creveld syndrome)*, however, in the latter polydactyly of hands is a constant feature, and upper lip and cardiac anomalies also seen in the Ellis-van Creveld syndrome help to make the differentiation. In *thanatophoric dysplasia* there is a reduction in the height of the vertebral bodies. In *metatropic dysplasia* and *mucolipidosis II* differences in the alterations in the vertebrae, pelvis, and long bones allow for distinction.

Prenatal Diagnosis Although this disorder has not been diagnosed prenatally it seems possible that current ultrasound techniques could detect the altered anatomy of the chest wall, polydactyly and shortened extremities.

Basic Defect, Genetics, and Other Considerations The basic defect in this rare autosomal recessive condition is not known, but it is postulated that the abnormal concentration of lipid seen in the costochondral biopsies of affected patients may reflect an inborn error of metabolism. Genetic heterogeneity is thought to exist because there are two forms of this disorder: one form with neonatal mortality and a nonlethal variety with subsequent renal disease. Each form appears to be consistent within families.

Prognosis and Treatment Early death resulting from asphyxia with or without pneumonia occurs in about half of the patients. In those patients who survive, the thoracic malformation persists but the respiratory problems are less severe. Chronic nephritis leading to renal failure is a serious feature of this condition. Mental retardation has been noted in a few patients. Respiratory infections should be treated promptly and vigorously. Successful thoracic reconstruction has been reported. Early detection of renal failure is of vital importance in the management of these patients.

REFERENCES

Cortina, H., Beltran, J., Olague, R. et al. The wide spectrum of asphyxiating thoracic dysplasia. *Pediatr. Radiol.*, 8: 93–99, 1979.

Oberklaid, F., Danks, D.M., Mayne, V. et al. Asphyxiating thoracic dysplasia: clinical, radiological and pathological information on 10 patients. *Arch. Dis. Child.* 52: 758–765, 1977.

Tahernia, A.C. and Stamps, P. "Jeune syndrome" (asphyxiating thoracic dystrophy): report of a case, a review of the literature and an editor's commentary. *Clin. Pediatr.* 16: 903–908, 1977.

M.R. [+ / few]

- **narrow thorax**
- **short limbs**
- **polydactyly hands / feet**
- **mildly dystrophic nails**

Asphyxiating Thoracic Dysplasia
[Jeune syndrome]

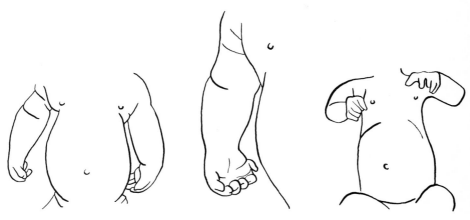

Marked narrowing of thoracic cage, lateral
displacement of the nipples, short upper
limbs, polydactyly and protuberance of abdomen

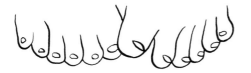

Polydactyly of toes and
hands, dystrophic nails

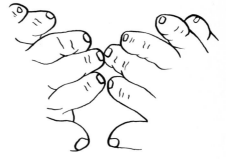

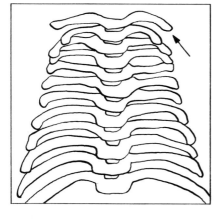

Note high position of
clavicles (arrow), narrow
thoracic cage, short,
wide, horizontal shape
to the ribs

155. CAMPOMELIC DYSPLASIA

Clinical Features The term campomelic dysplasia has been used nondiscriminately to include various conditions with congenitally bent or bowed legs. However, a distinct entity does exist for which this term was coined and its clinical features include the following: a low-to-normal weight term newborn with a large dolichocephalic head, disproportionate shortness mainly of the lower extremities, micrognathia, small mouth, cleft palate, long philtrum, flat nasal bridge, hypertelorism, narrow palpebral fissures, and dysplastic ears. The chest is bell-shaped and small, giving the abdomen the appearance of being large and protuberant. The lower extremities show symmetrical anterior bowing with pretibial dimples and talipes equinovarus, while the upper extremities are rarely bowed but may be mildly short. The hands commonly show mild brachydactyly and clinodactyly. Other findings may include hypotonia, medial deviation of the hallux, and dislocations of the hips, elbows, or fingers.

Specific Diagnosis The above clinical features in conjunction with certain radiographic findings make for easy recognition of this disorder. Radiographic findings include bowing of the lower extremities, absent or hypoplastic scapulae, nonmineralization of the thoracic pedicles, narrow vertical ilial bones, hypoplastic cervical vertebrae, widely spaced ischial bones, and absence of the distal femoral and proximal tibial epiphyses. Postmortem studies have shown absent or hypoplastic olfactory bulbs, hypoplastic trachea or cartilaginous rings, brain anomalies, hydronephrosis (38%), and congenital heart disease (21%).

Differential Diagnosis During the neonatal period this disorder may be confused with *diastrophic dysplasia, hypophosphatasia, osteogenesis imperfecta,* and the *Larsen syndrome,* but comparison of the scapulae, thoracic pedicles, and iliac bone changes among these conditions should allow for a distinct diagnostic separation. Other bone dysplasias presenting with congenital bowing of the extremities and early death must be ruled out.

Prenatal Diagnosis Possible in those pregnancies at risk using ultrasound to measure fetal femoral length, and perhaps to detect other associated skeletal anomalies.

Basic Defect, Genetics, and Other Considerations The basic defect is not known. Endochondral ossification has been shown to be defective primarily due to hypoplasia and vacuolar degeneration of cartilage cells in the growth zone. The mode of transmission has not been definitely established, but current evidence suggests autosomal recessive inheritance. Genetic heterogeneity is probably present, for in the long-limbed type about half the affected males have female external genitalia, with vagina, uterus, and fallopian tubes. Such patients have XY gonadal dysgenesis. Two very rare short-limbed forms have been termed (a) the short-bone craniosynostotic type, and (b) the short-bone normocephalic type. Whether or not these are really true variants of campomelic dysplasia remains to be clarified.

Prognosis and Treatment The prognosis in this disorder is poor as most die soon after birth or during infancy from a respiratory cause, usually aspiration pneumonia.

REFERENCES

Hall, B.D. and Spranger, J.W. Campomelic dysplasia: further elucidation of a distinct entity. *Am. J. Dis. Child. 134:* 285–289, 1980.

Hobbins, J.C., Grannum, P.A.T., Berkowitz, R.L., et al. Ultrasound in the diagnosis of congenital anomalies. *Am. J. Obstet. Gynecol. 134:* 331–345, 1979.

Khajavi, A. et al. Heterogeneity in the campomelic syndromes: long and short bone varieties. *Radiology 120:* 641–647, 1976.

- **large head /
  dolichocephaly**
- **short, bowed
  lower limbs**
- **small chest /
  protuberant abdomen**
- **small mouth /
  large philtrum**

Campomelic Dysplasia

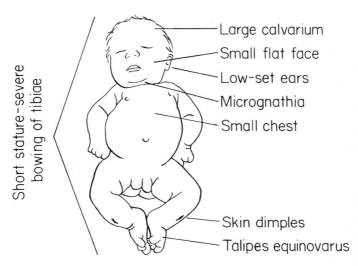

Short stature-severe bowing of tibiae

Large calvarium
Small flat face
Low-set ears
Micrognathia
Small chest

Skin dimples
Talipes equinovarus

Some phenotypic females are genotypic males
with XY gonadal dysgenesis

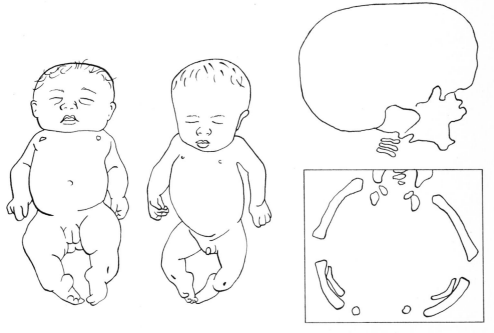

Similar features in two other infants — underdeveloped facial
structures, large skull, marked bowing of femur, tibia and fibula

156. CARTILAGE-HAIR HYPOPLASIA

Clinical Features Prenatal history is not remarkable and these infants are usually full term with normal birth weight. Various observers have commented that these infants tend to be "floppy" babies. As these patients develop, short-limbed dwarfism with fine, sparse, light-colored hair on the scalp and over other parts of the body become the main physical findings. The legs are relatively short with mild bowing of the femurs. The fingers and toes show brachydactyly with small nails. Limited extension of the elbow is noted despite a tendency toward hyperextensibility of the fingers, wrists, and feet. Pes planus and a prominent heel are commonly observed. Other skeletal abnormalities may include a mild flaring of the lower rib cage with a conspicuous sternum and lumbar lordosis. In most instances the head is of normal size and shape, but brachycephaly has been reported.

Specific Diagnosis The clinical features of this disorder are quite characteristic, which permits a precise diagnosis. The normal caliber of the hair shaft is reduced by about half and there is no central pigment core which can be seen on microscopic examination. Radiographically there are: irregularly scalloped metaphyses with sclerotic margins, flattened epiphyses, mild hypoplasia of the odontoid, normal or increased vertebral height, and a tibia characteristically shorter than the fibula. A cartilage biopsy shows hypoplastic changes with failure of the cartilage cells to form orderly columns. There is no specific laboratory test for this disorder, but because of an increased susceptibility to varicella and other infections some patients exhibit abnormal laboratory findings. While some display a chronic noncyclic neutropenia with maturation arrest, others may show persistent lymphopenia, diminished skin hypersensitivity, and diminished responsiveness of their lymphocytes to phytohemagglutinin in vitro. Serum immunoglobulin levels may be either normal or elevated.

Differential Diagnosis This disorder should be differentiated from the other genetic forms of *metaphyseal dysplasia* based on clinical and radiographic findings. The various *immunodeficiency diseases* can also be readily distinguished from cartilage-hair hypoplasia syndrome. Other conditions to be ruled out include *hypohidrotic ectodermal dysplasia, achondroplasia, vitamin-D resistant rickets,* and *hypophosphatasia.*

Prenatal Diagnosis Not presently available.

Basic Defect, Genetics, and Other Considerations The basic defect in this relatively rare autosomal recessive disorder is not known. Although originally described in the old-order Amish, this syndrome is now known not to be isolated to a single ethnic group, since an increased incidence has also been found in Finland. Over 100 cases have been reported. Genetic heterogeneity is thought to exist as there are three types: (a) typical; (b) mild; and (c) severe with an immune defect.

Prognosis and Treatment Since those with the severe form may have extreme susceptibility to varicella, a thorough immunologic examination is indicated before immunization is even considered. In these patients proper caution should be given to avoid other types of infection. In some infants there is a history of intestinal malabsorption but this tends to improve with age. Hirschsprung disease has been observed in a few patients. Adult height ranges from 107 to 150 cm. Orthopedic care is indicated for problems related to early osteoarthritic changes and equinovarus deformity of the feet. Because of an altered pelvic outlet, Cesarean section is necessary for female patients giving birth.

REFERENCES

Kelling, C., Goldsmith, C.A., and Baden, H.P. Biophysical and biochemical studies of the hair in cartilage-hair hypoplasia. *Clin. Genet. 4:* 500–506, 1973.

McKusick, V.A., Eldridge, R., Hostetler, J.A. et al. Dwarfism in the Amish. II. Cartilage-hair hypoplasia. *Bull. Johns Hopk. Hosp. 116:* 285–326, 1965.

Virolainen, M., Savilahti, E., Kaitila, I., et al. Cellular and humoral immunity in cartilage-hair hypoplasia. *Pediatr. Res. 12:* 961–966, 1978.

- **fine, sparse, light-colored hair**
- **short legs / bowing of femur**
- **brachydactyly / small nails**
- **limited extension of elbow / prominent heel**

Cartilage-Hair Hypoplasia

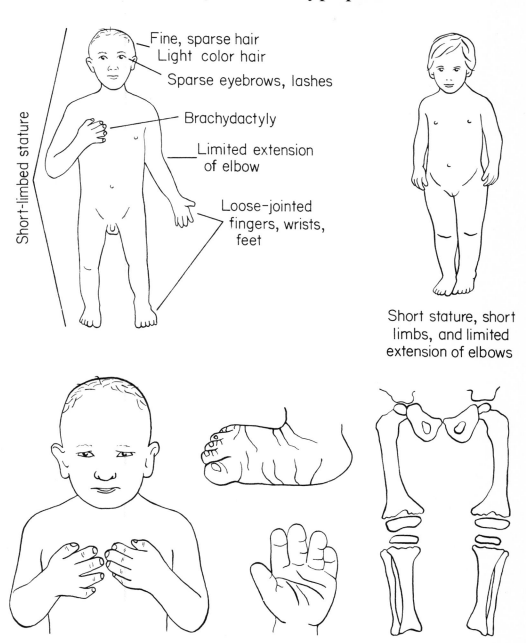

Short-limbed stature

Fine, sparse hair
Light color hair
Sparse eyebrows, lashes

Brachydactyly

Limited extension of elbow

Loose-jointed fingers, wrists, feet

Short stature, short limbs, and limited extension of elbows

Note sparse hair, eyebrows, lashes, posterior projection of heel, short and pudgy hands and the long bones are short with flared ends and metaphyseal irregularity

335

157. CHONDRODYSPLASIA PUNCTATA SYNDROMES

Clinical Features This condition has two distinct genetic types which share certain clinical features that have varying degrees of severity, such as stippled areas of calcification about the epiphyses, congenital cataracts, and various skeletal alterations. In both types the facies tends to be somewhat similar, showing a prominent forehead, hypertelorism, upward slant to the palpebral fissures, flat nasal bridge, anteverted nares, and flat face. In the recessive form congenital cataracts are present in about 70% of the patients, whereas only about 20% of those with the dominant form are born with cataracts. Cleft palate and submucous palatal cleft have been reported in the recessive type along with lymphedema of the cheeks, convergent strabismus, nystagmus, and microcephaly. In both forms the scalp hair is commonly sparse and coarse while the overall skin tends to be dry, scaly, and atrophic. Eczematoid dermatitis is common in the recessive form, while atrophoderma follicularis is seen in the dominant type. In the dominant form the height is reduced, there is a disproportionate limb length with mild or asymmetric shortening of the tubular bones, scoliosis, and frequently talipes calcaneovalgus. Contractures of the large joints have also been reported. In the recessive type there is severe rhizomelic shortening of the extremities and contractures are more common than in the dominant form.

Specific Diagnosis The diagnosis of each type can be distinguished by the above clinical findings. Notably the rhizomelic recessive form tends to be symmetrical, while the dominant form is frequently asymmetric and the findings are less severe. In the recessive form the epiphyseal and extraepiphyseal calcifications are usually severe, while in the dominant the calcifications are less and are seen in the vertebral column, epiphyses, flat and round bones, and at times in the larynx and tracheal rings.

Differential Diagnosis The types of calcification seen in infants with this condition are nonspecific and may be seen in a variety of disorders such as the *cerebrohepatorenal syndrome, multiple epiphyseal dysplasia, Warfarin embryopathy, chondritis secondary to bacteremia, G_M^1 gangliosidosis, Smith-Lemli-Opitz syndrome, trisomies 18 and 21, hypothyroidism,* and others.

Prenatal Diagnosis With ultrasonic methods, it would seem that measuring lengths of fetal long bones could detect the rhizomelic type prenatally. Such methods would be much more difficult in the dominant form.

Basic Defect, Genetics, and Other Considerations The basic defect is not known. In the dominant form the endochondral bone formation may be normal or mildly affected while in the recessive it is severely altered. It is thought that the epiphyseal and growth plate changes represent injury during development with subsequent healing by fibrosis, calcification, and ossification. These are relatively rare disorders and there may be heterogeneity within the dominant form. In the dominant type most cases are due to new mutations. Parental consanguinity has been recorded in the autosomal recessive type. A higher ratio of females to males in a form of chondrodysplasia punctata with widespread atrophic and pigmentary lesion of the skin has suggested to some that these patients may have an X-linked dominant form which is lethal in hemizygous males.

Prognosis and Treatment Few patients with the dominant form die in infancy and most go on to have a good prognosis. In contrast, more than half of those with the recessive form die during the first year and few survive puberty. Mental retardation is usually present in the recessive type. Treatment is symptomatic but proper care must be given for scoliosis, other orthopedic problems, and cataracts.

REFERENCES

Manzke, H., Christophers, E., and Wiedemann, H.R. Dominant sex-linked inherited chondrodysplasia punctata: a distinct type of chondrodysplasia punctata. *Clin. Genet. 17(2):* 97–107, 1980.

Spranger, J.W., Opitz, J.M., and Bidder, U. Heterogeneity of chondrodysplasia punctata. *Humangenetik 11:* 190–212, 1971.

Viseskul, C., Opitz, J.M., Spranger, J.W. et al. Pathology of chondrodysplasia punctata—rhizomelic type. *Birth Defects 10 (12):* 327–333, 1974.

M.R. [+ / most,
recessive
form]

- prominent forehead
- sparse, coarse scalp
  hair / dry scaly skin
- flat nasal bridge /
  anteverted nares
- short stature

Chondrodysplasia Punctata Syndromes

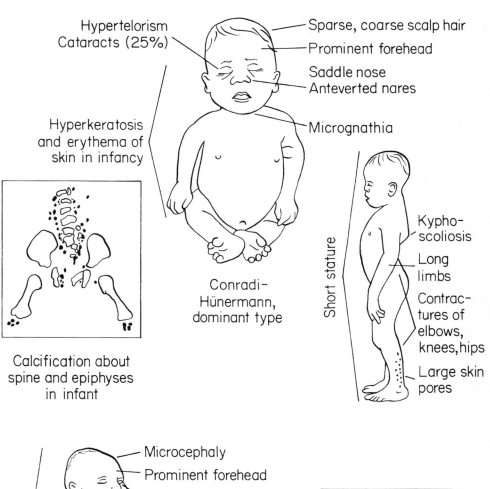

Hypertelorism
Cataracts (25%)

Sparse, coarse scalp hair
Prominent forehead
Saddle nose
Anteverted nares

Micrognathia

Hyperkeratosis
and erythema of
skin in infancy

Conradi–
Hünermann,
dominant type

Short stature

Kypho-
scoliosis
Long
limbs
Contrac-
tures of
elbows,
knees, hips
Large skin
pores

Calcification about
spine and epiphyses
in infant

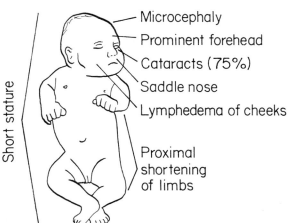

Short stature

Microcephaly
Prominent forehead
Cataracts (75%)
Saddle nose
Lymphedema of cheeks

Proximal
shortening
of limbs

Eczematoid dermatitis

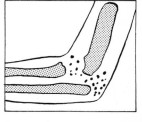

Rhizomelic, recessive type
with shortening of humerus
and calcification about elbow

158. CHONDROECTODERMAL DYSPLASIA
(Ellis-van Creveld syndrome)

Clinical Features The characteristic features are present at birth and include (a) bilateral postaxial polydactyly of the hands, (b) chondrodysplasia of the long bones, (c) dysplastic nails and teeth, and less often, (d) congenital heart malformations. The facies is usually normal except for a mild defect in the middle of the upper lip. This anomaly is due to fusion of the middle portion of the upper lip to the maxillary gingival margin so that no mucobuccal fold or sulcus exists anteriorly. Natal teeth have been noted in about 25%. The teeth are usually small and irregularly spaced. Oligodontia is a constant finding mainly in the mandibular anterior region. The crown form of many teeth is distinctive and bizarre. Those that are not conical are bicuspid with accentuated cuspal height and deep fissures. The enamel is hypoplastic in about 50%. The extremities are usually plump and markedly and progressively shortened distally, i.e. from the trunk to the phalanges. Polydactyly is common with the extra digit being on the ulnar side. Only rarely are there extra toes but postaxial heptadactyly has been noted. Other skeletal anomalies observed include genu valgum, talipes equinovarus, and calcaneovalgus, pectus carinatum with thoracic constriction, and curvature of the humerus. Most patients have severe dystrophy of the fingernails. The hair of the scalp, eyebrows, and pubis is sparse and thin. Approximately half the patients have congenital heart disease, most commonly a single atrium and endocardial cushion defect. About a third of the males have genital anomalies consisting of cryptorchidism, hypospadias, and mild epispadias. Other alterations occasionally seen are congenital cataract, internal strabismus, and hydrocephalus.

Specific Diagnosis Diagnosis is clinical based on the abovementioned findings in combination with certain radiographic alterations. In infancy the pelvis is dysplastic with low iliac wings and a hook-like downward projection of the medial acetabulum. The capital femoral epiphysis may ossify prematurely. The tubular bones are short and thickened. The fibula is severely shortened, being only half the normal length. Phalangeal bones are often missing, syncarpalism (hamate and capitate), synmetacarpalism, and polymetacarpalism are common. A particular pattern of cone-shaped epiphyses of the hands is apparently pathognomonic for the syndrome.

Differential Diagnosis This syndrome must be differentiated from *asphyxiating thoracic dysplasia* and other chondrodysplasias such as *achondroplasia, chondrodysplasia punctata, cartilage-hair hypoplasia,* and *Morquio syndrome.*

Prenatal Diagnosis This has been achieved in pregnancies at risk using fetoscopy for visualization of postaxial polydactyly. More recently it has been shown that such a diagnosis is possible by measuring fetal femoral length using ultrasonography.

Basic Defect, Genetics, and Other Considerations The basic defect is not known. Biopsy of cartilage plate shows a decrease in cartilage cells with disorganization of columnar chondrocytes. The syndrome has autosomal recessive transmission and parental consanguinity is present in approximately a third of the cases. The largest pedigree known is in the Old Order Amish in Pennsylvania. Almost as many persons are affected in this one family as have been reported in the entire medical literature.

Prognosis and Treatment A significant proportion of patients die from the consequences of congenital heart disease and cardiorespiratory problems. Adult height is quite variable and some affected individuals reach normal stature. Surgical intervention must be considered for repair of the cardiac malformation, genu valgum, amputation of extra digits, and correction of the oral problems.

REFERENCES

Filly, R.A., Golbus, M.S., Carey, J.C. et al. Short-limbed dwarfism: ultrasonographic diagnosis by mensuration of fetal femoral length. *Ultrasound 138:* 653–656, 1981.

Mahoney, M.J. and Hobbins, J.C. Prenatal diagnosis of chondroectodermal dysplasia (Ellis-van Creveld syndrome) with fetoscopy and ultrasound. *N. Engl. J. Med. 297:* 258–260, 1977.

McKusick, V.A., Egeland, J.A., Eldridge, R. et al. Dwarfism in the Amish I. The Ellis-van Creveld syndrome. *Bull. Johns Hopk. Hosp. 115:* 306–336, 1964.

M.R. [−]

Chondroectodermal Dysplasia
[Ellis-van Creveld syndrome]

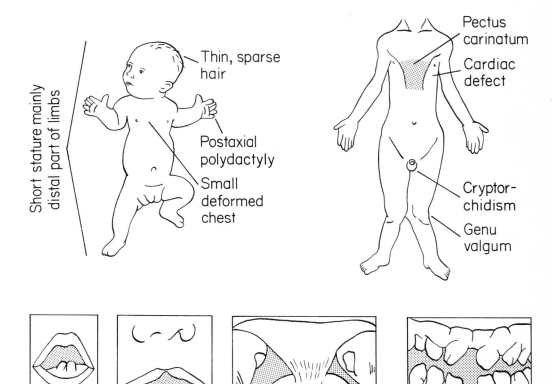

Short stature mainly distal part of limbs

Thin, sparse hair

Postaxial polydactyly

Small deformed chest

Pectus carinatum

Cardiac defect

Cryptor-chidism

Genu valgum

Neonatal teeth, short upper lip with midline defect, upper lip bound by frenulum, malformed, absent and irregularly spaced teeth

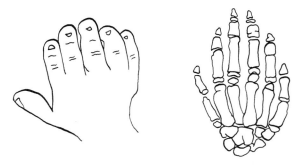

Postaxial polydactyly, hypoplastic nails, malformed middle phalanges and 5th metacarpal, fusion of capitate and hamate

159. CLEIDOCRANIAL DYSPLASIA

Clinical Features The appearance of affected individuals is usually so marked that they can be recognized early in infancy. On palpation the clavicle may be unilaterally (more often the right) or bilaterally absent due to total aplasia. More frequently it is hypoplastic at the acromial end. The clavicular deficiency is responsible for the long appearance of the neck and narrow shoulders. The range of shoulder movements made possible by this anomaly and associated muscle defects is remarkable, frequently allowing individuals to approximate their shoulders in front of their chest. The skull is brachycephalic with marked frontal and parietal bossing causing the face to appear small. The nose is broad at the base with a depressed nasal bridge. Frequently there is a groove overlying the metopic suture extending from the nasion to the sagittal suture. Closure of the fontanels and sutures is delayed and they may remain permanently open. Mild exophthalmus associated with a depressed orbital roof may be seen. Other skeletal anomalies described are asymmetric length of fingers with long second metacarpals, tapering distal phalanges, accessory proximal metacarpal epiphyses, delayed ossification of pubic bone, coxa vara or valga, genu valgum, scoliosis, cervical ribs, vertebral malformations, and small scapula. Oral findings include highly arched palate, submucous cleft or complete palatal cleft, relative prognathism, delayed eruption or failure of eruption of deciduous and permanent teeth, cyst formation around impacted or displaced teeth, and supernumerary teeth. Extracted teeth have been noted to be severely deformed. Conduction deafness has been reported in several patients. Short stature is common with males averaging 156 cm and females 144 cm.

Specific Diagnosis The diagnosis of this disorder is clinical based on the above features in combination with a variety of skeletal findings as noted by radiographic studies: brachycephaly and bossing of the cranium, delay in closure of the fontanels

and sutures, Wormian bones, aplasia or hypoplasia of one or both clavicles, and various dental anomalies including supernumerary dentition.

Differential Diagnosis Wide skull sutures and delayed closure of the fontanels are seen in *pyknodysostosis* but this disorder is also characterized by acroosteolysis and generalized skeletal sclerosis. A hypoplastic maxilla is also seen in *Apert syndrome* and in *craniofacial dysostosis*. Aplasia or hypoplasia of the clavicles may be seen in *mandibuloacral dysplasia, focal dermal hypoplasia* and *cleidofacial dysplasia*. Recently, cleidocranial dysplasia has been reported in a new autosomal recessive syndrome associated with severe micrognathia, absence of thumbs and first metatarsal bone, and distal aphalangia.

Prenatal Diagnosis Prenatal diagnosis of this disorder has not yet been achieved.

Basic Defect, Genetics, and Other Considerations Cleidocranial dysplasia is a diffuse disease involving the formation and development of cartilage and bone. The basic defect is not known. The disorder has autosomal dominant transmission with a wide range of expressivity. Approximately one-third of the cases represent new mutations. A recessive form has been described in two families in which the parents were normal and consanguineous and the affected children were more severely dwarfed with extensive skeletal changes.

Prognosis and Treatment This is not considered to be a life-threatening disorder. Intellect is usually normal. Pregnancy in affected females may require Caesarean section because of pelvic dysplasia. Treatment is symptomatic consisting of proper dental care and surgical closure of the cleft palate when indicated. Protective head gear may be useful while the fontanels are widely open.

REFERENCES

Goodman, R.M., Tadmor, R., Zaritsky, A. et al. Evidence for an autosomal recessive form of cleidocranial dysostosis. *Clin. Genet. 8:* 20–29, 1975.

Jackson, W.P.U. Osteo-dental dysplasia (cleido-cranial dysostosis). The "Arnold head." *Arch. Med. Scand. 139:* 292–307, 1951.

Tan, K.L. and Tan, L.K.A. Cleidocranial dysostosis in infancy. *Pediatr. Radiol. 11:* 114–116, 1981.

- increased shoulder movement / narrow shoulders
- brachycephaly / frontal and parietal bossing
- depressed nasal bridge
- supernumerary teeth

Cleidocranial Dysplasia

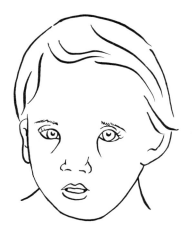
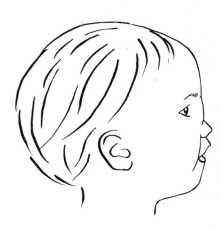

Hypertelorism, broad nasal bridge with paranasal bossing

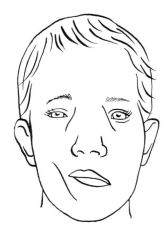
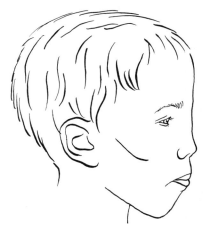

Broad, flat nasal bridge, hypertelorism, facial palsy and scaphocephaly

Sclerotic base of skull

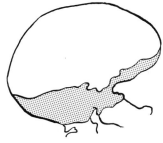
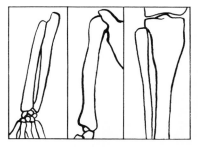

Meta-physeal flaring of long bones

160. CRANIOMETAPHYSEAL DYSPLASIA

Clinical Features Two genetic forms (autosomal dominant and recessive) of this disorder are known. In general the dominant type is less severe in its clinical manifestations and far more common than the recessive. Both types can usually be recognized during the first year of life by bizarre facies due to broadening of the root of the nose with resulting hypertelorism. The skull becomes scaphocephalic in shape with prominent frontal and parietal bossing. Increasing bony sclerosis narrows the nasal lumen leading to obstruction with resultant mouth breathing. Dental malocclusion is common. Alterations in the temporal bone and pyramid account for disturbances of sound conduction or perception. Deafness usually becomes evident before puberty. Defective vision with optic atrophy and facial paralysis may be found in more severely affected patients. Other findings may include a relatively small nose, variable proptosis of the eyes, limitation of motion at the elbows, and widening of the metaphyseal areas of long bones.

Specific Diagnosis Diagnosis is based on the above clinical features in conjunction with certain radiographic findings which include hyperostosis and sclerosis of the frontal and occipital regions of the skull. Most marked is frontonasal hyperostosis. Increased bone deposition on the walls of the paranasal sinuses and mastoid cells with variable degrees of obliteration and underpneumatization have been noted. The long tubular bones show some degree of midshaft sclerosis and thickening (club-shaped) more prominent in the upper extremities. Diaphyseal sclerosis is observed in the young but disappears with age. The short tubular bones exhibit the same changes as those noted in long bones. The ribs may be mildly widened. In general, the skeletal changes are related to age and are progressive in nature.

Differential Diagnosis This disorder must be differentiated from *Pyle disease* and *craniodiaphyseal dysplasia*. In *Pyle disease* the skull involvement is minimal or absent and the facial bones do not show hyperostosis; furthermore, the modeling defect in the tubular bones is much more marked. In *craniodiaphyseal dysplasia* there is a massive and generalized hyperostosis and sclerosis of the craniofacial bones, while the tubular bones show no metaphyseal widening but rather a diaphyseal endostosis. Both Pyle disease and craniodiaphyseal dysplasia are autosomal recessive disorders while craniometaphyseal dysplasia may be either autosomal dominant or recessive.

Prenatal Diagnosis To the best of our knowledge prenatal diagnosis of this disorder has not yet been achieved.

Basic Defect, Genetics, and Other Considerations The basic defect is not known, but it is thought to be a defect in bone modeling due to failure of resorption of the secondary spongiosa which would lead to increased bone deposition in the membranous bones of the cranium, base of skull, face, and mandible, and to widening of the metaphyses of the long bones. Although several cases have been sporadic, distinct autosomal dominant and recessive forms are known—the dominant type being more common. In a recent review it has been shown that both forms have essentially the same progressive bone alterations and clinical manifestations. However, the dominant type has a wider phenotypic expression than the recessive, and the more severely affected cases have recessive inheritance.

Prognosis and Treatment The disease tends to be progressive and serious complications may arise from compression of the cranial nerves resulting in facial paresis, external ophthalmoplegia, optic atrophy, sensorineural deafness, and other neurologic deficits; however the incidence of the complications seems to be low. Neurosurgical intervention may be necessary for relief from the above complications. Patients are of normal intelligence.

REFERENCES

Beighton, P., Hamersma, H., and Horan, F. Craniometaphyseal dysplasia—variability of expression within a large family. *Clin. Genet. 15:* 252–258, 1979.

Gorlin, R.J., Spranger, J., and Koszalka, M.F. Genetic craniotubular bone dysplasias and hyperostoses. A critical analysis. *Birth Defects 5 (4):* 79–95, 1969.

Penchaszadeh, V.B., Gutierrez, E.R., and Figueroa, E.P. Autosomal recessive craniometaphyseal dysplasia. *Am. J. Med. Genet. 5:* 43–55, 1980.

- **scaphocephaly / frontal / parietal bossing**
- **broad nasal root**
- **hypertelorism / proptosis**
- **facial paralysis / decreased vision / hearing**

Craniometaphyseal Dysplasia

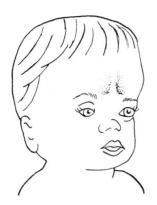
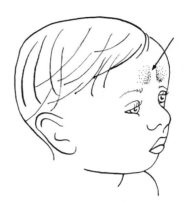

Note brachycephaly, frontal bossing with groove along metopic suture (arrow), broad nose, depressed nasal bridge and narrow shoulders

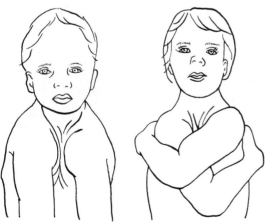
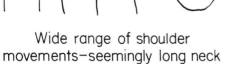
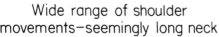

Wide range of shoulder movements—seemingly long neck

Large head, Wormian bones and deficient ossification of ischiopubic segments

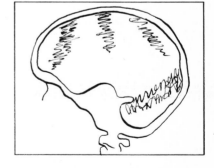
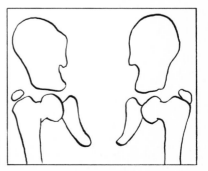

161. DIASTROPHIC DYSPLASIA

Clinical Features This disorder of short-limbed dwarfism can be recognized at birth and is characterized by the pathognomonic triad of pinnal calcification, hitch-hiker thumbs, and severe clubfoot. Mesomelic dwarfism is a constant feature and the mean birth length is approximately 33 cm. There is shortening of all limbs with severe bilateral talipes equinovarus which becomes worse with age. The patients bear their weight on their toes and walking is limited. The hand findings characteristically show short, broad fingers which may be deviated in an ulnar direction due to shortening of the ulna. The fingers are widely spaced with absence of flexion (symphalangism) at multiple interphalangeal joints, particularly the proximal interphalangeal ones. The thumbs, in contrast to the fingers, are hypermobile and broad. The first metacarpals are short, giving the clinical appearance of proximal insertion of the thumbs. Proximal insertion plus the abducted positioning of the thumbs accounts for the typical "hitch-hiker" configuration. Scoliosis is not present at birth but often appears within the first few years of life and is progressive. Kyphosis is occasionally observed and lordosis is frequent. Flexion contracture and/or subluxation or dislocation of the hips, knees, and shoulders are common and progressive. Swelling of the pinnae can be noted a few days to six weeks after birth; they become reddened, often fluctuant, and may feel cystic. After a three to four week period resolution ensues with subsequent thickening and deformity. The external auditory canals may be narrowed. The facies of these patients tends to be square, with a narrow nasal bridge, broad nose, and flared nostrils. The mouth is commonly full and broad with the lower lip slightly larger than the upper. Cleft palate is found in more than 30% of the patients. The mandible is usually small. Inguinal hernia has been reported.

Specific Diagnosis The clinical features involving the ears, hands, and feet described above make for relative ease in the recognition of this disorder. Skeletal radiograms show that the long bones are reduced in length, are thick, and have broad metaphyses and flattened irregular epiphyses which may be late in mineralizing. The first metacarpal is oval or triangular in shape and is set low on the carpus. Other radiographic findings include clubfeet, progressive scoliosis, distortion of the pelvic bones, deformed femoral heads, coxa vara with dislocation or subluxation and calcification and ossification in the pinnae. The epiphyses may have a stippled appearance during infancy. Precocious calcification of laryngeal and costal cartilages has been described. Characteristic histopathologic changes have been observed in resting cartilage consisting of focal death of chondrocytes with subsequent cyst formation and intracartilaginous ossification.

Differential Diagnosis This disorder has been confused with such conditions as *achondroplasia, arthrogryposis multiplex congenita,* and *cartilage-hair hypoplasia syndrome.* However, it can easily be differentiated from them by its unique and prominent features involving the hand and ear.

Prenatal Diagnosis Early prenatal diagnosis of this disorder has been achieved using ultrasound for the detection of the various skeletal anomalies.

Basic Defect, Genetics, and Other Considerations The basic defect in this chondroosseous disorder is not known. Ultrastructural analysis of cartilage has shown a paucity of chondrocytes which were poorly preserved and had a poor organellar development. This condition is transmitted as an autosomal recessive and parental consanguinity has been observed. A so-called "diastrophic variant" has been reported on several occasions in which the affected individuals are taller and have a less severe form of the disorder. Current thinking is that this is not a true variant but part of the single entity of diastrophic dysplasia showing a wide range of clinical variability.

Prognosis and Treatment Approximately 25% of these patients die in infancy from aspiration pneumonia or respiratory distress. Intelligence is normal. Mean adult height is about 112 cm. The talipes equinovarus is frequently resistant to treatment and tends to recur after therapy. Nevertheless, proper orthopedic management is indicated for a number of bony alterations associated with this disorder, especially subluxation of the second and third cervical vertebrae. This is frequent and may result in spinal cord compression. Surgical repair of the cleft palate is indicated.

REFERENCES

Horton, W.A., Rimoin, D.L., Lachman, R.S. The phenotypic variability of diastrophic dysplasia. *J. Pediatr. 93:* 609–613, 1978.

O'Brien, G.D., Rodeck, C., and Queenan, J.T. Early prenatal diagnosis of diastrophic dwarfism by ultrasound. *Br. Med. J. 280:* 1300, 1980.

Walker, B.A., Scott, C.I., Hall, J.G. et al. Diastrophic dwarfism. *Medicine 51:* 41–60, 1971.

- **clubbed hands / feet**
- **hitchhiker thumb**
- **deformed external ear**
- **very short stature**

Diastrophic Dysplasia

Marked shortness of stature

Micromelia, clubfeet and hands

Cystic swelling of auricles in infancy

Brachydactyly, thumb proximally placed (hitchhiker's thumb)

Marked shortness of stature

Flexion contracture and/or subluxation or dislocation of hips and knees, kyphoscoliosis, lordosis, clubfeet and hand deformity

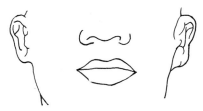

Broad full mouth, lower lip larger than upper, deformed ears

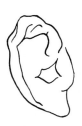

Cauliflower-like deformity of ear in adult

162. DYGGVE-MELCHIOR-CLAUSEN SYNDROMES

Clinical Features At birth affected infants often show a short neck, protruding sternum with barrel chest, and microcephaly. During the first year of life signs of mental retardation are common and by the time these patients begin to walk a severe degree of short trunk type dwarfism is clearly observable. They have a waddling gait, lumbar hyperlordosis, flexion at the hips, knees, and ankles, and genu valgum. All joint movements with the exception of the wrist tend to be restricted. Chest movements are also frequently limited. By the age of two to three years, shortness of trunk and neck, and pectus carinatum are prominent.

Specific Diagnosis Skeletal radiograms show characteristic changes with flat, anteriorly pointed vertebral bodies. Earlier in life the superior and inferior endplates of the vertebral bodies are notched. Congenital dysplasia of the odontoid process with atlantoaxial dislocation frequently has been observed. Other findings include short, broad ilia with defective ossification of their basilar portions and irregularly ossified "lacelike" crests; laterally displaced capital femoral epiphyses; irregular carpal bones, shortened metacarpals, and phalanges with accessory ossification centers. An abnormal peptidoglycan has been demonstrated in the urine of some patients. Histopathologic studies of the chondroosseous tissue show a specific abnormality which is completely different from that observed in the mucopolysaccharidoses. In affected adults the chondrocytes from the iliac crest are arranged in clusters, irregularly disposed with a markedly fibrous matrix. Throughout the relatively acellular matrix are scattered areas of amorphous appearing ossification which apparently result in the lacy appearance of the iliac crest seen radiographically.

Differential Diagnosis Patients with this disorder somewhat resemble those with the *Morquio syndrome* in skeletal alterations but do not have corneal clouding, do not excrete keratan sulfate in the urine, and most are mentally retarded.

Prenatal Diagnosis Early prenatal diagnosis of this syndrome is not yet possible.

Basic Defect, Genetics, and Other Considerations The basic defect is not known. Recent studies suggest that collagen aggregation is disturbed, as chondrocytes accumulate rather than secrete a regulatory factor and these cells undergo dystrophic calcification. Genetic heterogeneity is now known to exist in this disorder and those with severe mental retardation (the majority) tend to show autosomal recessive inheritance, while those with normal intelligence may display X-linked recessive transmission. It has been suggested that the X-linked recessive form may not show as severe a skeletal dysplasia as the autosomal recessive type. This is a rare syndrome with only about 45 cases of both types reported.

Prognosis and Treatment Life expectancy is not known. The oldest patients with mental retardation are in their twenties, while several with normal intelligence are in their forties. Spinal cord injury due to defects of the odontoid process and atlantoaxial dislocation is possible in both types and prophylactic spinal fusion should be considered.

REFERENCES

Rastogi, S.C., Clausen, J., Melchior, J.C. et al. Biochemical abnormalities in Dyggve-Melchior-Clausen syndrome. *Clin. Chim. Acta 84:* 173–178, 1978.

Toledo, S.P.A., Saldanha, P.H., Lamego, C. et al. Dyggve-Melchior-Clausen syndrome: genetic studies and report of affected sibs. *Am. J. Med. Genet. 4:* 255–261, 1979.

Yunis, E., Fontalvo, J., and Quintero, L. X-linked Dyggve-Melchior-Clausen syndrome. *Clin. Genet. 18:* 284–290, 1980.

M.R. [+ / most]

- microcephaly
- short neck / trunk
- protruding sternum / barrel chest
- restricted joint mobility

Dyggve-Melchior-Clausen Syndromes

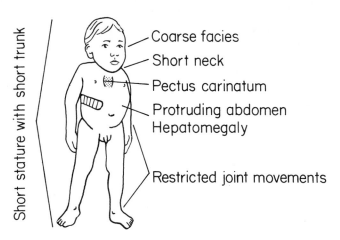

Short stature with short trunk

- Coarse facies
- Short neck
- Pectus carinatum
- Protruding abdomen
- Hepatomegaly
- Restricted joint movements

Autosomal recessive with mental retardation

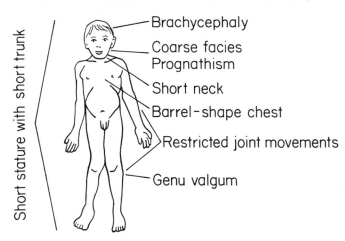

Short stature with short trunk

- Brachycephaly
- Coarse facies
- Prognathism
- Short neck
- Barrel-shape chest
- Restricted joint movements
- Genu valgum

X-linked recessive without mental retardation

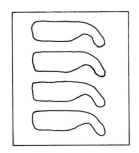
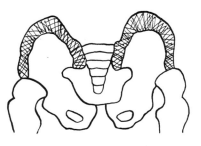
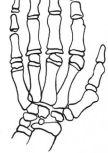

Platyspondyly, lacy periphery of iliac wings, short phalanges and irregular epiphyses

163. DYSCHONDROSTEOSIS

Clinical Features Dyschondrosteosis is the most common form of mesomelic dwarfism. The most consistent and characteristic finding is Madelung deformity of the wrist which is usually symmetrically involved but may be unilateral. This deformity is not commonly recognized clinically until it is accentuated by early epiphyseal fusion in the preadolescent period, however, radiographic features of dyschondrosteosis can be present from birth. Mild disproportionate short stature with mesomelia of the upper and lower limbs is common. Other skeletal anomalies may include short hands and feet with metaphyseal flaring in metacarpal and metatarsal bones, short fourth metacarpal and metatarsal bones, curvature of tibia, exostoses of proximal tibia and/or fibula, abnormal femoral neck, and abnormal tuberosity of humerus. One family has been reported with middle ear deformities and conductive hearing loss, while another family had associated paramyotonia. It remains to be determined whether these findings are part of the disorder.

Specific Diagnosis The clinical features described above in the presence of Madelung deformity make possible the diagnosis of this condition. The radiographic criteria for the recognition of Madelung deformity are as follows: a double (lateral and dorsal) bowing of the radius which involves the entire diaphysis but is most marked at the distal end; variable widening of the interosseous space; shortening of the radius; alteration in contour of the distal radius so that the articular surface of the epiphysis faces in an ulnar and palmar direction; premature fusion of the ulnar half of the epiphyseal line of the distal radius; dislocation or subluxation of the inferior radio–ulnar articulation with the distal ulna dorsal to the distal radius; decreased bone density on the ulnar border of the radius; small bone excrescences sometimes condensed into an exostosis along the inferior ulnar border of the radius; triangularization of the normally quadrangular shaped outline of the distal radial epiphysis; hypercondensation of the ulnar head; a change in the inferior radial articular surface with modification of the relationship of the carpal bones, wedging them between the deformed radius and protruding ulna and giving them a triangular configuration with the lunate at the apex and an arched curvature of the carpal bones.

Differential Diagnosis The Madelung deformity must be differentiated from other possible causes such as *infection* and *trauma*. There is some dispute as to whether Madelung deformity may be distinct and heritable in the absence of the generalized bone dysplasia.

Prenatal Diagnosis This has not been achieved. In the severe form ultrasonography could possibly detect the short, hypoplastic changes in the long bones of the limbs.

Basic Defect, Genetics, and Other Considerations Dyschondrosteosis should be thought of as a generalized bone dysplasia. The basic defect in this autosomal dominant disorder is not known. It has been thought that females are more affected but this may be bias of ascertainment. A more severe form of dyschondrosteosis is due to homozygosity for the gene (*mesomelic dysplasia, Langer type*).

Prognosis and Treatment Adult height varies from 137 to 152 cm. Affected individuals are of normal intelligence. Limitation of movement has been noted to involve the wrist, elbow, or both. Orthopedic surgery may be indicated for severe deformity of the wrist.

REFERENCES

Carter, A.R. and Currey, H.L.F. Dyschondrosteosis (mesomelic dwarfism)—a family study. *Br. J. Radiol.* 47: 634–640, 1974.

Langer, L.O. Jr. Dyschondrosteosis, a hereditable bone dysplasia with characteristic roentgenographic features. *Am. J. Roentgenol.* 95: 178–188, 1965.

Langer, L.O. Jr. Mesomelic dwarfism of the hypoplastic ulna, fibula, mandible type. *Radiology* 89: 654–660, 1967.

- **Madelung deformity**
- **short hands / feet**
- **coxa valga**
- **mesomelic dwarfism**

Dyschondrosteosis

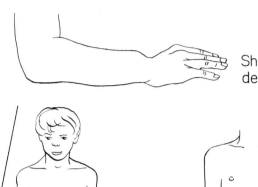

Short forearm with Madelung deformity of wrist

Short stature - short limbs

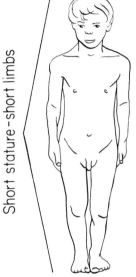

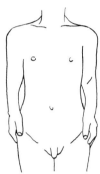

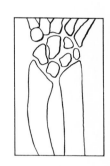

Varying degrees of shortening of forearms and lower legs – short radius with bowing – wedging of carpal bones

Markedly short stature

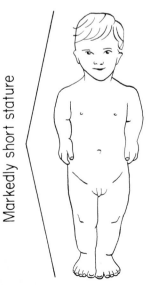

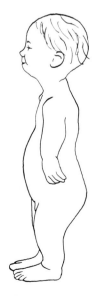

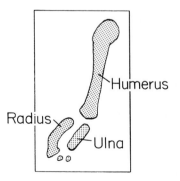

Radius, Humerus, Ulna

Langer type – homozygous form

Marked mesomelic shortening with small mandible and altered forearm bones

164. HAJDU-CHENEY SYNDROME
(arthrodentoosteodysplasia)

Clinical Features The onset of signs in this disorder occurs during early childhood commonly with hand manifestations. Most striking are shortening and clubbing of the distal portion of fingers and toes, primarily the former. The terminal portion of the thumb is especially short. The interphalangeal joints are frequently hyperflexible. With motion, pain or paresthesia may be noted in the joints. The skull may be dolichocephalic and have an unusual protuberance of the squamous portion of the occipital bone. There is delayed closure of the anterior fontanel. The hair is frequently thick and coarse. Early loss of teeth with marked atrophy of the alveolar process of the maxilla and mandible is a constant feature. Some patients have been prognathic while others have had a very small mandible. Unusual facies is characterized by midfacial hypoplasia, fullness of outer supraorbital ridges, mild ocular hypertelorism, small mouth, long nose and short philtrum. Other features include short stature in adulthood, progressive kyphosis, valgus deformity of the elbows and knees, conductive deafness, 6th nerve palsy, blurred vision, headache, hirsutism, long nose, and hypogonadism.

Specific Diagnosis Diagnosis is clinical based on the above features in association with certain radiographic findings, the most striking of which is lysis of the terminal phalanges. Other skeletal roentgenographic findings include widening of the metopic, coronal, and lambdoidal sutures with Wormian bones, absent frontal sinusus, enlarged sella turcica, dolichocephaly, bathrocephaly, and basilar impression of the skull, vertebrae concave on their superior and inferior surfaces, straight cervical spine, kyphosis, marked osteoporosis, and valgus deformation of elbows and knees. Elevated levels of serum alkaline phosphatase and lactic dehydrogenase have been reported.

Differential Diagnosis Acroosteolysis can be observed in a number of disorders such as *pyknodysostosis, mandibuloacral dysplasia, Puretic syndrome, epidermolysis bullosa, scleroderma, psoriasis, hyperparathyroidism,* and various *sensory neuropathy-acroosteolysis syndromes.* An *autosomal dominant form of acroosteolysis* involving just the phalanges, mainly the terminal portion, has been described.

Prenatal Diagnosis Prenatal diagnosis of this disorder is not yet possible.

Basic Defect, Genetics, and Other Considerations The basic defect in this disorder is not known but appears to involve some component of connective tissue affecting the development and persistence of skeletal tissues. Inheritance is autosomal dominant with sporadic cases presumably representing new gene mutations. Originally it was thought that this condition was less severe in females but this has not been substantiated.

Prognosis and Treatment Adults seldom reach a height greater than 157 cm. Multiple fractures may involve the spine, long bones, hands, or feet. Osseous compression may result in a basilar compression which can be life threatening. Most patients have an early loss of teeth. The use of fluoride and sex hormones may be beneficial in the treatment of the osteoporosis, thus lessening the chance for fractures.

REFERENCES

Cheney, W.D. Acro-osteolysis. *Am. J. Roentgen. 94:* 595–607, 1965.

Herrmann, J., Zugibe, F.T., Gilbert, E.F. et al. Arthro-dento-osseous dysplasia (Hajdu-Cheney syndrome). *Z. Kinderheilkd. 14:* 93–110, 1973.

Weleber, R.G. and Beals, R.K. Hajdu-Cheney syndrome—report of 2 cases and review of literature. *J. Pediatr. 88:* 243–249, 1976.

- dolichocephaly / thick coarse hair
- clubbing of fingers and toes / short terminal phalanges
- small mouth / midface hypoplasia
- large nose / short philtrum

Hajdu-Cheney Syndrome
[arthrodentoosteodysplasia]

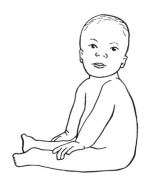

Infant with wide face, flat nose, hypertelorism

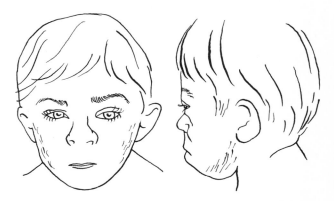

Older child with broad nose, heavy eyebrows, lashes, facial hair, small mouth, hypertelorism, midfacial hypoplasia, micrognathia

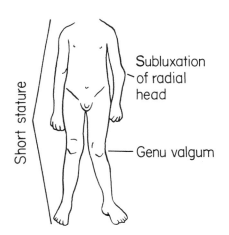

Short stature

Subluxation of radial head

Genu valgum

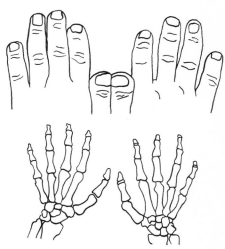

Short terminal phalanges due to osteolysis

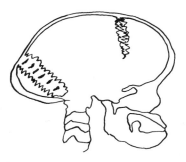

Bathrocephaly, Wormian bones in suture lines

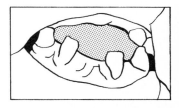

Early loss of teeth

351

165. HOLT-ORAM SYNDROME

Clinical Features The upper extremity anomalies are usually visible at birth. Although such abnormalities of the upper limb may vary extensively, the characteristic findings are a thumb anomaly and atrial septal defect. The thumb may be absent, rudimentary, finger-like, or triphalangeal. Frequently the radius may be absent or hypoplastic. Patients with severe phocomelia have been reported, the most affected having phocomelia of both upper limbs, complete on the left, with one finger only directly attached to the shoulder. At the other end of the spectrum some patients have clinically normal hands but abnormal upper limbs and an inability to oppose the thumbs completely. The most common cardiac defect is ASD, ostium secundum type. Other defects include patent ductus arteriosus, pulmonary hypertension, VSD, and transposition of great vessels. The P-R interval may be prolonged on ECG. Like the upper limb malformations, the cardiovascular anomalies are also variable and may be absent in some patients.

Specific Diagnosis It is important to know that in this disorder the lower limbs are normal and other associated anomalies involving the visceral and skeletal systems are not known to occur. In addition to confirming obvious upper limb anomalies, radiograms of the wrist frequently show alterations in size, number, and shape of carpal bones. Particularly common are abnormally shaped scaphoid bones, additional carpal bones (mainly os centrale, which is the remnant of an ossicle that is normally present in the fetus but normally fuses with the scaphoid before birth) and carpal fusions. In general all metacarpals are longer while the middle phalanges are shorter. The most striking increase is in the first metacarpal and the greatest shortening is of the fifth phalanx. However, such changes may not be specific for this syndrome. Dermatoglyphic studies usually show multiple deviations from the normal. Proper cardiac studies are indicated in all patients, as the congenital heart defect may be so minimal that it is not suspected from physical examination.

Differential Diagnosis Since the Holt-Oram syndrome is not associated with abnormal facies, deafness, ear malformations, mental retardation, and hematologic disorders, the differentiation from other syndromes is relatively easy where upper limb anomalies and congenital heart disease may be part of the syndrome complex. A nonfamilial condition called *ventriculoradial-dysplasia* should be differentiated from the Holt-Oram syndrome. The former is characterized by aplasia of the radius with absent or residual thumbs, VSD, and severe or moderate pulmonary hypertension.

Prenatal Diagnosis Depending on the degree of severity of the limb and cardiac anomalies, this syndrome theoretically should be diagnosable in some cases prenatally by ultrasound and fetoscopy.

Basic Defect, Genetics, and Other Considerations The basic defect in this uncommon condition is not known. It is transmitted in an autosomal dominant mode with a high degree of penetrance and variable expressivity. While most patients have both cardiac and limb anomalies, some have one without the other.

Prognosis and Treatment Life span may be altered due to cardiac involvement, while hand function may be impaired. Intelligence is normal. Treatment consists of surgery for congenital heart disease and skeletal anomalies.

REFERENCES

Holt, M. and Oram, S. Familial heart disease with skeletal malformations. *Br. Heart J. 22:* 236–242, 1960.

Kaufman, R.L., Rimoin, D.L., McAlister, W.H. et al. Variable expression of Holt-Oram syndrome. *Am. J. Dis. Child. 127:* 21–25, 1974.

Pozanski, A.K., Gall, J.C. Jr., and Stern, A.M. Skeletal manifestations of the Holt-Oram syndrome. *Radiology 94:* 45–54, 1970.

- **absent or altered thumbs**
- **upper limb anomalies / phocomelia**
- **atrial septal defect**
- **other cardiac defects**

Holt-Oram Syndrome

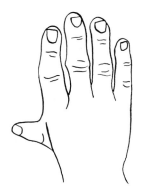

Small, low-set thumb

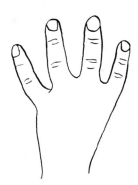

Absence of thumb

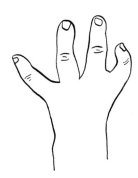

Ectrodactyly, small thumb

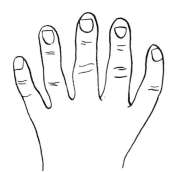

Triphalangeal thumbs

Degrees of phocomelia and ectrodactyly

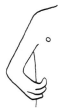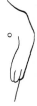

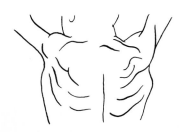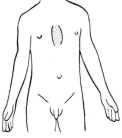

Hypoplasia of shoulder muscles, pectus excavatum, long forearms, congenital heart disease, ASD and VSD

166. HYPOCHONDROPLASIA

Clinical Features This disorder resembles achondroplasia but all features are much milder. At birth, weight and length are commonly within the lower limits of normal and thus short stature is usually not recognized until the age of three to six years. Patients exhibit small stature with disproportionately short limbs. The hands and feet are short and broad. No trident hand deformity is present. Limitation of motion at the elbow is common. Genu varum has been noted in some patients. The head is macrocephalic in 50%. It is brachycephalic in shape with a prominent forehead. There are no facial abnormalities. Lordosis occurs in about 30%.

Specific Diagnosis Diagnosis is clinical based on the above features and certain radiographic findings, the most prominent of which is shortening of the long bones, especially the humerus and femur. Other features include ball-in-socket appearance of the epiphyses of the long bones, flaring of the metaphyses, disproportionately long fibula, prominent styloid process of the ulna, champagne glass configuration of pelvic inlet, short femoral necks, narrow sacrum with a horizontal tilt, and caudal narrowing of the lumbar interpedicular distances. No abnormal laboratory findings are known.

Differential Diagnosis This disorder must be differentiated from *achondroplasia*. This can be done by noting its less severe clinical and radiographic changes. The face is almost always involved in achondroplasia while it appears normal in hypochondroplasia. There are other forms of *short-limbed dwarfism* which might be considered such as *dyschondrosteosis,* where the face is normal but the patients have a Madelung deformity of the wrist.

Prenatal Diagnosis Ultrasound studies might be able to detect a shortening of the humerus or femur in those pregnancies at risk for this disorder; however, such a prenatal diagnosis has not yet been made.

Basic Defect, Genetics, and Other Considerations The basic defect is not known. Histologic studies show regular chondroosseous tissue and thus the defect may be due to a quantitative decrease in the rate of endochondral ossification. Hypochondroplasia is an autosomal dominant condition with varying expressivity. It should not be considered a rare disorder, for it probably occurs more frequently than achondroplasia. It has been postulated that hypochondroplasia may represent an allelic mutation to achondroplasia.

Prognosis and Treatment This is not a life-threatening disorder and the neurological complications associated with achondroplasia are rare. The average height in these patients ranges from 130 to 145 cm. Cesarean section is usually necessary for delivery in pregnant patients. About 10% have mild mental retardation. Treatment is supportive.

REFERENCES

Frydman, M., Hertz, M., and Goodman, R.M. The genetic entity of hypochondroplasia. *Clin. Genet.* 5: 223–229, 1974.

Hall, B.D. and Spranger, J. Hypochondroplasia: clinical and radiological aspects in 39 cases. *Radiology 133:* 95–100, 1979.

McKusick, V.A., Kelly, T.E., and Dorst, J.P. Observations suggesting allelism of the achondroplasia and hypochondroplasia genes. *J. Med. Genet. 10:* 11–16, 1973.

- **small stature / disproportionately short limbs**
- **brachycephaly / prominent forehead**
- **short, broad hands and feet**

Hypochondroplasia

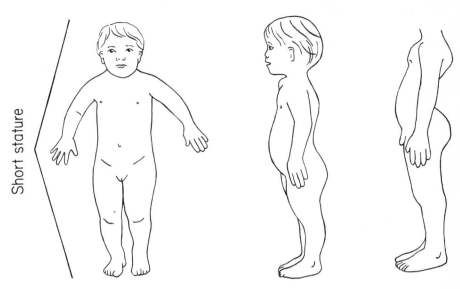

Short stature

Child with normal facies, mild bowing of legs and lumbar lordosis – with age greater lumbar lordosis

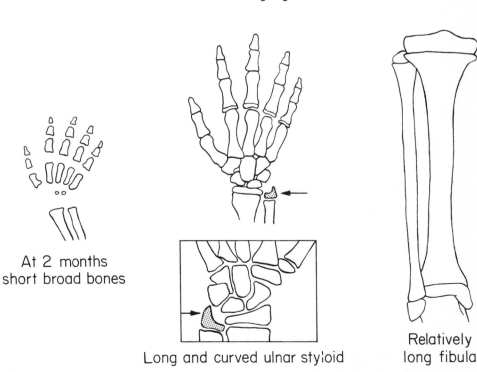

At 2 months short broad bones

Long and curved ulnar styloid

Relatively long fibula

355

167. INFANTILE OSTEOPETROSIS

Clinical Features This disorder is characterized by increased density and brittleness of the bones. Clinical manifestations are evident during infancy. Brittleness predisposes the bones to fracture and such may occur during delivery. Although the fractures tend to heal satisfactorily, deformities frequently develop during childhood. During the first year of life the head becomes enlarged and square in shape with a prominent forehead. Vision is usually disturbed early in life and diminishes progressively as the child grows older. Ocular ptosis, strabismus, cataracts, optic atrophy, and retinal degeneration are commonly observed. Progressive deafness is a frequent finding. The teeth develop abnormally and have a tendency to decay. An agonized facial expression may be seen early in the disease and this may be altered by the development of facial palsy. Patients usually have a hypochromic anemia and in the final stage of the disease develop a pancytopenia. Hepatosplenomegaly and enlargement of the lymph nodes have been observed. General growth is retarded and some patients are dwarfed.

Specific Diagnosis In addition to the above clinical features the diagnosis must be confirmed by the radiographic finding of a generalized bone sclerosis of the entire skeleton. Roentgenograms of the tubular bones show transverse bands in the metaphyseal regions and longitudinal striations in the shafts. The vertebrae show the classical prominent anterior vascular notches. As the condition progresses the proximal humerus and distal femur develop a flask-shaped configuration. The skull becomes progressively thickened with encroachment upon the foramina of the cranial nerves. Serum chemistries are usually normal but hypophosphatemia, hypocalcemia, and tetany have been reported. Histologic examination of bone shows obliteration of the medullary cavity with a lattice-like network of hyaline cartilage surrounded by thick bone which exhibits a paucity of fibrils. Foci of osteoblastic and osteoclastic activity can be seen.

Differential Diagnosis This disease must be distinguished from other disorders in which osteosclerosis occurs such as *pycnodyosostosis, van Buchem disease, craniometaphyseal dysplasia, Engelmann disease, osteopoikilosis, fluorosis,* and *heavy metal intoxication.*

Prenatal Diagnosis This disorder has been recognized in the third trimester of pregnancy by skeletal radiographs of the fetus, and it would seem that recognition could be made with present-day ultrasonographic methods much earlier based on comparative fetal bone density.

Basic Defect, Genetics, and Other Considerations The basic defect is not known. Many theories have been proposed such as faulty resorption of primary spongiosa, poorly formed hypofibrillar bone, and thyrocalcitonin hypersecretion, but none has been substantiated. Transmission is by autosomal recessive inheritance and parental consanguinity has been noted in many families. This is a relatively rare disorder but an unusually high frequency has been observed in Costa Rica. The autosomal dominant form of the disease is essentially benign.

Prognosis and Treatment The prognosis is poor. Most patients die during childhood usually due to anemia or secondary infection. Osteomyelitis is a frequent complication, particularly in the mandible or maxilla. Mentality is normal but chronic illness, blindness, and deafness interfere with development. Treatment is symptomatic. The use of steroids has been reported to be of some value. A few patients have been reported to have had successful bone marrow transplantation.

REFERENCES

Coccia, P.F., Krivit, W., Cervenka, J. et al. Successful bone-marrow transplantation for infantile malignant osteopetrosis. *N. Eng. J. Med. 302:* 701–708, 1980.

Lehman, R.A., Reeves, J.D., Wilson, W.B., et al. Neurological complications of infantile osteopetrosis. *Ann. Neurol. 2:* 378–384, 1977.

Loria-Cortés, R., Quesada-Calvo, E., and Cordero-Chaverri, C. Osteopetrosis in children: a report of 26 cases. *J. Pediatr. 91:* 43–47, 1977.

- **enlarged square-shaped head**
- **agonized facies**
- **ptosis / decrease in vision**
- **brittle bones / progressive deafness**

Infantile Osteopetrosis

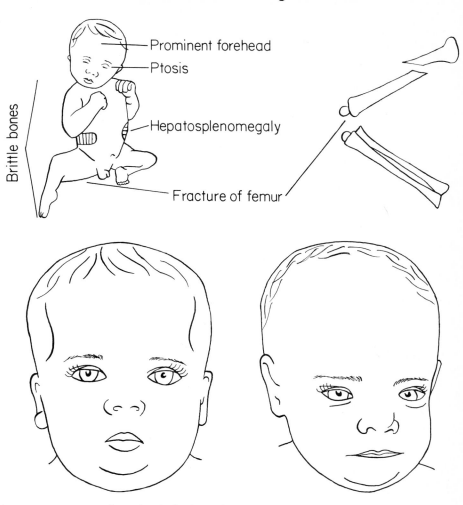

Prominent forehead

Ptosis

Hepatosplenomegaly

Brittle bones

Fracture of femur

Agonized facies with large, square-shaped heads, prominent foreheads, ptosis and strabismus

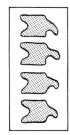 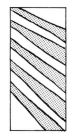 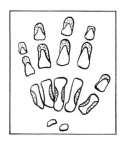

Dense bones with anterior notching of vertebrae, thick ribs, bone within bone appearance of hand

168. KNIEST DYSPLASIA

Clinical Features At birth affected infants frequently have cleft palate, clubfoot, and prominent knees. Marked lumbar lordosis and/or kyphoscoliosis and tibial bowing usually develop within the first few years of life resulting in a disproportionate shortening of the trunk. The child may not sit and walk until the age of two and three years, respectively. Walking is difficult and flexion contractures in the hips produce a characteristic stance. The long bones are short and bowed and the joints are enlarged. Adult height ranges between 105 and 145 cm. There is limitation of joint motion with pain, stiffness, and flexion contractures of the major joints. The fingers are long and knobby and flexion is limited resulting in an inability to form a fist. The face is round, with the midface flat and the nasal bridge depressed, which gives the eyes an exophthalmic appearance. The neck is short and the head appears to sit upon the thorax. Severe myopia, fluid vitreous, and lattice degeneration with or without retinal detachment and/or cataract formation are frequent eye findings. Congenital unilateral ptosis has been reported in one patient. Conduction and/or sensorineural deafness may develop before puberty. Umbilical and inguinal hernias are common.

Specific Diagnosis Characteristic radiographic changes can be observed at birth and these include dumbbell-shaped femora, hypoplastic pelvic bones, vertical clefts of the vertebrae, and platyspondyly. During childhood the findings consist of a dessert-cup shaped pelvis, increased soft tissue densities around the joints, enlarged epiphyses, cloud-like calcifications near the epiphyseal plates, and flat elongated vertebral bodies with cloud-like calcifications. The bones of the upper limbs are short. The metaphyses of long bones flare and the epiphyses are large, irregular, and punctate. The proximal row of carpal bones is small but the bone age is normal or advanced. The pelvic bones are also markedly small. The femoral capital epiphysis forms late, the neck is wide and short with a poorly ossified central area, and there may be coxa vara. The trochanter is prominent. The chondroosseous histopathology is distinctive. Resting cartilage contains large cells, a loosely woven matrix with irregular staining, and many holes resembling "swiss cheese cartilage." The growth plate contains hypercellular cartilage with ballooned chondrocytes and sparse matrix.

Differential Diagnosis This condition has been confused with the *Morquio syndrome, metatropic dysplasia,* and *spondyloepiphyseal dysplasia.* These disorders can be readily distinguished on the basis of skeletal roentgenograms and clinical features.

Prenatal Diagnosis This disorder has not yet been diagnosed prenatally.

Basic Defect, Genetics, and Other Considerations The basic defect is not known. Increased urinary excretion of keratan sulfate has been reported in several patients. Ultrastructural studies have shown chondrocytes filled with dilated cisternae of endoplasmic reticulum. Most cases have been sporadic, however, more than one generation of affected has been reported, which suggests autosomal dominant inheritance. Parental consanguinity has not been noted and multiple affected sibs of unaffected parents have not been observed.

Prognosis and Treatment Motor milestones and speech development may be delayed, but intelligence usually is normal. Recurrent respiratory distress with tracheomalacia may occur in infancy. These patients have a normal life span. Orthopedic surgery is usually indicated for the various skeletal problems. Appropriate care for cleft palate, the hearing disorder, and regular eye examinations for detection and prevention of retinal detachment are all important aspects of treatment.

REFERENCES

Horton, W.A. and Rimoin, D.L. Kniest dysplasia. A histochemical study of the growth plate. *Pediatr. Res. 13:* 1266–1270, 1979.

Kim, H.J., Beratis, N.G., Brill, P. et al. Kniest syndrome with dominant inheritance and mucopolysacchariduria. *Am. J. Hum. Genet. 27:* 755–764, 1975.

Lachman, R.S., Rimoin, D.L., Holister, D.W. et al. The Kniest syndrome. *Am. J. Roentgenol. 123:* 805–814, 1975.

- **large head / short neck**
- **round face / cleft palate / short nose**
- **bowing / shortening of long bones**
- **enlarged joints**

Kniest Dysplasia

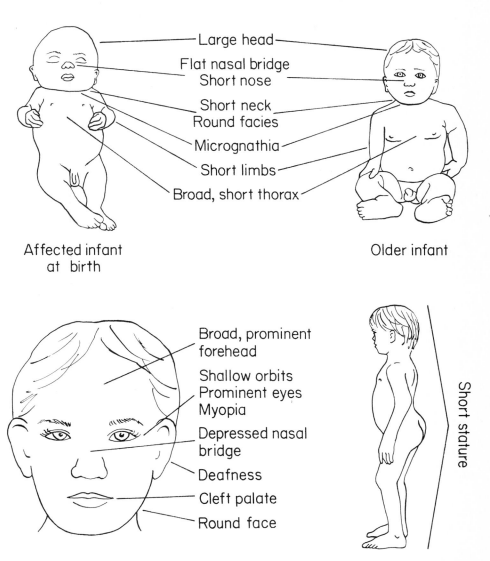

Large head
Flat nasal bridge
Short nose
Short neck
Round facies
Micrognathia
Short limbs
Broad, short thorax

Affected infant
at birth

Older infant

Broad, prominent forehead

Shallow orbits
Prominent eyes
Myopia

Depressed nasal bridge

Deafness

Cleft palate

Round face

Older child with flat midface

Short stature

Short trunk, dorsal kyphosis,
lumbar lordosis, flexion
deformities and enlarged joints

169. LANGER-GIEDION SYNDROME

Clinical Features Certain facial features in this syndrome may be recognizable at birth: bulbous pear-shaped nose with tented alae, prominent elongated philtrum, apparent mandibular micrognathia, thin upper lip, and large laterally protruding ears. Mild microcephaly is a common finding. The scalp hair tends to be thin but the eyebrows may be normal. During infancy and early childhood, the skin is loose. This feature disappears with age. Brown to black maculopapular nevi are frequently located on the upper part of the trunk, neck, scalp, and face. They are not present before four years and they increase in number with age. Other features include the following: multiple cartilaginous exostoses with onset in childhood, asymmetric limb growth, scoliosis, joint hypermobility, hypotonia, hearing deficit, short stature of postnatal onset, winged scapulae, exotropia, and syndactyly.

Specific Diagnosis In addition to the various clinical features noted above, all patients have multiple exostoses which are present by the third or fourth year of life. These exostoses have the same distribution as those found in familial multiple exostoses. Other roentgenographic findings include scoliosis, thin ribs, and cone-shaped epiphyses and clinobrachydactyly.

Differential Diagnosis This syndrome shares many features with the *trichorhinophalangeal syndrome,* but multiple exostoses, loose skin, joint hypermobility, microcephaly, skin nevi, and delay in onset of speech are not found in the latter. Short stature, sparse hair, and brachydactyly may be observed in *cartilage-hair hypoplasia.*

Multiple cartilaginous exostoses in the absence of other anomalies is a recognized autosomal dominant disorder.

Prenatal Diagnosis At present this disorder has not been diagnosed prenatally.

Basic Defect, Genetics, and Other Considerations The basic defect in this relatively rare syndrome is not known. Most cases have been sporadic although occurrence in a father and daughter has been reported. No advanced parental age or consanguinity has been observed. Some patients have been shown to have a deletion of the long arm of chromosome 8, however, the chromosomal alteration was not identical in all. Because of the physical similarities with the trichorhinophalangeal (TRP) syndrome, some refer to this disorder as TRP syndrome Type II.

Prognosis and Treatment Mild to moderate mental retardation has been noted in all cases. A significant delay in onset of speech is common. Upper respiratory tract infections are frequent in infancy but abate in childhood. The overall prognosis in this disorder remains unclear. The risk of malignancy at the site of exostoses is not known for this syndrome but is definitely increased during adulthood in hereditary multiple exostoses. Multiple fractures have been reported in some patients. Treatment is mainly symptomatic consisting of special education for the mental retardation with emphasis on speech development. Orthopedic surgery is indicated for impinging exostoses.

REFERENCE

Hall, B.D., Langer, L.O., Giedion, A. et al. Langer-Giedion syndrome. *Birth Defects 10 (12):* 147–164, 1974.

Gorlin, R.J., Cervenka, J., Bloom, B.A. et al. No chromosome deletion found on prometaphase

banding in two cases of Langer-Giedion syndrome. *Am. J. Med. Genet. 13:* 345–347, 1982.

Wilson, W.G., Herrington, R.T., and Aylsworth, A.S. The Langer-Giedion syndrome: report of a 22-year-old woman. *Pediatrics. 64:* 542–545, 1979.

- microcephaly [mild] / sparse scalp hair
- bulbous nose / tented alae / long philtrum
- thin upper lip
- palpable exotoses

Langer-Giedion Syndrome

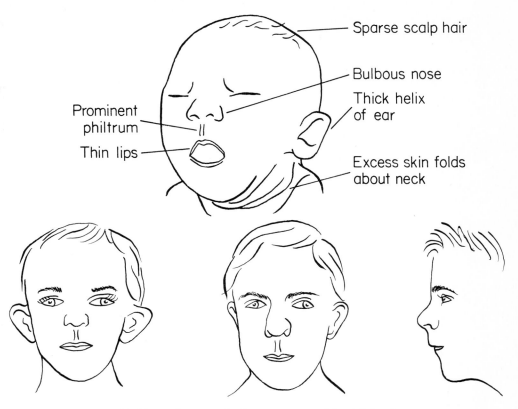

Sparse scalp hair

Bulbous nose

Thick helix of ear

Prominent philtrum

Thin lips

Excess skin folds about neck

Full eyebrows, bulbous nose with thick alae, superiorly tented nares, long, prominent philtrum, thin lips, strabismus and large, protruding ears

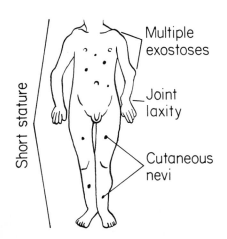

Short stature

Multiple exostoses

Joint laxity

Cutaneous nevi

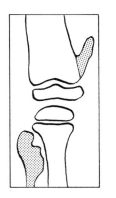
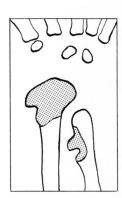

Multiple exostoses

170. McCUNE-ALBRIGHT SYNDROME

Clinical Features The characteristic features consist of polyostotic fibrous dysplasia, abnormal pigmentation of the skin, and sexual precocity. The pigmentary finding is an early manifestation of the disorder appearing from the fourth month to the second year of life, however, in a few patients it has been observed a few weeks postnatally. Well defined, generally unilateral, irregular macular spots (cafe-au-lait type) are scattered over the forehead, nuchal area, and buttocks. Oral pigmentation on the lips and mucosa has been observed but is infrequent. There appears to be a correlation between the amount of pigmentation and the degree of bone involvement. Although any bone may be involved, the long bones are more commonly affected, especially the upper end of the femur. Most patients are initially seen for a limp, leg pain, or fracture. A bowing resembling a hockey stick may result in a leg-length discrepancy. Other bones affected include the tibia, fibula, pelvis, humerus, radius, and ulna. Bilateral involvement occurs in approximately half the cases. Single bone (monostotic) involvement has been reported. Incipient bowing of the legs may be seen as early as the first year of life and nearly always before the age of ten years. Facial asymmetry is found in about 25% of the patients. The jaws may be enlarged and distorted. Protrusion of the eye with associated visual disturbances has been noted. The bony lesions of the skull and facial skeleton, in contrast to the cystic lesions of the long bones, are hyperostotic. Thus overgrowth of bone around the foramens may result in deafness and/or blindness. Skeletal maturation is frequently rapid, producing accelerated growth in childhood and short stature in adulthood. Sexual precocity occurs mainly in females but has been described in affected males. About half of all females with this syndrome have precocious puberty. It usually first presents as vaginal bleeding which may occur as early as three months or, more commonly, between one and five years. It is usually irregular, lasts from 2 to 4 days and may, at times, be profuse. There is no evidence that ovulation takes place early. Breast development and other secondary sex characteristics appear after the menarche, usually from the fifth to the tenth year but have been described as early as birth. Hypertrophy of the external genitalia has been noted. In males precocious puberty may be accompanied by gynecomastia and spermatogenesis. Hyperthyroidism is seen in 20% of patients and, rarely, the Cushing syndrome is found.

Specific Diagnosis Skeletal radiographs show hypo- or hypersclerotic cysts which may be scattered throughout the skeleton. They have a ground-glass appearance due to myriad thin, calcified trabeculae. Serum calcium level is usually normal while the serum phosphorus is diminished in 40% of cases. Serum alkaline phosphatase levels are elevated in about 50%. Elevated steroid excretion and increased urinary luteinizing hormone and estrogen levels have been reported.

Differential Diagnosis The bony lesions in children should be distinguished from those of *hyperparathyroidism, giant cell tumors,* and *neurofibromatosis*. With regard to skin pigmentation, the giant pigment granules seen in *neurofibromatosis* are rare in this syndrome. Precocious puberty may be caused by the *adrenogenital syndrome* or an *ovarian granulosa cell tumor.*

Prenatal Diagnosis This is not yet possible.

Basic Defect, Genetics, and Other Considerations The basic defect is not known. All reported cases have been sporadic except perhaps one case in a mother and daughter and a report in monozygotic twins, suggesting a possible genetic origin.

Prognosis and Treatment Life span can be normal but when fibrous dysplasia is extensive early in life, the prognosis is poor. Sarcomatous degeneration has been reported in a few patients. Orthopedic intervention is frequently indicated for bony deformity and nonunion of fractures. Medroxyprogesterone may be used for control of sexual precocity.

REFERENCES

Albright, F., Butler, A.M., Hampton, A.O., et al. Syndrome characterized by osteitis fibrosa, disseminata, areas of pigmentation and endocrine dysfunction with precocious puberty in females. Report of five cases. *N Engl. J. Med. 216:* 727–746, 1937.

Firat, D. and Stutzman, L. Fibrous dysplasia of the bone. Review of twenty-four cases. *Am. J. Med. 44:* 421–429, 1968.

Lemli, L. Fibrous dysplasia of bone: report of female monozygotic twins with and without the McCune-Albright syndrome. *J. Pediatr. 91:* 947–949, 1977.

- **hyperpigmentation**
- **lower limb deformity / bowing of leg**
- **facial asymmetry / protrusion of eye**
- **sexual precocity, mainly female**

McCune-Albright Syndrome

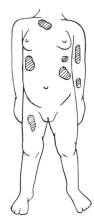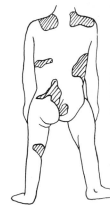

Precocious puberty, pigmentary changes in a young child

Hockey-stick deformity of left leg, irregular areas of pigmentation

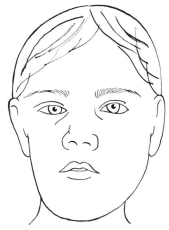

Facial asymmetry and fullness of left cheek

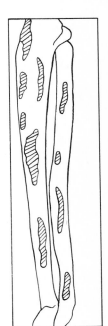

Pseudocystic involvement of tibia and fibula

Pigmentation of oral mucosa and lips

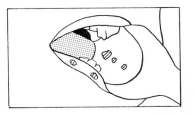

171. MELNICK-NEEDLES SYNDROME

Clinical Features The syndrome is characterized by a diffuse bone dysplasia and abnormal facies. Early in childhood affected patients tend to have recurrent respiratory and ear infections. There is failure to gain in weight and height and the anterior fontanel closes late. The facial appearance is unusual and consists of a high forehead, full cheeks, micrognathia, prominent eyes, large ears, and marked malocclusion. The body shape is altered due to a long neck, narrow shoulders, and short upper arms. An abnormal gait, dislocation of the hips, and mild scoliosis are common.

Specific Diagnosis Diagnosis is clinical based on the above features in combination with specific radiographic findings. Most striking are the changes in the long bones with bowing of the radius and tibia producing a S-shaped configuration. The metaphyses at the proximal and distal ends of the humerus, fibula, and tibia are flared. Coxa valga is marked. The ribs are ribbon-like with cortical irregularities. The iliac bones are flared at the crest and constricted in the supraacetabular area, while the ischial bones are tapered. All vertebral bodies are unusually tall, especially those of the axis, atlas, and occipital condyles. The thoracic vertebrae show an anterior concavity with double beaking. Delayed closure of the anterior fontanel and sclerosis of the skull base and mastoid processes are common along with hypoplastic changes in the mandibular coronoid process. In adults bony changes may be mild.

Differential Diagnosis Radiographic findings are distinctive enough to differentiate this syndrome from other conditions in which there is delayed closure of the anterior fontanel.

Prenatal Diagnosis This syndrome has been recognized in the last trimester of pregnancy by skeletal radiographs of the fetus. Although distinct skeletal changes can be noted late in pregnancy, no information is available as to the earliest gestational date that such skeletal defects would be diagnosable with present-day techniques.

Basic Defect, Genetics, and Other Considerations The basic defect is not known. This relatively rare syndrome appears to be an X-linked dominant, lethal in males, however, a few affected males have been reported. The large number of isolated female cases representing new mutations suggests reduced fertility, but more information is needed.

Prognosis and Treatment Affected individuals tend to be of normal intelligence and have a normal life span. With age, arthritic changes may involve the spine and hips. Normal childbirth may not be possible due to pelvic deformities. Treatment consists of appropriate dental care and orthopedic intervention to correct the scoliosis if severe.

REFERENCES

Gorlin, R.J. and Knier, J. X-linked or autosomal dominant, lethal in male, inheritance of the Melnick-Needles syndrome (osteodysplasty)? *Am. J. Med. Genet. 13:* 453–456, 1982.

Melnick, J.C. and Needles, C.F. An undiagnosed bone dysplasia. A two family study of 4 generations and 3 generations. *Am. J. Roentgen 97:* 39–48, 1966.

Perry, L.D., Edwards, W.C., and Bramson, R.T. Melnick-Needles syndrome. *J. Pediatr. Ophthalmol. Strabismus, 15:* 226–230, 1978.

- **high forehead**
- **full cheeks / micrognathia**
- **prominent eyes / large ears**
- **long neck / narrow shoulders**

Melnick-Needles Syndrome

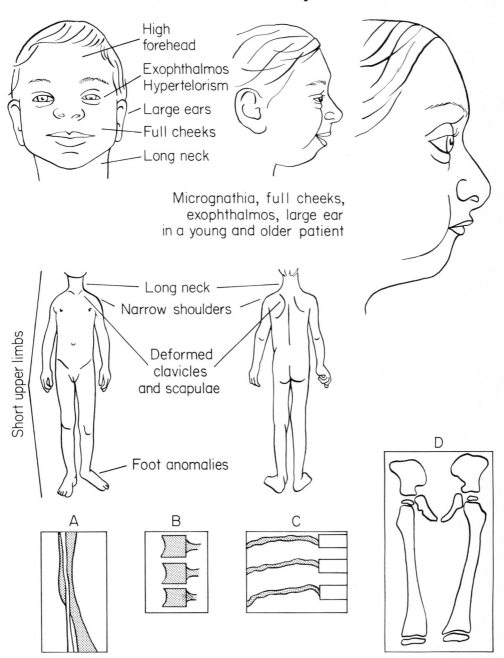

High forehead

Exophthalmos
Hypertelorism

Large ears

Full cheeks

Long neck

Micrognathia, full cheeks, exophthalmos, large ear in a young and older patient

Long neck

Narrow shoulders

Deformed clavicles and scapulae

Foot anomalies

Short upper limbs

A   B   C   D

(A) S-shaped tibia, (B) tall vertebral bodies with anterior concavity, (C) thin ribs with cortical irregularities, (D) flared ilia, tapered ischial bones, coxa valga, metaphyseal flare

172. METATROPIC DYPLASIA

Clinical Features This disorder is suggested in infants who have normal craniofacial features but short extremities and a relatively long narrow trunk. During the neonatal period, body length is usually within the normal range, but late in infancy kyphoscoliosis develops and rapidly progresses, resulting in short-trunk dwarfism. Because of the change in body proportions with age the term "metatropic" dysplasia was coined from the Greek *metatropos* meaning "changing pattern." The extremities are short with bulbous enlargements of the metaphyses and limited joint movement. The hands and feet are short and hyperextensible. Some patients have a peculiar tail-like skin fold over the sacrum.

Specific Diagnosis The diagnosis is made from the above clinical features in association with characteristic radiographic changes which include marked platyspondyly with tongue-like flattening of the vertebrae and relatively large intervertebral spaces. The long bones are short with irregular expanded metaphyses resembling barbells. The epiphyses are deformed, flattened, and irregular with a delay in ossification. The tubular bones of the hands are short and broad with irregular epiphyses and metaphyses. The ribs are short with flared and cupped costochondral junctions. There is marked flaring of the iliac crest.

Differential Diagnosis This disorder must be differentiated from *Morquio disease, Kniest dysplasia,* and *achondroplasia. Morquio disease* has distinguishing craniofacial findings, including clouding of the cornea and excess excretion of keratansulfate in the urine. In *Kniest dysplasia* there are flat facies with prominent eyes, cleft palate, hearing loss, myopia, and limited joint motion. *Achondroplastic* infants tend to have frontal bossing and a depressed nasal bridge. Each of these disorders also has skeletal findings which can be helpful in differentiating them from metatropic dysplasia.

Prenatal Diagnosis Prenatal diagnosis of this disorder may be possible using sonography to measure the length of fetal long bones in the extremities.

Basic Defect, Genetics, and Other Considerations The basic defect is not known, but from various histopathologic studies it has been postulated that the alteration may be in ossification rather than in chondrogenesis. This relatively rare skeletal disorder is transmitted in an autosomal recessive fashion.

Prognosis and Treatment Many patients with metatropic dysplasia die in infancy, but survival into adulthood is common. Adult height varies from 110 to 120 cm. Scoliosis becomes quite severe and incapacitating with age and is resistant to treatment. Intellect does not seem to be altered.

REFERENCES

Larose, J.H. and Gay, B.B. Jr. Metatropic dwarfism: *Am. J. Roentgenol. 106:* 156–161, 1969.

Maroteaux, P., Spranger, J.W., and Wiedemann, H.R. Der metatropische Zwergwuchs. *Arch. Kinderheilkd. 173:* 211–226, 1966.

Rimoin, D.L., Siggers, D.C., Lachman, R.S. et al. Metatropic dwarfism, the Kniest syndrome and the pseudoachondroplastic dysplasias. *Clin. Orthop. and Rel. Res. 114:* 70–82, 1976.

- **short extremities / long trunk**
- **kyphoscoliosis**
- **short feet and hands / hyperextensible**
- **skin fold over sacrum**

Metatropic Dysplasia

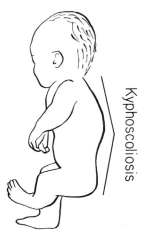

Kyphoscoliosis

Long narrow
trunk, short limbs
and enlarged joints

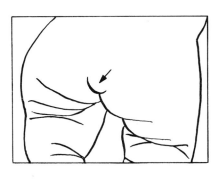

Tail-like appendage
overlying sacrum (arrow)

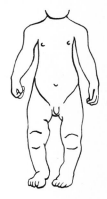

Narrow thorax,
prominent joints
with restricted
mobility

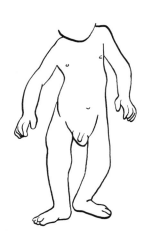
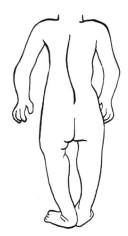

Older child with
narrow thorax, severe
kyphoscoliosis with
altered posture

Platyspondyly, wide intervertebral space at birth-
"Halberd" appearance of
iliac wings, broad metaphyses
with dumb-bell shape
femurs in a newborn

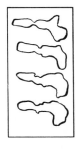
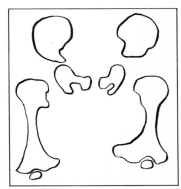

173. NAIL-PATELLA SYNDROME

Clinical Features This disorder can be recognized at birth by the absence or hypoplasia of the nails and patellae. When present, the nails are markedly reduced in size, with the ulnar half missing and never reaching the fingertips. The thumbnails are most commonly involved with changes in the other nails diminishing progressively from the index to the fifth finger. Fingernails are more frequently affected than toenails. Triangular lunulae, absent skin creases of the distal fingers, clinodactyly, and camptodactyly are other hand findings that have been observed. If the patella is present it is hypoplastic and dislocation is common. The elbow joints may show limited supination and incomplete extension. Numerous other skeletal anomalies have been observed some of which include iliac horns, hypoplastic scapulae, cervical ribs, pectus carinatum, scoliosis, and hyperostosis frontalis. Eye findings may show ptosis, cataracts, paralysis of the internal rectus, and heterochromia with a clover-leaf deformity of the iris. A nephropathy resembling glomerulonephritis or congenital nephrosis has been noted in some affected persons. Cancer of the colon has also been seen in association with this syndrome.

Specific Diagnosis The combination of nail and patellar findings is quite distinct and makes for ease in the diagnosis. Although there can be many skeletal changes observed in this condition the presence of iliac horns and absence or hypoplasia of the patellae are the most characteristic radiographic features. Electron microscopic findings in the kidney may show focal thickening and wrinkling of the glomerular basement membrane, focal fusion of the foot processes of the visceral epithelial cells, and occasional erythrocytes in Bowman spaces.

Differential Diagnosis Absence of nails or *anonychia* may be an isolated genetic defect or associated with *ectrodactyly* or a syndrome with areas of *flexural pigmentation*. Both *anonychia* and *onychodystrophy* may also occur in the same family. Hypoplastic nails may also be noted with *genetic forms of deafness* and may be seen in infants of mothers taking *anticonvulsant drugs* during pregnancy. *Aplastic* or *hypoplastic patellae* may be associated with *aniridia* or *coxa vara* and *tarsal synostosis. Familial dislocation of the patella* has been described.

Prenatal Diagnosis Since the ABO blood group locus and the nail-patella locus are linked, under the right circumstances linkage studies may be helpful in making a prenatal diagnosis of the disorder. Certain skeletal anomalies may be detectable using sonography in those pregnancies at risk.

Basic Defect, Genetics, and Other Considerations The basic defect in this disorder involving ectodermal and mesodermal structures is not known. The gene for this autosomal dominant syndrome is located on the terminal portion of the long arm of chromosome 9, linked to the ABO blood group locus. The recombination fraction is about 10% but is higher in females than males. The familial aggregation of the renal aspects suggests two separate genes—one for the nephropathic form and one for the non-nephropathic type. They might be allelic since no heterogeneity has been detected in linkage with the ABO locus.

Prognosis and Treatment In general, the prognosis for this disorder is good but renal complications can shorten life. Death as early as eight years has been reported. Approximately 10% of the patients die of renal disease. Treatment is symptomatic with efforts to diagnose the renal disease early.

REFERENCES

Daniel, C.R. III, Osment, L.S., and Noojin, R.O. Triangular lunulae: A clue to nail-patella syndrome. *Arch. Dermatol. 116:* 448–449, 1980.

Silverman, M.E., Goodman, R.M., and Cuppage, F.E. The nail-patella syndrome: clinical findings and ultrastructural observations in the kidney. *Arch. Int. Med. 120:* 68–74, 1967.

Zimmerman, C. Iliac horns: a pathognomonic roentgen sign of the familial onycho-osteodysplasia. *Am. J. Roentgenol. 86:* 478–483, 1961.

- **absent / hypoplastic nails**
- **absent / hypoplastic patellae**
- **limited mobility of elbows**
- **eye and skeletal anomalies**

Nail-Patella Syndrome

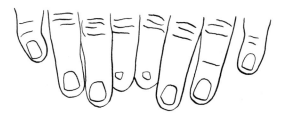

Hypoplasia of nails of index fingers and thumbs, clinodactyly, and decrease in creases over distal joints

Triangular lunula and nail dystrophy tends to involve the ulnar side of nail

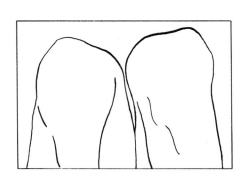

Knees with absence of patellae

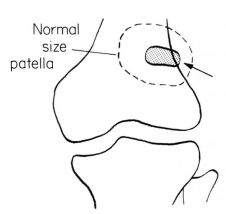

Normal size patella

Size of hypoplastic patella (arrow)

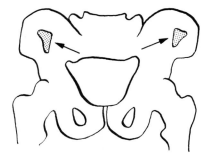

Iliac horns (arrows)

369

174. PYCNODYSOSTOSIS

Clinical Features The term for this disorder is derived from the Greek "pyknos" referring to the increased density of the bones. Affected individuals have a characteristic facies due to underdeveloped facial bones, a relatively large head with frontal and occipital prominence, pinched nose with upturned tip, blue sclerae, mild exophthalmos, receding chin, and obtuse mandibular angle. The palate tends to be high, narrow, and grooved. Due to persistence of deciduous teeth, there is an appearance of a double row of teeth. Dental caries is common. Because of shortness of the extremities adult height is reduced, being 134 to 152 cm. The trunk is not shortened but often exhibits marked pectus excavatum with underdeveloped breasts in females. The shoulders tend to be narrow with partial aplasia of acromial ends of the clavicles. Kyphosis, scoliosis, increased lumbar lordosis, and a narrow thorax have been reported. The terminal phalanges of fingers and toes are reduced and widened, causing the tips to appear bulbous. The nails may be flat, thin, and hypoplastic. The skin over the dorsal surface of the fingers is frequently wrinkled.

Specific Diagnosis Many of the facial features described above are present at birth. Radiographically there is generalized skeletal sclerosis without significant disturbance of modelling. The sclerosis may be of a minor degree in infancy but increases progressively during growth. Radiograms of the skull show separation of sutures, an open anterior fontanel, hypoplastic paranasal sinuses, small facial bones, Wormian bones in lambdoidal sutures and lack of mandibular angle. The terminal phalanges of the fingers and toes show fragmentation of the heads with preservation of the bases, osteolysis of the unguiculate portions, or narrowing of the ends of otherwise normal terminal phalanges. Brachymesophalangy of the fifth fingers, less often the index fingers, is a common finding. Reduced serum alkaline phosphatase has been found in a few cases. Intermittently high plasma calcitonin levels have been reported.

Differential Diagnosis *Mandibuloacral dysplasia* resembles pycnodysostosis, but there is no increase in bone density or aplasia of the mandibular angle. The open cranial fontanels and sutures might suggest *cleidocranial dysplasia*. In *acroosteolysis* the alveolar process is often markedly atrophic, but the angle is not missing as in pycnodysostosis, furthermore, the former is inherited as an autosomal dominant disorder.

Prenatal Diagnosis This is presently not available.

Basic Defects, Genetics, and Other Considerations The precise nature of the basic defect in pycnodysostosis is not known. Morphologically the defect in mature bone appears to be primarily one of disorganization of bone structure at the level of lamellar bone formation and of the osteon, although whether there is a biochemical defect in one or more of the matrix components has not been determined. Although this condition is relatively uncommon (100 patients in 50 kindreds) it has wide geographic distribution. It may be particularly common in Japan. There have been many reports of parental consanguinity and affected sibs with normal parents; thus autosomal recessive inheritance is well established. Genetic heterogeneity is most probably present as there have been several reports of atypical forms of this condition.

Prognosis and Treatment In general, this is not a life threatening disorder, but osteomyelitis is a common complication following fracture, especially of the mandible, and as such the prognosis may be guarded. Approximately two-thirds of the patients have fractures involving mainly the lower extremities, mandible, and clavicle. There may be a progressive loss of bone in the distal phalanges and outer clavicle and persistent open fontanels, especially the posterior. Special dental care is frequently indicated.

REFERENCES

Maroteaux, P. and Lamy, M. Deux observations d'une affection osseuse condensante: la pycnodysostose. *Arch. Franc. Pediat., 19:* 267–274, 1962.

Meredith, S.C., Simon, M.A., Laros, G.S. et al. Pycnodysostosis. A clinical, pathological and ultra-microscopic study of a case. *J. Bone Joint Surg. 60-A:* 1122–1127, 1978.

Sedano, H.O., Gorlin, R.J., and Anderson, V.E. Pycnodysostosis. Clinical and genetic considerations. *Am. J. Dis. Child. 16:* 70–77, 1968.

- **frontal / occipital prominence**
- **pinched / anteverted nose**
- **prominent eyes**
- **short stature / narrow shoulders**

Pycnodysostosis

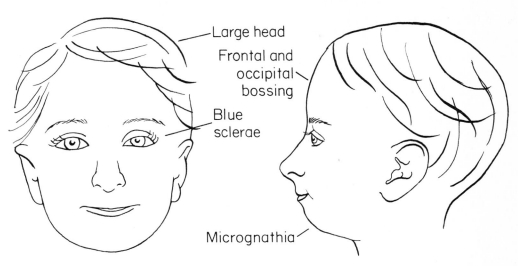

Large head

Frontal and occipital bossing

Blue sclerae

Micrognathia

Note small face, prominent eyes, pinched nose with anteverted nares

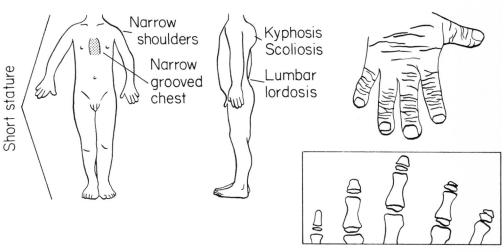

Short stature

Narrow shoulders

Narrow grooved chest

Kyphosis
Scoliosis

Lumbar lordosis

Wrinkled skin of hands, short terminal phalanges due to acroosteolysis

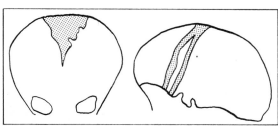

Open anterior fontanel, separation of sutures

175. THANATOPHORIC DYSPLASIA

Clinical Features Thanatophoric (death-carrying) dysplasia is incompatible with life. In approximately 70% of cases there is a history of polyhydramnios. At least 35% are premature and born by breech presentation. The skull is large (up to 40 cm) with prominent frontal bossing. A clover-leaf skull deformity has been described in some affected infants. The nasal bridge is depressed. Bulging of the eyes is common. The extremities are severely shortened and bowed. Redundant skin folds are present about the arms and legs. The chest is markedly narrow in contrast to a large protruding abdomen. The extremities extend outward from the trunk with the thighs abducted and externally rotated in a frog-like position. Total body length ranges from 29 to 47 cm (40 cm average). There is hypotonia and the primitive and deep tendon reflexes are absent.

Specific Diagnosis Distinct radiologic features include a narrow thorax, high clavicles, and very short ribs flared at the costochondral junctions. The interpediculate distance of the lower lumbar vertebrae is reduced. Due to reduced vertebral height, the intervertebral spaces are greatly enlarged (2–3 times the height of the vertebral body). The scapulas are incompletely developed. The pelvis is short and broad. The ilia appear rectangular with transverse measurement larger than vertical. The iliac bones articulate low on the sacrum and the sacrosciatic notches are narrow. The pubic and ischial bones are short and broad. The acetabular roofs are flattened and horizontal. There is striking micromelia of the long bones which are short, broad, and bowed. At the knees, the epiphyses are not ossified. The metaphases are cupped and flared, especially at the proximal end of the femurs. Pear-shaped translucencies are seen at the proximal end of the femur. The total configuration is that of a "telephone receiver." The development of the vault of the skull is excessive, contrasting with reduction in size of the skull base and foramen magnum. Histopathologic studies have shown disorganization of endochondral ossification, while electron microscopy has revealed large conspicuous homogeneous intracytoplasmic vacuoles in chondrocytes.

Differential Diagnosis Thanatophoric dysplasia mainly must be differentiated from *achondroplasia,* especially the homozygous form. In *achondrogenesis* the head is larger; ossification is severely deficient in the vertebral bodies, especially in the lumbar region and absent in the sacral, pubic, and ischial bones.

Prenatal Diagnosis This disorder has been diagnosed late in pregnancy using sonography and radiographs but now with improved sonographic methods it is possible to recognize this condition earlier (16–20 weeks of gestation) by measuring head size, and the lengths of the long bones of the extremities.

Basic Defect, Genetics and Other Considerations The basic defect is not known; however, there is a generalized disruption of endochondral bone formation. It has been observed there is little attempt at column formation and no orderly progression of chondrocytes at the growth plate. The genetics is poorly understood at present because of heterogeneity. Birth order seems to be elevated and some think that autosomal recessive inheritance is likely in those cases with a clover-leaf skull deformity. Nearly all cases have been sporadic. There appears to be male predilection.

Prognosis and Treatment Most die shortly after birth from respiratory insufficiency due to the small thoracic cage.

REFERENCES

Nissenbaum, M., Chung, S.M.K., Rosenberg, H.K. et al. Thanatophoric dwarfism: two case reports and survey of the literature. *Clin. Pediatr. 16:* 690–697, 1977.

Rimoin, D.L. The chondrodystrophies. In: Harris, H. and Hirschhorn, K. (eds.), *Adv. Hum. Genet. 5:* 1–118, 1975.

Shaff, M., Fleischer, A.C., Battino, R. Antenatal sonographic diagnosis of thanatophoric dysplasia. *J. Clin. Ultrasound 8:* 363–365, 1980.

- large head / frontal bossing
- depressed nasal bridge
- redundant skin folds arms / legs
- short, bowed limbs / narrow chest

Thanatophoric Dysplasia

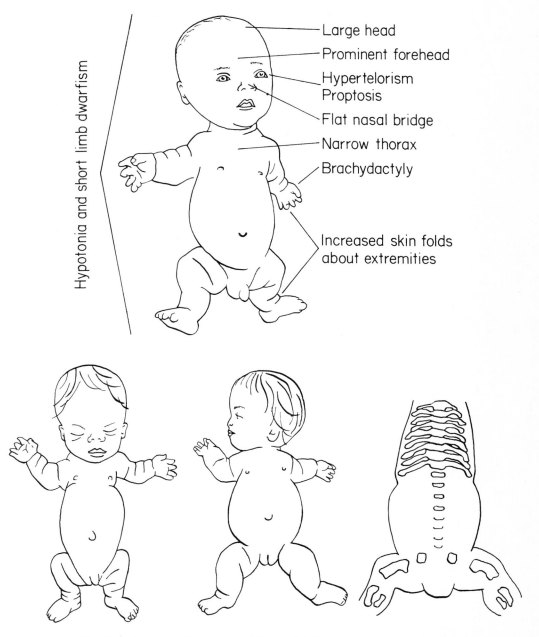

Hypotonia and short limb dwarfism

Large head
Prominent forehead
Hypertelorism
Proptosis
Flat nasal bridge
Narrow thorax
Brachydactyly

Increased skin folds about extremities

Similar features in other affected infants—note short ribs, platyspondyly, short long bones and bent femurs

176. THROMBOCYTOPENIA–APLASIA OF RADIUS
(TAR Syndrome)

Clinical Features The main features present at birth are hypomegakaryocytic thrombocytopenia and bilateral aplasia of the radius. Other hematologic findings include absence of megakaryocytes, "leukemoid" granulocytosis, eosinophilia, and anemia out of proportion to apparent blood loss. Bilateral aplasia of the radius is a consistent finding and ulnar and humeral deformities have frequently been noted. The presence of thumbs in the absence of the radius is an important differentiating feature. Lower limb anomalies have been reported in some cases and these include hip dislocation, coxa valga, femoral and tibial torsion, abnormal tibiofibula joints, ankylosis of the knee, patella dislocation, small feet, valgus and varus foot deformity, abnormal toe placement, and hypoplasia or aplasia of the lower limbs. Other associated anomalies are asymmetric first rib, cervical rib, cervical spina bifida, fused cervical spine, mandibular and/or maxillary hypoplasia, cardiac anomalies (most commonly tetralogy of Fallot or atrial septal defect), decreased IQ, low-set ears, and Meckel's diverticulum.

Specific Diagnosis This syndrome is easily recognizable when the above clinical features are present (mainly involving the upper limbs) in conjunction with a bone marrow examination showing an absence or decrease in megakaryocytes.

Differential Diagnosis This syndrome can be differentiated from *Fanconi anemia* by the absence of thumbs, late onset of hematologic manifestation, and chromosomal changes observed in the latter. In the *Aase syndrome* triphalangeal thumbs, VSD, and leukopenia are helpful differentiating findings. Patients with *pseudothalidomide* or *Holt-Oram syndrome* have normal platelets and other distinguishing characteristics.

Prenatal Diagnosis Theoretically a prenatal diagnosis could be made using ultrasound and fetoscopy to demonstrate the upper limb anomalies.

Basic Defect, Genetics, and Other Considerations The basic defect in the syndrome is not known. The vast majority of reported cases fit the criteria for autosomal recessive inheritance. Some families have shown scattered cases in more than one generation but not fitting a Mendelian pattern, thus suggesting multifactorial transmission with environmental factors interacting to determine the phenotype. For some unknown reason, the syndrome occurs more frequently in females.

Prognosis and Treatment Approximately 40% of the patients expire in early infancy due to hemorrhage. The severity of the hematological disorder usually becomes less with age and therefore vigorous early management is indicated. Orthopedic procedures should be considered when necessary to improve function and cosmetic needs of the patient.

REFERENCES

Edelberg, S.B., Cohn, J., and Brandt, N.J. Congenital hypomegakaryocytic thrombocytopenia associated with bilateral absence of radius—the TAR syndrome: intra-family variation of the clinical picture. *Hum. Hered. 27:* 147–152, 1977.

Hall, J.G., Lewin, J., Kuhn, J.P. et al. Thrombocytopenia with absent radius (TAR). *Medicine, 48:* 411–439, 1969.

Ray, R., Zorn, E., Kelly, T. et al. Lower limb anomalies in the thrombocytopenia absent-radius (TAR) syndrome. *Am. J. Med. Genet., 7:* 523–528, 1980.

- **bilateral aplasia of radius**
- **lower limb anomalies [in some]**
- **small feet**
- **anemia**

Thrombocytopenia-Aplasia of Radius
[TAR syndrome]

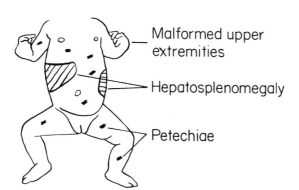

Malformed upper extremities

Hepatosplenomegaly

Petechiae

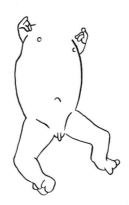

Both upper and lower limbs deformed plus small penis

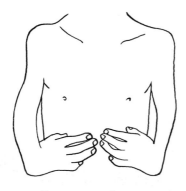
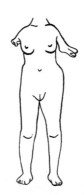

Degrees of upper limb involvement

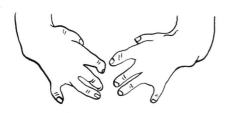
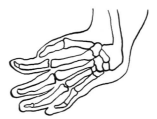

Syndactyly, camptodactyly, small, low-set thumbs, absent radius, malformed ulna and carpal bones

C. Genetic Syndromes

f. Skin / Hair

177. ACRODERMATITIS ENTEROPATHICA

Clinical Features Skin lesions, hair loss, nail changes, and gastrointestinal disturbances are noted between the ages of three weeks and ten years with an average age at onset of nine months. Many patients exhibit the full syndrome by one year. The cutaneous features consist of irregular plaques of vesicles and bullae on erythematous bases. Satellite vesicles, bullae, and pustules may occur on the skin about the plaques. Characteristically, the lesions are localized at the mucocutaneous orifices and on the peripheral parts of the extremities (mouth, eyelids, elbows, knees, nails, anogenital area). Hair loss occurs early in the disease and involves the scalp, eyebrows, and eyelashes. Affected children show a striking uniformity of appearance due to the alopecia and the orificial location of the lesions. These children tend to hold their head at an angle with their face downward. After a short period of time the vesicular lesions begin to dry and crust, subsequently developing into sharply marginated lesions. When the lesions heal they leave no scars. Gastrointestinal disturbances consist of bouts of diarrhea with increased excretion of fat. Many of these children suffer from thrush. *C. albicans* may be recovered in the stools, oral cavity, skin, and nails. The thrush appears as a white coating on the oral mucosa which is firmly attached to underlying structures. On the buccal mucosa and borders of the tongue, there may be numerous small papillomas with a whitish, thickened epithelial covering. Severe halitosis is common. Delayed eruption of deciduous teeth has been reported.

Specific Diagnosis This is mainly a clinical diagnosis based on the previously described features. Biopsy of skin lesions has not revealed specific changes. Low serum zinc levels have been found in some patients. Duodenal and jejunal biopsies have shown a decrease in leucine aminopeptidase and succinic dehydrogenase activity.

Differential Diagnosis This condition should be differentiated from *generalized moniliasis* where the course is not intermittent and there is no total alopecia or familial background. Skin lesions, nail changes, and total alopecia are rarely seen in *celiac disease*. Other disorders having similar features to acrodermatitis enteropathica are *dystrophic epidermolysis bullosa, acrodermatitis continua Hallopeau,* and *Kawasaki disease.* Extensive *parenteral feeding* or prolonged *diuresis* may produce a similar clinical condition probably due to a *zinc deficiency.*

Prenatal Diagnosis This has not yet been achieved.

Basic Defect, Genetics, and Other Considerations The basic defect is not known. It has been suggested that absence of a low molecular weight zinc-binding factor may be the cause of deficient zinc absorption. The binding factor is present in human breast milk which has been known to ameliorate the disorder. Furthermore, it has been noted that the onset of the syndrome often coincides with the time of weaning. There are many reports of affected sibs and an autosomal recessive mode of transmission seems plausible. Although rare, the disorder is evenly distributed worldwide.

Prognosis and Treatment In the past the majority of cases have ended fatally. Body growth is retarded in most patients and approximately half suffer from mental changes often in the form of schizoid features associated with exacerbations. Successful treatment with the oral administration of zinc sulfate has been achieved. The standard dose is 50 mg three times daily in the form of tablets or powder dissolved in fruit juice.

REFERENCES

Barnes, P.M. and Moynahan, E.J. Zinc deficiency in acrodermatitis enteropathica. *Proc. R. Soc. Med.* 66: 327–329, 1973.

Danbolt, N. and Closs, K. Acrodermatitis enteropathica. *Acta Derm-venerol. (Stockh.)* 23: 127–169, 1943.

Neldner, K.H. and Hambidge, K.M. Zinc therapy of acrodermatitis enteropathica. *N. Engl. J. Med.* 292: 879–882, 1975.

- **skin lesions / vesicles and bullae**
- **lesions at muco-cutaneous orifices / extremities**
- **hair loss / scalp, eyebrows, lashes**
- **diarrhea**

Acrodermatitis Enteropathica

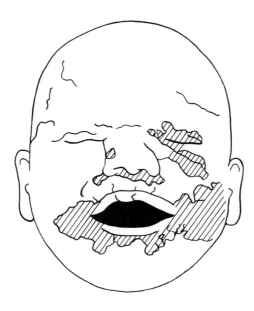

Inflammatory skin changes involving perioral area
and other parts of face – alopecia present

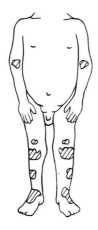
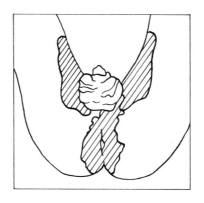

Symmetric skin lesions (vesiculobullous) in
areas of natural body creases

379

178. BLOOM SYNDROME

Clinical Features The key features are growth retardation, sun-sensitive telangiectatic eruptions on the face, altered immune function, and a predisposition to cancer. Full-term infants tend to have low mean birth weight (males 2094 g and females 1841 g). Although the skin is normal at birth, late in infancy or early in childhood telangiectatic erythematous lesions begin to develop about the nose, lips, and malar area. In about half of the patients, lesions also involve the forearms, dorsa of hands, back of the neck and ears. Exposure to sunlight exacerbates the skin lesions. The erythema tends to fade after puberty, followed by scarring, atrophy, and depigmentation. Cafe-au-lait spots are observed in more than half the patients. During childhood these patients may present with dwarfism, although by the late teens sufficient growth has usually taken place and they are not true dwarfs. Adult height rarely exceeds 145 cm. Body proportions are normal but they appear delicate and slender. They show a striking resemblance to one another due to their small, narrow faces, dolichocephalic heads, protruding ears, facial skin lesions, and short stature. A high-pitched voice has been noted. Older patients may have reduced muscle strength accompanied by ultrastructural changes in skeletal muscle. Some affected males have disproportionately small testes. Azoospermia has been demonstrated in a few cases. Menstrual periods are often irregular and infrequent in affected females.

Specific Diagnosis By childhood the clinical features are usually characteristic and combined with chromosomal studies and the demonstration of diminished immunoglobulins, allow for relatively easy diagnosis. The most characteristic chromosomal aberration is a quadriradial configuration. Chromatid gaps, breaks, interchanges, and numerous sister-chromatid exchanges are observed.

Differential Diagnosis The Bloom syndrome should be differentiated from *ataxia-telangiectasia, Cockayne syndrome, Rothmund-Thomson syndrome, dyskeratosis congenita, Fanconi anemia,* and *xeroderma pigmentosum* since all these disorders are characterized by growth retardation, increased incidence of neoplasia, immunologic deficiency, late-onset diabetes, and premature senility of the skin and conjunctiva. Increased chromosomal breaks have also been reported in Fanconi anemia, ataxia-telangiectasia and dyskeratosis congenita, but the changes are unlike those seen in Bloom syndrome.

Prenatal Diagnosis Since affected infants are small at birth, prenatal detection through the use of ultrasound may be of value in determining fetal size. Amniocentesis has been done in a few pregnancies known to be at risk. Here the previously mentioned chromosomal changes can serve as a diagnostic aid.

Basic Defect, Genetics, and Other Considerations The basic defect in this autosomal recessive syndrome is not known. Attempts to find an enzymatic alteration involving the repair mechanism of DNA using ultraviolet light have been unproductive. Approximately 45% of all patients are of Ashkenazi Jewish origin. It has been estimated that the heterozygote frequency in the Ashkenazi Jewish community is greater than 1 in 120. Parental consanguinity is rare among affected Jewish families and high in non-Jewish affected families. Males seem to be more often affected than females. A possible explanation for the relatively low incidence in females is the disproportionately high death rate among females during fetal and early postnatal life. There is no evidence to suggest that the course of this disorder in non-Jews is different from that in Jews.

Prognosis and Treatment Intelligence appears to be normal in most patients. The fact that married males have not had children raises the question of possible sterility in the male. More studies are needed to assess the fertility of female patients. All patients have a propensity to develop neoplasias and these include acute leukemia, reticulum cell sarcoma, squamous cell carcinoma of the tongue, and various neoplastic lesions of the gastrointestinal tract. As a result, life span is shortened for these patients. Early detection of cancer obviously is of prime importance as well as proper treatment of all infections during infancy and childhood. Patients should avoid exposure to sunlight. The use of various protective creams tends to reduce the severity of the facial lesions.

REFERENCES

Bloom, D. The syndrome of congenital telangiectatic erythema and stunted growth. *J. Pediatr. 68:* 103–113, 1966.

German, J. Bloom's syndrome II. The prototype of human genetic disorders predisposing to chromosome instability and cancer. In: *Chromosomes and Cancer,* ed. J. German, pp. 601–617. New York, Wiley, 1974.

German, J. Bloom's syndrome. In: *Genetic Diseases Among Ashkenazi Jews,* eds. R.M. Goodman and A.G. Motulsky, pp. 121–139. New York, Raven Press, 1979.

M.R. [+ / few]

- **telangiectatic erythematous lesions about face**
- **dolichocephaly**
- **small, narrow face / protruding ears**
- **slender, short habitus**

Bloom Syndrome

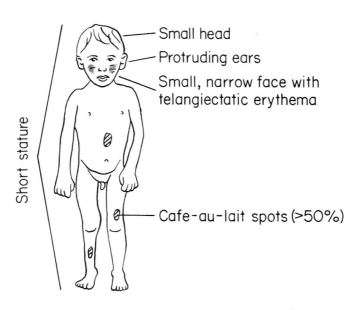

Short stature

Small head
Protruding ears
Small, narrow face with telangiectatic erythema

Cafe-au-lait spots (>50%)

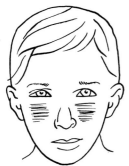
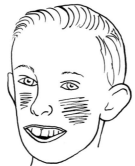
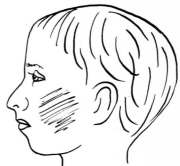

Similar facial and skin findings along with
mild dolichocephaly and prominent nose

Normal 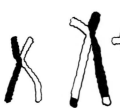 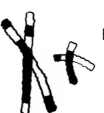 Bloom

Chromosomes showing almost no sister chromatid
exchange in the normal but marked in the Bloom cell

381

179. DYSKERATOSIS CONGENITA

Clinical Features This disorder is characterized by hyperpigmentation of the skin, nail dystrophy, and mucous membrane changes, as well as pancytopenia (50%) and solid tumors (17%). Skin changes appear around puberty and are well-developed by the second decade. The skin develops a gray-brown color with a reticulate lacy pattern simulating poikiloderma which involves the face, neck, and trunk, but at times becoming more widespread. Generalized hyperpigmentation is common. Later findings include deforming atrophic changes of the hands, elbows, knees, and feet with traumatic formation of bullae. Acrocyanosis of the hands and feet along with palmoplantar hyperkeratosis and hyperhidrosis have been frequently noted. In most cases the nails become dystrophic around puberty. Sparse hair has been noted in about 20% of cases. Crops of vesicles and bullae appear on the oral mucosa most frequently around the age of six years, although in some cases earlier. These flaccid bullae are recurrent and painless. After several attacks the mucosa becomes atrophic and the tongue loses its papillae and becomes smooth. Mucosal atrophy or stenosis has been reported in the mouth, esophagus, anus, urethra, and vagina. Chronic blepharitis, ectropion, profuse tearing due to keratinization with obstruction of the lacrimal points, and loss of eyelashes are common eye findings in this disorder. Other features occasionally described include the following: thinning of the ear drum, malformation of the middle ear, small testes, enlarged thyroid, mental retardation, schizophrenia, malformed teeth, frail skeletal structure, splenomegaly, and premature graying of hair.

Specific Diagnosis The clinical picture is quite characteristic with the oral changes appearing first in early childhood followed by the cutaneous alterations around puberty. The histologic appearance of the skin is not diagnostic. Demonstration of pancytopenia, low serum gamma globulins, thymic dysplasia, and increased sister chromatid exchange may aid in the diagnosis.

Differential Diagnosis Although there are similarities between this disorder and *Fanconi anemia*

they can be distinguished clinically by the absence of renal and skeletal anomalies in dyskeratosis congenita. In *focal dermal hypoplasia* there is also a poikiloderma-like condition but missing digits, scoliosis, and hypohidrosis are associated with this syndrome. Dyskeratosis congenita should be differentiated from a number of other disorders such as *xeroderma pigmentosum, pachyonychia congenita,* several *palmar-plantar hyperkeratotic syndromes, epidermolysis bullosa, incontinentia pigmenti,* etc.

Prenatal Diagnosis The finding of increased sister chromatid exchange in chromosomes from lymphocytes of patients with this disorder may be a diagnostic aid in the prenatal recognition of this condition. In families where this syndrome is obviously X-linked recessive, prenatal sex determination may be considered. Further knowledge is needed before the disorder can be precisely diagnosed prenatally.

Basic Defect, Genetics, and Other Considerations The basic defect in this condition is not known. It has been shown that the oral lesions are characterized by a decreased number of keratinosomes associated with a decreased epithelial cell turnover. Thus, the disorder is not really a dyskeratosis. Although most patients are males and there is well documented evidence for X-linked recessive inheritance, there are apparently other genetic forms transmitted as autosomal dominant (Scoggins type) and recessive. In the X-linked recessive form, linkage studies have been unrewarding.

Prognosis and Treatment Several reports describe an increased frequency in carcinomatous lesions involving the buccal and cervical mucosa. Premalignant and carcinomatous changes have also been reported in the urethral and anal mucosa. Aplastic anemia and hypersplenism have been described in many patients. Thus, the prognosis is guarded in this disorder. Patients should be kept under close observation for early detection of malignant changes and appropriate therapy instituted. The teeth are subject to early decay and periodontal disease secondary to noncare, as it is painful to brush.

REFERENCES

Burgdorf, W., Kurvink, K., and Cervenka, J. Sister chromatid exchange in dyskeratosis congenita lymphocytes. *J. Med. Genet. 14:* 256–257, 1977.

Sirinavin, C. and Trowbridge, A.A. Dyskeratosis congenita: clinical features and genetic aspects. Report of family and review of the literature. *J. Med. Genet. 12:* 339–354, 1975.

Trowbridge, A.A., Sirinavin, C., and Linman, J.W. Dyskeratosis congenita: hematologic evaluation of a sibship and review of the literature. *Am. J. Hematol. 31:* 143–152, 1977.

- vesicles / bullae on oral mucosa
- smooth tongue
- generalized hyper-pigmentation
- dystrophic nails

Dyskeratosis Congenita

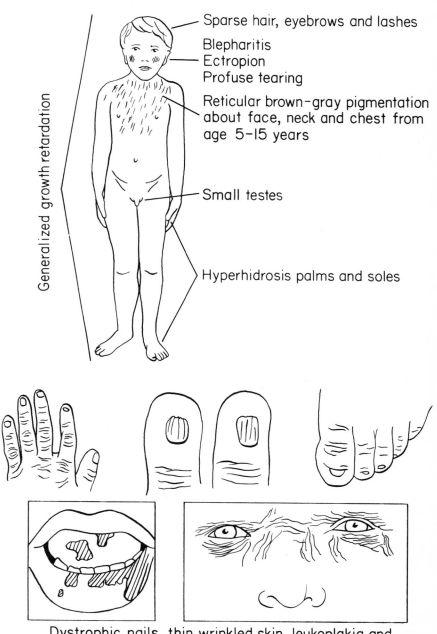

Generalized growth retardation

Sparse hair, eyebrows and lashes

Blepharitis
Ectropion
Profuse tearing

Reticular brown-gray pigmentation about face, neck and chest from age 5–15 years

Small testes

Hyperhidrosis palms and soles

Dystrophic nails, thin wrinkled skin, leukoplakia and mucosal atrophy of lips and tongue, atrophic skin about eyes, absence of eyebrows and lashes

180. ENDOCRINE-CANDIDOSIS SYNDROMES

Clinical Features This group of disorders is generally characterized by certain endocrine diseases that also exhibit superficial candidosis. Candidosis commonly involving the oral and perioral areas is usually the first feature of the syndrome to appear within the first six years of life. These children may also exhibit diminished, brittle scalp hair, sparse eyebrows, dry skin, and thin altered nails. Anal and/or vaginal candidosis may also be present. These findings are then followed from three months to thirteen years later by the various endocrine components. The most common endocrine associations are juvenile hypoparathyroidism, Addison disease, and hypothyroidism. However, in some patients one or more of the following conditions may be present: a celiac-like syndrome, chronic liver disease, achlorhydria, pernicious anemia, malfunction of the thyroid gland (Hashimoto disease), and pulmonary infiltrates of undetermined cause. Not all the features of the syndrome are present in the same patient or in a single family.

Specific Diagnosis The diagnosis is clinical based on the presence of superficial candidosis associated with one of the various conditions previously mentioned. Culture studies should be done to document the presence of *Candida albicans* and endocrine and other investigations are required to prove the diagnosis of any of the suspected associated disorders. Immunologic abnormalities may include hypergammaglobulinemia, selective IgA deficiency, anergy, autoimmune endocrinopathies, and chronic hepatitis. Defective suppressor T-cell function has been noted in both affected and clinically normal sibs.

Differential Diagnosis Candidosis may be seen in association with a number of conditions such as *various neoplasms* (*leukemia* and *lymphoma*), *prolonged antibiotic* and *corticosteroid therapy,* and *acrodermatitis enteropathica.* Increased susceptibility to chronic mucocutaneous candidosis may also be seen in *familial chronic mucocutaneous candidiasis, Di George syndrome,* and *Swiss type agammaglobulinemia.*

Prenatal Diagnosis This has not yet been achieved.

Basic Defect, Genetics, and Other Considerations The basic defect is not known, but in familial candidiasis endocrinopathy the immunologic abnormalities suggest defective immunoregulation, rather than disordered effector mechanisms. Family studies favor autosomal recessive inheritance. Genetic heterogeneity is probably present in this group of disorders. Familial chronic mucocutaneous candidiasis is a distinct entity also inherited as an autosomal recessive disorder and frequently associated with iron deficiency. An autosomal dominant form of mucocutaneous candidosis has been reported in association with increased susceptibility to bacterial infection, hyperkeratosis follicularisis, alopecia universalis, keratoconjunctivitis, and diarrhea in infancy. This disorder has been shown to have B-cell abnormalities.

Prognosis and Treatment In general the prognosis is good, but it is dependent on the other associated conditions and the degree to which each can be properly treated.

REFERENCES

Arulanantham, K., Dwyer, J.M., and Genel, M. Evidence for defective immunoregulation in the syndrome of familial candidiasis endocrinopathy. *N. Engl. J. Med., 300:* 164–168, 1979.

Myllärniemi, S. and Perheentupa, J. Oral findings in the autoimmune polyendocrinopathy-candidosis syndrome (APECS) and other forms of hypoparathyroidism. *Oral Surg. 45:* 721–729, 1978.

Spinner, M.W., Blizzard, R.M., and Childs, B. Clinical and genetic heterogeneity in idiopathic Addison's disease and hypoparathyroidism. *J. Clin. Endocr. 28:* 795–804, 1968.

- **moniliasis / face, scalp, mouth, nails**
- **alopecia / sparse eyebrows**
- **dry skin**
- **associated with endocrine disorder**

Endocrine-Candidosis Syndromes

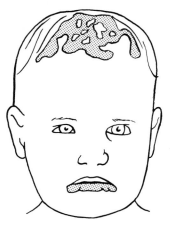
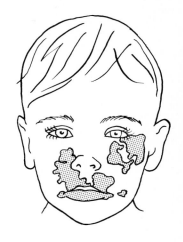
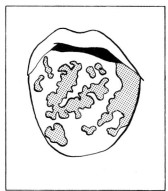
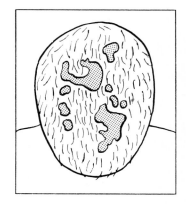
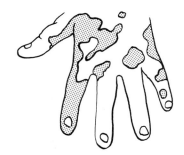
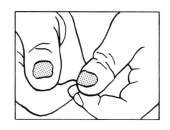
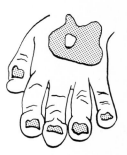

Moniliasis involving corners of mouth, face,
tongue, scalp, hands and nails – for a specific
diagnosis, various associated endocrine
and other conditions must be considered

181. EPIDERMOLYSIS BULLOSA SYNDROMES

Clinical Features Epidermolysis bullosa is composed of various genetic disorders characterized by blistering of the skin and involving the oral and other mucosae. The conditions are grouped on the basis of whether or not they lead to scarring and also by their mode of inheritance. The main types will be discussed separately.

Dominant Simplex This form usually appears neonatally or during infancy when the child begins to crawl. The hands and feet are most commonly involved, rarely other parts of the body, but the nails are normal. Heat appears to be an important precipitating factor in blister formation.

Dominant Dystrophic This form usually presents itself in early childhood with 20% showing changes before the age of one year. The ankles, knees, hands, elbows, and feet are involved with flat, pink, scar-producing bullae. In most instances the nails are thick and dystrophic. Oral bullae have been noted in about one-fifth of the patients. Hyperhidrosis of the palms and soles has been reported in some patients.

Recessive Dystrophic There are probably many subtypes in this form, but in general the disorder begins shortly after birth. The bullae can arise spontaneously or be due to pressure or trauma. In infants, the feet, buttock, scapulae, elbows, hands, and occiput are commonly involved. In other children the hands, feet, and elbows tend to be the more common sites; however, the eyes, teeth (pockmarked alteration of the enamel, delayed eruption, and dental caries), oral mucosa, and esophagus are also commonly affected. Scarring may result in a clawhand deformity, laryngeal stenosis, and partial or complete obstruction of the esophagus.

Recessive Lethal or Herlitz Type Some consider this to be a more severe form of the recessive dystrophic type. Its features appear at birth with absence of pigmentary changes and death by the age of three months. A few hours after birth there may be hemorrhagic vesicles at the base of the fingernails. Later the nails become loose and fall away. Sites of skin lesions include the trunk, face, scalp, extremities, and umbilicus. The palms and soles are not affected. These fragile and hemorrhagic bullae are commonly found in the mouth between the hard and soft palates.

Specific Diagnosis The above forms can usually be recognized by their sites of involvement, severity of clinical manifestations, mode of genetic transmission, and histopathological findings. Microscopically the bullae are subepithelial in the recessive dystrophic and lethal forms, while in the simple form, they are usually within the epidermis beneath the stratum corneum.

Differential Diagnosis In children this condition must be differentiated from other disorders which produce skin lesions such as *congenital syphilis* and *porphyria, bullous impetigo, bullous dermatitis herpetiformis, Ritter disease,* and *drug eruptions*.

Prenatal Diagnosis This is possible in the lethal form using fetoscopy for obtaining a fetal skin biopsy which shows separation of the epidermis from the dermis at the lamina lucida along with reduced number of malformed hemidesmosomes. The dominant dystrophic type has also been diagnosed in utero by detecting an elevated level of α-fetoprotein in the maternal serum and amniotic fluid.

Basic Defect, Genetics, and Other Considerations The basic defect in this group of disorders is not known. In the simplex form it has been postulated that there may be an activation by mechanical trauma of cytolytic enzymes within the epidermal cells. Ultrastructural studies in the lethal form have shown fewer hemidesmosomes and tonofilaments in the skin. The mode of genetic transmission in the above forms is either autosomal dominant or autosomal recessive as indicated. There is much heterogeneity in epidermolysis bullosa and the exact status of many of these variants remains to be clarified in terms of classification.

Prognosis and Treatment In the lethal recessive form patients die early in infancy while in the dystrophic recessive type death is not unusual during childhood. In the dominant simple type the lesions often show marked improvement by puberty, while in the dominant dystrophic form some improvement is common with age. Treatment in all forms tends to be symptomatic with avoidance of trauma and mechanical factors that may lead to blistering.

REFERENCES

Gedde-Dahl, T. *Epidermolysis bullosa: a clinical genetic, and epidemiologic study.* Johns Hopkins Press, Baltimore, 1971.

Rodeck, C.H., Eady, R.A.J., and Gosden, C.M. Prenatal diagnosis of epidermolysis bullosa letalis. *Lancet 1:* 949–952, 1980.

Yacoub T. et al. Maternal serum and amniotic fluid concentrations of alphafetoprotein in epidermolysis bullosa simplex. *Br. Med. J. 1:* 307, 1979.

- **bullae over skin**
- **scarring**
- **dysplastic nails**
- **contractures of fingers**

Epidermolysis Bullosa Syndromes

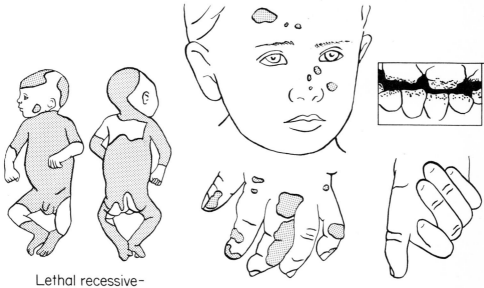

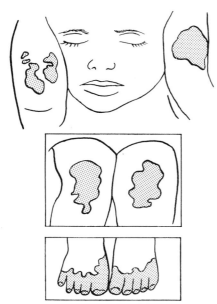

Lethal recessive–
bullae and denuded
areas over body

Dystrophic recessive–bullae, pitting of teeth,
later contracture of fingers and loss of nails

Dystrophic dominant –limbs and nails
involved with residual scarring

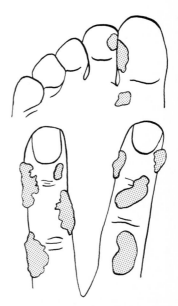

Simple dominant –usually only
hands and feet involved

182. FAMILIAL LYMPHEDEMA SYNDROMES

Clinical Features Familial lymphedema may have its onset at birth or anytime thereafter to adulthood. It generally involves the lower extremities bilaterally, but unilateral involvement is known. The upper limbs may also be affected. It can occur as an isolated finding presenting as a nontender chronic swelling of the extremities, or it may be a transient or permanent feature associated with a number of syndromes. Some attempt has been made to classify the various types of familial lymphedema by either time of onset or mode of genetic transmission. One of the more common forms of isolated lymphedema has its onset at birth and is transmitted as an autosomal dominant trait. This has been called Milroy disease or congenital hereditary lymphedema. It usually involves the lower limbs and expressivity varies from minimal swelling of an ankle to greatly enlarged feet, legs, and thighs. There is usually slow progression in the severity of the edema.

In the late-onset form or Meige type of lymphedema, the swelling may appear during the teens but usually presents between the ages of 20 and 40 years. The course is usually chronic with slow progression involving the lower extremities; however upper limb and unilateral involvement have been reported. Autosomal dominant inheritance has been noted in several families, recessive transmission in a few, and in others the genetic transmission remains unclear.

Transient congenital lymphedema of the hands and feet may be observed in both the Turner syndrome and the Noonan syndrome, and at times the lymphedema may be chronic in the latter.

Syndromes associated with lymphedema include: (a) dystrophic yellow nails and pleural effusion (auto. dominant), (b) extra row of eyelashes, ectropion lower lid, webbing of neck, and vertebral anomalies (auto. dominant), (c) cerebrovascular malformation and pulmonary hypertension (auto. dominant), (d) recurrent cholestatic jaundice (auto. recessive), and (e) ptosis of eyelids (auto. dominant).

Specific Diagnosis In general the diagnosis for each of the various types is dependent on the clinical features, associated findings, family history, and when indicated chromosomal studies (e.g., Turner syndrome). Lymphangiographic studies are seldom diagnostic in these primary forms and often quite difficult to perform.

Differential Diagnosis Secondary forms of lymphedema due to *bacterial* or *parasitic infections, neoplasia, postphlebitic* and *postlymphangitic* causes must be ruled out. Other causes of peripheral edema due to *renal, cardiac,* or *liver* diseases must also be excluded.

Prenatal Diagnosis In a pregnancy at risk for congenital lymphedema ultrasound studies may be helpful in detecting an altered thickness or diameter of an affected limb or limbs. A fetal skin biopsy taken from an extremity may show hypoplastic lymphatic vessels. However, most cases of congenital lymphedema do not lend themselves to an accurate prenatal diagnosis at present.

Basic Defect, Genetics, and Other Considerations The basic defect is not known, but in most instances there seems to be a hypoplasia of the lymphatic vessels. This hypoplasia may be transient or permanent. The genetics of the various forms have been discussed under clinical features.

Prognosis and Treatment The lymphedema per se does not alter life span. However, such complications as lymphangitis or the development of lymphangiosarcoma may result in an early death. The prognosis for each form must be considered individually. With extreme edema, problems in ambulation coupled with various emotional difficulties are common. Resection of subcutaneous tissues with subsequent skin autografts have been done with variable results. Diuretics, elevation of the limb, and bed rest are not effective.

REFERENCES

Adam, A.H. et al. Prenatal diagnosis of fetal lymphatic system abnormalities by ultrasound. *J. Clin. Ultrasound 7:* 361–364, 1979.

Goodman, R.M. Familial lymphedema of the Meige type. *Am. J. Med. 32:* 651–656, 1962.

Miller, M. and Motulsky, A.C. Noonan syndrome in an adult family presenting with chronic lymphedema. *Am. J. Med. 65:* 379–383, 1978.

- edema of distal limb or limbs
- variable onset

Familial Lymphedema Syndromes

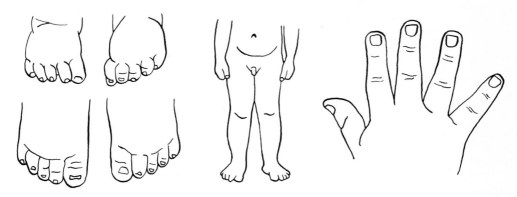

Milroy disease – lymphedema onset at birth involving mainly feet and lower limbs but also hands and arms

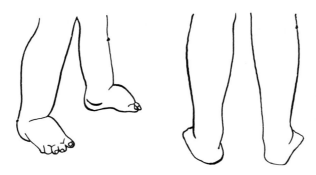

Meige type-onset during teens

A   B   C   D

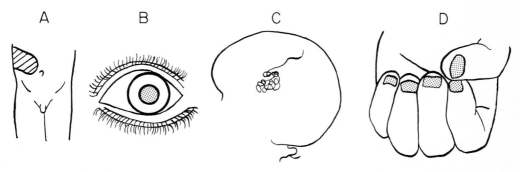

Lymphedema associated with A) neonatal cholestasis and cirrhosis, B) distichiasis (extra rows of eyelashes), C) extracranial vascular malformation and D) yellow dystrophic nails

183. FOCAL DERMAL HYPOPLASIA
(Goltz syndrome)

Clinical Features The disorder is characterized by the presence of atrophy and linear hyperpigmentation of the skin, localized deposits of superficial fat, multiple papillomas of mucous membranes or periorificial skin, abnormalities of the extremities, and anomalies of the nails. At birth asymmetric skin lesions are usually present in the form of scar-like abnormalities, streaky hyperpigmentation, atrophy, and telangiectasia. Some infants may show isolated areas of total absence of skin. A rather pathognomonic finding is the presence of soft, yellow, baggy herniations of subcutaneous fat mainly in the regions of the iliac crest, groin, and posterior aspect of the thigh. Papillomas frequently develop on the lips, gums, base of tongue, circumoral area, anogenital and inguinal regions, axillae, and around the umbilicus. The scalp hair is usually sparse and brittle or there may be areas where hair is absent. The nails may be absent, dystrophic, spooned, grooved, or hypopigmented. The most common eye anomalies are chorioretinal and iris colobomata. Other defects include strabismus, nystagmus, obstructed tear ducts, microphthalmia, and unilateral anophthalmia. The external ears may be hypoplastic and deafness has been reported. A frequent hand anomaly is bilateral syndactyly between the third and fourth fingers. Other findings include clinodactyly, polydactyly, oligodactyly, and adactyly. Brachydactyly can be present due to shortened phalanges, metacarpals, or metatarsals. Midclavicular aplasia or hypoplasia occurs principally on the right side. Rib anomalies, scoliosis, and spina bifida occulta are common. A constant finding is osteopathia striata. Other findings include microcephaly, mental and growth retardation, hypoplasia of the genital system, small breasts, hypodontia, oligodontia, microdontia, fragility of the enamel and cleft lip and palate. Very rarely cardiac anomalies (aortic stenosis, ASD with pulmonary hypertension) and abnormalities of the kidney and ureter have been described.

Specific Diagnosis In conjunction with the above clinical features the diagnosis is made by the characteristic histology with fat cells replacing connective tissue in the corium. Linear striations of the metaphyseal regions of the long bones (osteopathia striata) as seen on radiographic studies are another diagnostic feature.

Differential Diagnosis This disorder should be differentiated from *incontinentia pigmenti* and *Rothmund-Thomson* syndrome. In *nevus lipomatosus superficialis* the neutral fat-containing cells are adjacent to blood vessels in the mid- and upper layers of the skin.

Prenatal Diagnosis Since this disorder predominantly affects females, prenatal sexing with possible interruption of pregnancy has been offered to those families at risk. A precise in utero diagnosis has not yet been made.

Basic Defect, Genetics, and Other Considerations The basic defect in this disorder is not known. Most consider this condition to be transmitted as an X-linked dominant trait due to the preponderance of affected females (only 11 affected males reported as of 1981). Furthermore, it is thought that this syndrome in its fullest expression is lethal in males and accounts for markedly reduced fertility in the female. An increase in spontaneous abortions is a recognized feature of this disorder in affected women.

Prognosis and Treatment The only risk to life may come from soft tissue defects involving mainly the heart and kidneys, but these are uncommon manifestations of the syndrome. Some individuals are severely handicapped by skeletal deformities as well as the cosmetic changes resulting from the cutaneous and ocular features. Ocular, dental, plastic, and orthopedic procedures are frequently indicated.

REFERENCES

Fjellner, B. Focal dermal hypoplasia in a 46,XY male. *Int. J. Dermatol. 18:* 812–815, 1979.

Goltz, R.W., Henderson, R.R., Hitch, J.M., et al. Focal dermal hypoplasia syndrome. A review of the literature and report of two cases. *Arch. Dermatol. 101:* 1–11, 1970.

Warburg, M. Focal dermal hypoplasia. Ocular and general manifestations with a survey of the literature. *Acta Ophthal. 48:* 525–536, 1970.

- atrophy / linear hyper-pigmentation of skin
- multiple mucosal papillomas
- herniation of sub-cutaneous fat
- eye and digital anomalies

Focal Dermal Hypoplasia
[Goltz syndrome]

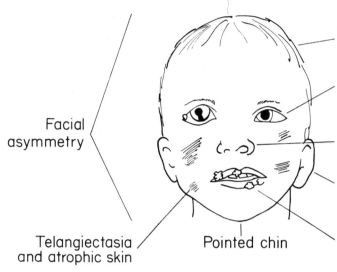

Sparse hair

Strabismus
Iris colobomas
Irregular pupil

Facial asymmetry

Notching of alae nasi
Deviation of septum

Thinning ear helix
Hearing loss

Papillomas of lips
Hypodontia
Defective teeth

Telangiectasia and atrophic skin

Pointed chin

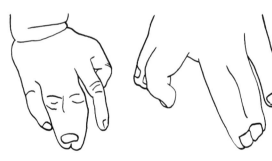

Syndactyly of digits with bizarre nail formation

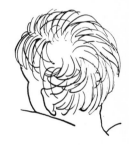

Sparse hair occiput

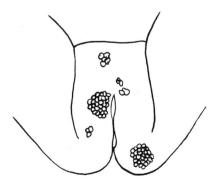

Papillomas in genital region

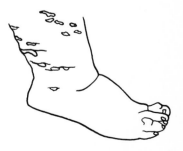

Herniations of subcutaneous fat and reticular hyperpigmentation

184. HYPERKERATOSIS PALMOPLANTARIS
AND PERIODONTOCLASIA
(Papillon-Lefevre syndrome)

Clinical Features Onset is usually between the first and fourth year of life when erythema and keratoderma appear on the palms and soles and extend to the sides of the hands and feet. The involved areas are sharply outlined. The soles are usually more severely involved. The Achilles tendon area, external malleoli, tibial tuberosities, and dorsal finger and toe joints may exhibit a scaly redness. Severity may decrease with age. Hyperhidrosis and malodor are frequent. Hyperkeratoses are common on the elbows and knees. The hair may be normal or sparse and the nails may show dystrophic changes. The deciduous teeth erupt normally. Then the gingiva becomes red and swollen. This progresses to destruction of the alveolar bone and loss of the deciduous teeth by the age of four to five years. The same process is repeated with the permanent teeth and after these teeth are lost the gingiva assumes its normal appearance. Only the third molars do not exfoliate. During the stage of active periodontal breakdown, the rest of the oral tissue appears normal. There may be a general increased susceptibility to infection (furunculosis, pyoderma). Other relatively uncommon findings may include calcific deposits in the attachment of the tentorium and choroid and retardation in somatic, mental, and skeletal development.

Specific Diagnosis The diagnosis is clinical based on the above features. No d'stinct laboratory findings have been described.

Differential Diagnosis Palmoplantar hyperkeratosis is part of *mal de Meleda disease,* but no dental anomalies are noted and the skin findings are usually present at birth. Numerous other genetic conditions have palmoplantar hyperkeratosis but these can be distinguished from the Papillon-Lefevre syndrome by their mode of inheritance, clinical appearance, and other associated abnormalities. Involvement of the elbows and knees may resemble *psoriasis.* Premature loss of deciduous and/or permanent teeth may be found in *acrodynia, histiocytosis X, hypophosphatasia, leukemia, acatalasia, Chediak-Higashi syndrome,* and *idiopathic periodontosis.*

Prenatal Diagnosis This is not yet possible.

Basic Defect, Genetics, and Other Considerations The basic defect in this relatively rare autosomal recessive disorder is not known. There may be a weakness in chemotactic activity of leukocytes. Parental consanguinity is common. Over 150 cases have been reported. There is a form with arachnodactyly and clawlike nails and terminal phalanges. This likely represents a different disorder.

Prognosis and Treatment The patients have a normal life span. Intellect has not been noted to be impaired. Extraction of teeth and use of dental prosthesis are indicated. There is no specific treatment for the hyperkeratosis.

REFERENCES

Djawari, D. Deficient phagocytic function in Papillon-Lefèvre syndrome. *Dermatologica 156:* 189–192, 1978.

Gorlin, R.J., Sedano, H., and Anderson, V.E. The syndrome of palmar-plantar hyperkeratosis and premature periodontal destruction of the teeth. A clinical and genetic analysis of the Papillon-Lefèvre syndrome. *J. Pediatr. 65:* 895–908, 1964.

Haneke, E. The Papillon-Lefèvre syndrome: keratosis palmoplantaris with periodontopathy, report of a case and review of the cases in the literature. *Hum. Genet. 51:* 1–35, 1979.

- **hyperkeratosis palms / soles**
- **hyperhidrosis hands / feet**
- **premature periodontitis / loss of teeth**
- **hyperkeratotic nails**

Hyperkeratosis Palmoplantaris and Periodontoclasia
[Papillon-Lefevre syndrome]

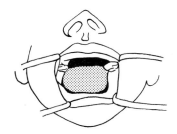

Child with loss of
all deciduous teeth,
except a few molars

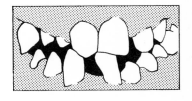

Severe periodontal
disease in a child

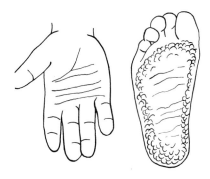

Hyperkeratosis of hand
and foot in child

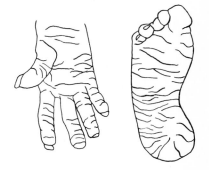

Severe hyperkeratotic lesions
with nails also involved
in an adult

185. HYPOHIDROTIC ECTODERMAL DYSPLASIA

Clinical Features The most characteristic feature of this disorder is hypohidrosis. Since the physical findings may not be apparent early in infancy, it is important to be aware that the male infant may present with fever of unknown origin. By the second year of life, the facies begins to assume a distinct appearance consisting of frontal bossing, depressed nasal bridge, and protruding lips and ears. Decreased tearing has been reported in some patients. The most striking oral manifestation is hypodontia or even anodontia in many patients. The incisors, canines, and premolars when present often have conical crowns. The pharyngeal and laryngeal mucosa may be atrophic resulting in dysphonia. Patients commonly have atrophy of the nasal mucosa associated with severe crusting and marked ozena. The skin is soft, thin, and dry. Fine, linear wrinkles and increased pigmentation are frequently seen about the eyes and mouth. Hyperkeratoses are common about the palms and soles. The scalp hair is usually blond, fine, stiff, and short. An anterior upsweep of the scalp hair has been noted in some affected patients during childhood. The eyelashes and eyebrows are sparse or even absent. The body is usually devoid of lanugo hair and after puberty, although the beard is normal, the axillary and pubic hair is scant. The nails may be normal or spoon-shaped. The mammary glands may be hypoplastic or aplastic. Eczema is common.

Specific Diagnosis The diagnosis should be suspected in an infant, usually male, who presents with fever of unknown origin and who shows some of the physical findings mentioned above. The triad of hypohidrosis, hypotrichosis, and hypodontia is of crucial importance. Dermatoglyphic studies will show a diminished number of sweat pores, while skin biopsy reveals a decreased number of sweat glands. Actual decreased secretion of sweat may be demonstrated using various methods. Dental radiograms may be helpful in ascertaining the presence of hypo- or anodontia and in ruling out pseudoanodontia.

Differential Diagnosis Several physical features in this syndrome can be found in other disorders. For example, conical teeth may also be seen in *idiopathic oligodontia, chondroectodermal dysplasia, incontinentia pigmenti,* and *Rieger syndrome.* Lack of eruption of permanent teeth is noted in *cleidocranial dysplasia* and as an *autosomal dominant trait.* Two forms of *autosomal dominant hidrotic ectodermal dysplasia* are known but in addition to normal sweating they have other findings not associated with hypohidrotic ectodermal dysplasia. An autosomal recessive form of hypohidrotic ectodermal dysplasia is known (see Genetics, below).

Prenatal Diagnosis This should theoretically be possible by using fetoscopy for obtaining a skin biopsy in a male fetus to determine the number of sweat glands.

Basic Defect, Genetics, and Other Considerations The basic defect in this ectodermal disorder is not known. Analysis of over 300 cases shows that this syndrome is usually transmitted as an X-linked recessive condition. Carrier mothers usually show minimal expression of the gene in the form of hypodontia and/or conical crowned teeth and reduced sweating, which can be documented by using dermatoglyphics and showing fewer sweat pores than normal. The rare autosomal recessive form is clinically indistinguishable from the X-linked type save that females are as severely affected as males, the nasal discharge tends to be more purulent, and the parents are normal.

Prognosis and Treatment In infants, bouts of hyperpyrexia can endanger life and thus once the diagnosis is made, they should be protected from exposure to excessive heat. Swimming should be encouraged as a sport. Atrophic rhinitis and eczema are often chronic problems. In adults life expectancy is seemingly unaffected. Dentures may be worn as early as three years of age and new ones made every two years. Synthetic tears are useful for dryness of the eyes.

REFERENCES

Gorlin, R.J., Old, T., and Anderson, V.E. Hypohidrotic ectodermal dysplasia in females. A critical analysis and argument for genetic heterogeneity. *Z. Kinderheilkd. 108:* 1–11, 1970.

Pinhiero, M. and Freire-Maia, N. Christ-Siemens-Touraine syndrome: a clinical and genetic analysis of a large Brazilian kindred. *Am. J. Med. Genet. 4:* 113–134, 1979.

Ramchander, V., Jankey, N., Ramkissoon, R. et al. Anhidrotic ectodermal dysplasia in an infant presenting with pyrexia of unknown origin. *Clin. Pediatr. 17:* 51–54, 1978.

- **hypohidrosis / hypotrichosis**
- **frontal bossing / depressed nasal bridge**
- **protruding lips / ears**
- **oligodontia**

Hypohidrotic Ectodermal Dysplasia

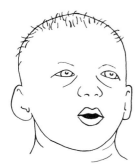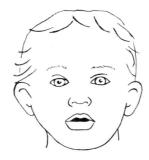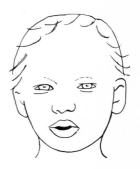

Infant and older male children with sparse hair,
eyelashes, and eyebrows, thick lips and protruding ears

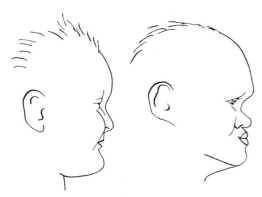

Child and adult with frontal bossing,
depressed nasal bridge
and prominent lips

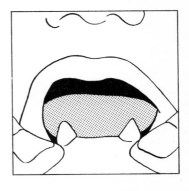

Hypodontia and conical
crown teeth in a child

Normal   Female carrier   Affected male

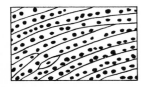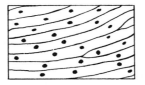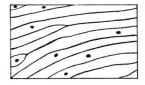

Number of sweat pores from palm prints

186. ICHTHYOSIS CONGENITA GRAVIS
(harlequin fetus)

Clinical Features This disorder with its profound morphologic features was first described in 1750, when it was noted in the diary of a South Carolina minister, Rev. Oliver Hart. His lucid outstanding description is as follows: "On Thursday, April ye 5, 1750, I went to see a most deplorable object of a child, born the night before of one Mary Evans in "Chas" town. It was surprising to all who beheld it, and I scarcely know how to describe it. The skin was dry and hard and seemed to be cracked in many places, somewhat resembling the scales of a fish. The mouth was large and round and open. It had no external nose, but two holes where the nose should have been. The eyes appeared to be lumps of coagulated blood, turned out, about the bigness of a plum, ghastly to behold. It had no external ears, but holes where the ears should be. The hands and feet appeared to be swollen, were crampt up and felt quite hard. The back part of the head was much open. It made a strange kind of noise, very low, which I cannot describe. It lived about eight and forty hours and was alive when I saw it."

Affected infants are usually born prematurely and are of low birth weight even for gestational age. The entire skin, including that of the scalp, is composed of horny plates as much as 5 mm in thickness; these are broken up by horizontal and vertical fissures and arranged transversely to the axis of the body. The general color is gray or yellow, but the intersecting furrows which tend to follow the body folds are red, purple or brown. The plaques tend to have a diamond-like configuration and thus the skin resembles a harlequin clown's suit. Ectropion extensive enough to obliterate the globe, eclabium, absent pinnae, and distortion of the alae nasi are constant features of the syndrome. A few hairs may appear in the fissures between the plaques but the scalp hair is sparse and the eyebrows and eyelashes are usually absent. The digits are atrophic and in a flexed position due to the tight keratinous skin. There are no consistent internal manifestations but in a few cases structural and

functional abnormalities of the thyroid and thymus have been reported.

Specific Diagnosis The clinical findings described above are so dramatic and uniform in all cases that the diagnosis is readily made at birth. Skin biopsy shows marked hyperkeratosis with a hyperplastic epidermis. Keratin plugs can also be seen distending hair follicles in the epidermis.

Differential Diagnosis This disorder should be differentiated from a more mild form of ichthyosis—the *lamellar exfoliative type* or the *collodion fetus*. In this condition the infant is enveloped with a shiny membrane likened to a thick coating of shellac or collodion which has been allowed to dry. Within a few hours after birth the infants begin to shed this membrane.

Prenatal Diagnosis This has been achieved by demonstrating altered skin histology as obtained by fetoscopic skin biopsies. The findings show the early pathologic changes of premature hyperkeratosis most marked around hair follicles and sweat ducts, and forming plugs of hyperkeratotic debris.

Basic Defect, Genetics, and Other Considerations The basic defect in this rare autosomal recessive condition is not known. An electron microscopic study has shown crystals resembling cholesterol and masses of autophagic vacuoles, many of them glutted with lipid, deposited within cells of the stratum corneum. Biochemically, cholesterol and triglyceride levels in the stratum corneum were markedly elevated. A defect in epidermal lipid metabolism is postulated. Fewer than 30 cases have been reported in the literature with at least six families having two affected sibs and in several the parents were consanguineous.

Prognosis and Treatment Most affected infants die during the first few weeks of life or earlier— one patient lived until the age of nine months. No adequate treatment is available.

REFERENCES

Baden, H.P. and Goldsmith, L.A. The structural proteins of the harlequin fetus: stratum corneum. *J. Invest. Dermatol. 61:* 25–26, 1973.

Buxman, M.M., Goodkin, P.E., Fahrenbach, W.H. et al. Harlequin ichthyosis with epidermal lipid abnormality. *Arch. Dermatol. 115:* 189–193, 1979.

Elias, S., Mazur, M., Sabbagha, R. et al. Prenatal diagnosis of harlequin ichthyosis. *Clin. Genet. 17:* 275–280, 1980.

- **thick skin with cracks**
- **ectropion**
- **flat nose / distorted nasal alae**
- **atrophic digits**

Ichthyosis Congenita Gravis
[harlequin fetus]

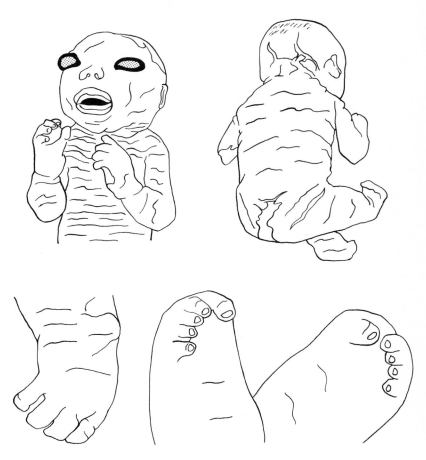

Entire skin covered by a thick layer of keratin
with cracks (like armor plating), ectropion
and hypoplastic digits with flexion deformity
and absence of digital creases

397

187. INCONTINENTIA PIGMENTI SYNDROME

Clinical Features A few days after birth, linear or grouped vesicles appear over the extremities. After a month these vesicles may be replaced by violaceous papules and inflammatory lesions. A few weeks later hyperkeratotic warty lesions appear on the dorsal surface of the digits and over the knuckles and joints. The inflamed areas eventually heal and may become atrophic. Frequently at birth or much later, brownish gray macules appear in streaks, whorls, or patches over the trunk and extremities. Fading of the pigmentation may begin at about the age of two years, but pigmented areas tend to remain minimal throughout life. Alopecia of the atrophic, scarring type involving the apex of the crown is noted in most patients. Hypoplasia of the eyebrows and eyelashes has been described. Common eye findings include strabismus, cataract, optic atrophy, retinal detachment, and changes like those seen in retrolental fibroplasia. Various anomalies of the teeth have been noted in most patients affecting both the primary and permanent dentitions, more frequently the latter. These anomalies include delayed tooth eruption, pegged or conical crowned teeth, oligodontia, and malformed teeth. CNS involvement is common with such manifestations as mental retardation, microcephaly, hydrocephaly, seizures, and spastic and lax paralysis. Other associated alterations include dystrophic changes of the fingernails, breast asymmetry, syndactyly, hemiatrophy, and shortening of an arm or leg.

Specific Diagnosis Eosinophilia is common during the vesicular stage and may reach over 50%. Chromosomal instability has been demonstrated. Ultrastructurally all three stages of the skin lesions show dyskeratosis, phagocytosis of dyskeratotic cells and melanosomes by macrophages, and the presence of melanophages in the upper dermis. These findings point to the relationship among all three stages of the disorder and suggest that pigmentary incontinence is a phagocytic phenomenon. Hemivertebrae and extra ribs may be seen radiographically.

Differential Diagnosis The skin lesions present in early infancy must be distinguished from those seen in *epidermolysis bullosa, bullous impetigo, contact dermatitis, dermatitis herpetiformis, verrucous nevus, Naegeli syndrome,* and *congenital syphilis. Hypomelanosis of Ito* or *incontinentia pigmenti achromians* superficially resembles classical incontinentia pigmenti as a negative image. Similar dental changes may be seen in *congenital syphilis* and various forms of *ectodermal dysplasia.*

Prenatal Diagnosis This is not yet possible.

Basic Defect, Genetics, and Other Considerations The basic defect is not known. Neutrophil and lymphocyte dysfunction has been demonstrated. Most investigators consider this condition to be transmitted as an X-linked dominant trait with lethality in the male. Over 700 cases have been reported, all females except for approximately 2% of the patients.

Prognosis and Treatment Disability may result from neurologic, ocular, osseous, or other lesions. Reproductive fitness may be reduced in some cases. Symptomatic treatment and control of secondary infections are recommended.

REFERENCES

Carney, R.G. Jr. Incontinentia pigmenti: a world statistical analysis. *Arch. Dermatol. 112:* 535–542, 1976.

Jessen, R.T., Van Epps, D.E., Goodwin, J.S. et al. Incontinentia pigmenti. Evidence for both neutrophil and lymphocyte dysfunction. *Arch. Dermatol. 114:* 1182–1186, 1978.

Wiklund, D.A. and Weston, W.L. Incontinentia pigmenti: a four generation study. *Arch. Dermatol. 116:* 701–703, 1980.

- **linear vesicles over extremities**
- **pigmented streaks trunk / extremities**
- **alopecia / sparse eyebrows and lashes**
- **eye and tooth anomalies**

Incontinentia Pigmenti Syndrome

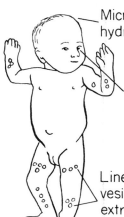

Microcephaly or hydrocephaly

Strabismus
Cataract
Blue sclerae
Myopia
Nystagmus
Microphthalmia
Optic atrophy

Linear or grouped vesicles over extremities few days after birth

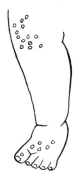
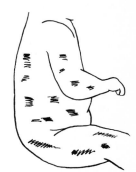

Hyperkeratotic lesions about knee and foot — later streaky changes over trunk and limbs

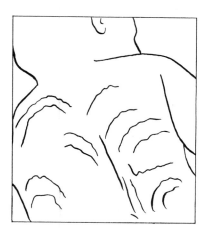

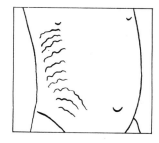

Whorls and splashes of macular pigmentation

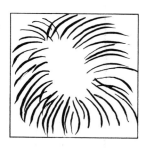

Alopecia at crown of head

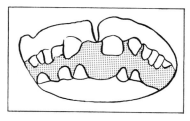

Missing teeth, some with conical crown form

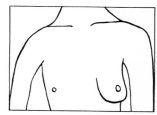

Hypoplasia of shoulder, arm and breast

188. JOHANSON-BLIZZARD SYNDROME

Clinical Features At birth these infants may present with hypotonia and hyperextensibility of the joints. The facial appearance is striking due to marked hypoplasia of the nasal alae. Multiple anomalies have been described which include mild to moderate microcephaly, midline posterior scalp defects, sparse hair, hypoplastic deciduous teeth, absent permanent teeth, dilation of renal calyx, hydronephrosis, imperforate anus, single urogenital orifice with infantile ovaries and double or septate vagina, aplasia of lacrimal puncta, hypoplastic nipples and areolas, skin dimples, and clitoromegaly. Pitting edema of the hands and feet has also been noted. Most of these patients suffer from severe mental and growth retardation, sensorineural deafness, hypothyroidism, and malabsorption.

Specific Diagnosis The diagnosis is clinical and can be made with ease due to the distinct facial features, mainly the hypoplastic nasal alae. The malabsorption is apparently due to a trypsinogen deficiency. Hypothyroidism in this syndrome is unusual in that cholesterol is not elevated. This may be due to the associated malabsorption.

Differential Diagnosis The severe oligodontia in this syndrome should be differentiated from that occurring in various genetic forms of *ectodermal dysplasia*. The etiology of the *hypothyroidism* and *malabsorption* must be differentiated from other causes.

Prenatal Diagnosis This is not available presently.

Basic Defect, Genetics, and Other Considerations The basic defect in this rare syndrome is not known. The first report of autopsy findings in an eight-year-old boy described a small thyroid filled with colloid, virtually complete replacement of the pancreas with adipose tissue, and a brain of normal size but with evidence of a cortical developmental defect manifested by abnormalities of gyral formation and of cortical neuronal organization. Although few cases have been reported, there is evidence to suggest that this syndrome may be inherited as an autosomal recessive disorder. Parental consanguinity and affected sibs have been observed. Most cases have been sporadic.

Prognosis and Treatment Mental deficiency may be of such a degree that these children are institutionalized. Improvement in growth rate may occur using thyroid and pancreatin replacement therapy.

REFERENCES

Daentl, D.L., Frias, J.L., Gilbert, E.F. et al. The Johanson-Blizzard syndrome: case report and autopsy findings. *Am. J. Med. Genet. 3:* 129–135, 1979.

Johanson, A. and Blizzard, R. A syndrome of congenital aplasia of the alae nasi, deafness, hypothyroidism, dwarfism, absent permanent teeth and malabsorption. *J. Pediatr. 79:* 982–987, 1971.

Mardini, M.K., Ghandour, M., Sakati, N.A. et al. Johanson-Blizzard syndrome in a large inbred kindred with three involved members. *Clin Genet. 14:* 247–250, 1978.

M.R. [+ / most]

- **microcephaly**
- **sparse hair / scalp defects**
- **hypoplasia nasal alae**
- **hypoplastic nipples / areolas**

Johanson-Blizzard Syndrome

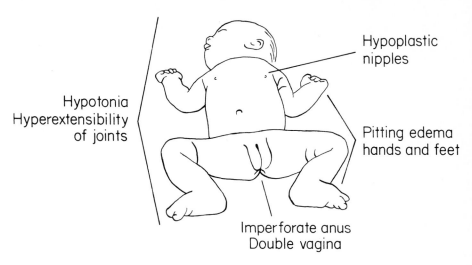

Hypoplastic nipples

Hypotonia
Hyperextensibility
of joints

Pitting edema
hands and feet

Imperforate anus
Double vagina

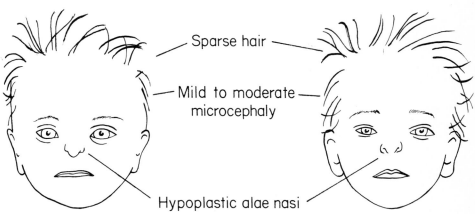

Sparse hair

Mild to moderate microcephaly

Hypoplastic alae nasi

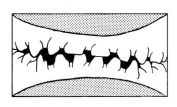

Cone-shaped crowns
of primary teeth

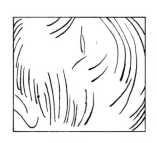

Occipital scalp defects

401

189. LEOPARD SYNDROME
(multiple lentigines syndrome)

Clinical Features The acronym *LEOPARD* stands for the main clinical features as they were originally reported, consisting of (a) Lentigines, (b) Electrocardiographic changes, (c) Ocular hypertelorism (d) Pulmonic stenosis, (e) Abnormal genitalia, (f) Retardation of growth, and (g) Deafness. Although multiple lentigines are a most striking finding in this syndrome, some patients do not develop these lesions. When present they appear at birth or in infancy and increase in number until puberty. The lentigines involve all parts of the body, except the mucosal surfaces, and are more numerous over the upper trunk and neck. A few large "cafe-noir" spots may appear in the truncal area. The face has a triangular shape due to biparietal bossing. Hypertelorism, ptosis of eyelids, epicanthal folds, low-set ears, and frequently mild pterygium colli are common facial findings. More than 75% of the patients exhibit growth retardation below the 25th percentile for both height and weight. Skeletal anomalies consist of pectus excavatum or carinatum, kyphoscoliosis, hyperflexible metacarpophalangeal joints, winging of the scapulas, spina bifida occulta, absent ribs, cubitus valgus, limitation in movement of elbows, and outer table deficiency of the temporal bone. Although a variety of cardiac lesions have been reported the most common is mild valvular pulmonic stenosis. Other anomalies include hypertrophic cardiomyopathy, atrial septal defect, infundibular or supravalvular pulmonic stenosis, aortic valvular dysplasia, and atrial myxoma. Frequently patients with no structural defect of the heart have a characteristic electrocardiographic pattern consisting of a superiorly oriented mean QRS axis in the frontal plane located between -60 and $-120°$. Complete bundle branch and heart block have also been reported. Sensorineural hearing loss of severe degree has been observed in approximately 15% of patients. Mild mental retardation and abnormal electroencephalographic findings have been described in some patients. Fifty percent of all affected males have hypospadias, while unilateral or bilateral cryptorchidism is frequent. Late menarche is common in affected females and hypoplasia or absence of an ovary has been found occasionally.

Specific Diagnosis Skin biopsy is helpful in differentiating lentigines from similar lesions. The classic histologic picture is that of elongated clubbed epidermal ridges with increased melanocytes and melanin in the basal cell layer. Packets of melanosomes are often seen within the melanocytes. The electrocardiographic changes of an S_1, S_2, S_3 pattern tend to characterize this syndrome. These findings together with the previously described clinical features make this a relatively easy syndrome to recognize.

Differential Diagnosis In the absence of lentigines the disorder shares many clinical features with the *Noonan syndrome*. The cardiac findings together with short stature, delayed puberty, and deafness are seen in the *rubella syndrome*, while hypertelorism, ptosis of eyelids, short stature, and cryptorchidism are found in the *Aarskog syndrome*.

Prenatal Diagnosis This has not yet been achieved in this syndrome.

Basic Defect, Genetics, and Other Considerations The basic defect is not known. This relatively rare syndrome is transmitted as an autosomal dominant with almost full penetrance and marked variability in expression.

Prognosis and Treatment There is a tendency for the lentigines to slightly fade in color after puberty. The prognosis is generally good and the pulmonary stenosis rarely disabling. Treatment is symptomatic. Some have reported good cosmetic results with facial dermabrasion.

REFERENCES

Gorlin, R.J., Anderson, R.C., and Blaw, M. Multiple lentigines syndrome. Complex comprising multiple lentigines, electrocardiographic conduction abnormalities, ocular hypertelorism, pulmonary stenosis, abnormalities of genitalia, retardation of growth, sensorineural deafness and autosomal dominant hereditary pattern. *Am J. Dis. Child.* *117*: 652–662, 1969.

Selmanowitz, V.J., Orentreich, N., and Felsenstein, J.M. Lentiginosis profusa syndrome (multiple lentigines syndrome). *Arch. Dermatol. 104:* 393–401, 1971.

Voron, D.A., Hatfield, H.H., and Kalkhoff, R.K. Multiple lentigines syndrome. Case report and review of the literature. *Am. J. Med. 60:* 447–456, 1976.

- multiple lentigines
- biparietal bossing /
  triangular face
- ptosis / epicanthal
  folds
- chest deformity /
  skeletal anomalies

Leopard Syndrome
[multiple lentigines syndrome]

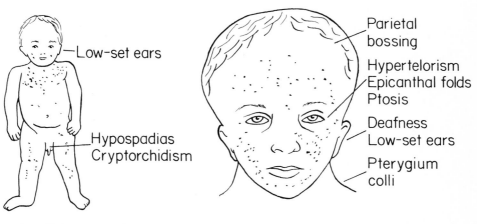

Low-set ears

Hypospadias
Cryptorchidism

Lentigines may be
present at birth

Parietal
bossing

Hypertelorism
Epicanthal folds
Ptosis

Deafness
Low-set ears

Pterygium
colli

Triangular face with
multiple lentigines

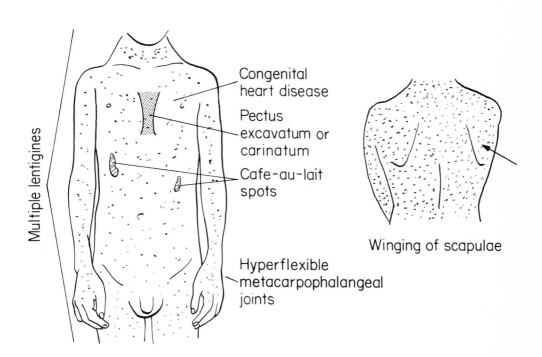

Congenital
heart disease

Pectus
excavatum or
carinatum

Cafe-au-lait
spots

Multiple lentigines

Hyperflexible
metacarpophalangeal
joints

Winging of scapulae

190. MONILETHRIX

Clinical Features In infancy the hair tends to break off on the occiput where it is rubbed against the pillow. The entire scalp and body hair may be affected or the condition may be more localized. In many areas both on the scalp and the body, the hair fails to appear at the surface, but instead folds on itself and is eventually pushed out of the follicle as a horny plug. The beading and fragility of the hairs leads to fracturing about 5 mm from the scalp. Follicular hyperkeratosis of the scalp, forehead, face, and nape also occur. Physical retardation, syndactyly, juvenile cataracts, nail and teeth anomalies, and other hair defects including pili torti and trichorrhexis nodosa have been reported. Keratosis pilaris and aminoaciduria of arginosuccinic acid with elevated plasma glutamic acid has been described.

Specific Diagnosis In monilethrix the hair consists of elliptical nodes 0.7 to 1.0 mm apart, separated by constricted inner nodes and an absent medulla through which the hair fractures. The condition may be recognized on inspection but confirmation by examination of the hair under the light microscope is necessary.

Differential Diagnosis By use of the scanning electron microscope, monilethrix can be differentiated from other congenital hair defects such as *pili torti, trichorrhexis nodosa,* and *bamboo hair.* Monilethrix has also been reported in a *syndrome* with mental retardation, epilepsy, schizophrenia, and neurodegenerative disease.

Prenatal Diagnosis Prenatal diagnosis is not available presently.

Basic Defect, Genetics and Other Considerations The basic defect is not known. A cuticular alteration with longitudinal ridging of the internodes has been described using the scanning electron microscope. A variation in the hair sulfur content has also been reported. This rare condition is transmitted as an autosomal dominant trait with incomplete penetrance and variable expressivity. Genetic heterogeneity may be present as some have noted autosomal recessive inheritance.

Prognosis and Treatment By itself monilethrix is not a life threatening disorder. The condition may improve around puberty and during pregnancy. Many forms of treatment have been used but long-term results have not been rewarding. Use of a wig for females is recommended.

REFERENCES

Brown, A.C. Congenital hair defects. *Birth Defects 7 (8):* 52–68, 1971.

Salamon, T. and Schnyder, U.W. Ueber die Monilethrix. *Arch. Klin. Exp. Dermatol. 215:* 105–136, 1962.

Solomon, I.L. and Green, O.C. Monilethrix: its occurrence in seven generations, with one case that responded to endocrine therapy. *N. Engl. J. Med. 269:* 1279–1282, 1963.

- sparse body and scalp hair
- short, broken hair / beading of hair
- follicular hyperkeratosis / scalp, face, nape

Monilethrix

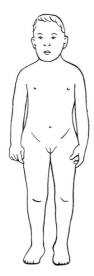
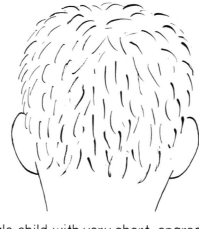

Female child with very short, sparse hair of scalp, eyebrows and lashes

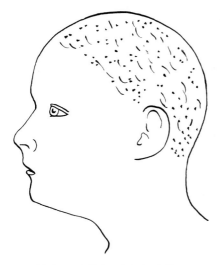

Older child with balding, very short, brittle hair, follicular hyperkeratosis, absent eyebrows and lashes

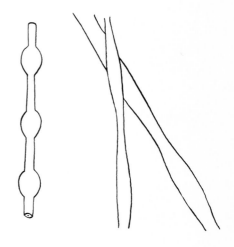

Schematic diagram of hair and scanning electron micrograph showing elliptical nodes and constricted internodes

191. MULTIPLE PTERYGIUM SYNDROME

Clinical Features Many of the anomalies in this syndrome are recognizable at birth. They include: pterygia of neck and axillary, antecubital, popliteal, digital, and intercrural areas; multiple joint contractures, rocker bottom feet; genital anomalies characterized by a small penis, hypoplastic scrotum, and cryptorchidism in males; and aplasia of labia majora with protrusion of the labia minora and normal clitoris in females. Other findings described are a sad and apparently emotionless face with dystopia canthorum, a long narrow nose, pointed receding chin, down-turned angles of mouth with or without cleft palate, low posterior hairline, and a crouched or semicrouched stance. There is often mild cutaneous syndactyly between the fingers and flexion deformity of the digits, the thumbs being flexed and apposed. Skeletal anomalies consist of fusion of cervical vertebrae, rib anomalies, scoliosis, lordosis, and vertical talus.

Specific Diagnosis The diagnosis is clinical, based on the above clinical features in a family setting compatible with autosomal recessive inheritance.

Differential Diagnosis The differentiation of this syndrome from the *popliteal pterygium* syndrome is not difficult due to the multiplicity of pterygia in the syndrome discussed here. An *autosomal dominant syndrome of multiple pterygia, ptosis, and skeletal anomalies* has been described. This condition differs from the multiple pterygium syndrome on the basis of normal stature, normal external genitalia, and absence of intercrural pterygium and cleft palate. An *X-linked dominant form of multiple pterygium* has been reported with the affected individuals also having normal external genitalia. The *Turner syndrome, leopard syndrome,* and the *Noonan syndrome* are all associated with pterygia about the neck.

Prenatal Diagnosis The extensive pterygia formation in this syndrome could lend itself to possible prenatal diagnosis using fetoscopy; however, to the best of our knowledge such a procedure has not been done in a pregnant woman at risk for this condition.

Basic Defect, Genetics, and Other Considerations The basic defect in this syndrome is not known. Biopsy has shown muscle degeneration and disorganization of the myofibrils compatible with lack of muscle use. The syndrome of multiple congenital pterygia plus other anomalies described here is transmitted in an autosomal recessive fashion; however, many patients with this disorder represent sporadic cases which are usually milder in their phenotypic expression. Other genetic syndromes having multiple pterygia are mentioned under Differential Diagnosis.

Prognosis and Treatment Growth is usually retarded below the third percentile and these patients rarely exceed 135 cm in height as adults. Surgical treatment may be necessary not only for cosmetic reasons but also for practical considerations as the popliteal pterygia may markedly inhibit walking.

REFERENCES

Chen, H., Chang, C.H., Misra, R.P. et al. Multiple pterygium syndrome. *Am. J. Med. Genet. 7:* 91–102, 1980.

Escobar, V., Bixler, D., Gleiser, S. et al. Multiple pterygium syndrome. *Am. J. Dis. Child. 132:* 609–611, 1978.

Norum, R.A., James, V.L., and Mabry, C.C. Pterygium syndrome in three children in a recessive pedigree pattern. *Birth Defects 5 (2):* 233–235, 1969.

- **multiple pterygium**
- **ptosis of lids**
- **flexion of fingers**
- **short stature**

Multiple Pterygium Syndrome

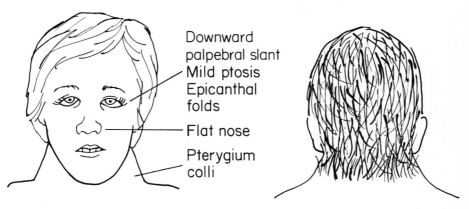

Downward palpebral slant
Mild ptosis
Epicanthal folds

Flat nose

Pterygium colli

Pterygium colli, low-set posterior hairline

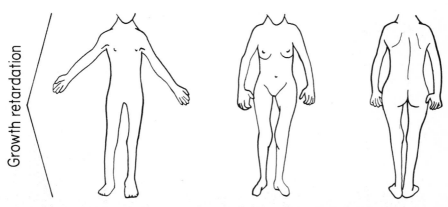

Growth retardation

Different aged females with pterygia of neck, axillae, antecubital and popliteal areas, poorly developed external genitalia, deformed hands

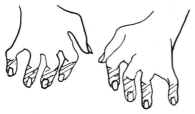

Syndactyly and flexion deformity of fingers

192. NEUROFIBROMATOSIS
(von Recklinghausen disease)

Clinical Features Approximately 40% of patients with this disorder show some manifestations at birth and more than half display findings by the second year of life. Smooth-edged pigmented (cafe-au-lait) spots appear during the first decade usually preceding the tumors. The spots are pale yellow to light brown, irregular in outline, and variable in size. They are frequently present at birth and constitute the earliest physical finding. Axillary and intertriginous freckling when present is a helpful, usually diagnostic, sign. Lisch nodules, or pigmented iris hamartomas are present in 94% of patients who are six years or older. Various types of tumors are associated with neurofibromatosis, the most common being plexiform neurofibroma. The tumors may be present at birth but usually appear during childhood or later in life. Some patients have hundreds of small skin tumors while others have large, unilateral pendulous masses. The tumors are of multiple cell origin. The tongue, stomach, intestine, kidney, bladder, larynx, and heart may be involved. Other tumors include fibromas, meningiomas, Schwannomas, neuromas mainly of the optic, acoustic, and spinal nerves, and gliomas (astrocytomas and ependymomas). Pheochromocytoma occurs in about 1% of cases. Numerous bony abnormalities have been described due frequently to subperiosteal erosive changes caused by pressure from proliferating tumor tissue in the periosteum and overlying soft parts. Macrocephaly, kyphoscoliosis, pseudoarthrosis (tibia, less often radius), hemihypertrophy of limb or digit, spina bifida, absent patella, and complete or partial absence of limb bones have been reported. Endocrine disturbances such as hypopituitarism, hypogonadism, gigantism, acromegaly, hypoglycemia, diabetes insipidus, myxedema, hyperparathyroidism, and others may occur in association with this condition. A commonly overlooked feature is the low frequency of a variety of cardiovascular anomalies such as pulmonic valvular stenosis, supravalvular aortic stenosis, coarctation of the aorta, atrial septal defect, congenital heart block, and renal artery stenosis.

Specific Diagnosis It is thought that any person with more than six cafe-au-lait spots exceeding 1.5 cm in diameter must be presumed to have neurofibromatosis even in the absence of a positive family history. Biopsy of individual lesions is useful for establishing the diagnosis in questionable cases.

Differential Diagnosis Cafe-au-lait spots may be seen in the *McCune-Albright syndrome* and in the *leopard syndrome*. However in the former disorder these patients often have associated bone cysts and no skin tumors. There is a *"central" form of neurofibromatosis* also transmitted as an autosomal dominant trait. It is characterized by later age of onset and more uniform clinical picture in which the CNS is mainly affected. These patients have *bilateral acoustic neuromas* and other CNS tumors. Most patients have 1 or 2 cafe-au-lait spots or subcutaneous neurofibromas. A number of conditions have been reported to be associated with neurofibromatosis, the most recent one being a *gammopathy with aorta outflow obstruction*.

Prenatal Diagnosis This has not yet been achieved in this syndrome.

Basic Defect, Genetics, and Other Considerations The basic defect in this autosomal dominant disorder is not known. This disorder has the highest mutation rate known in man (1×10^{-4} per gamete per generation) and 50% of cases represent a new mutation. Patients with neurofibromatosis (peripheral form) have increased levels of a functional beta-nerve growth factor (NGF) activity that can be detected in radioreceptor assay but they lack the antigenic determinants which are scored in the radioimmunoassay. In contrast, patients with bilateral acoustic neuromas (central form) have raised levels of beta-NGF antigenic activity on radioimmunoassay, but only low-to-normal levels of beta-NGF functional activity with the radioreceptor assay. The changes in NGF in these two distinct hereditary disorders suggest different alterations in NGF synthesis or regulation.

Prognosis and Treatment Intellectual handicap is present in about 40% with frank mental retardation in 2–5%. Seizures are found in 3%. Prognosis depends on the degree and site of involvement. Neurofibrosarcomatous transformation has been reported in 3–7% of cases. Surgical removal of tumors is indicated when they cause mechanical damage, are severely disfiguring or when malignant. Often the patient needs psychological support.

REFERENCES

Brasfield, R.D. and Das Gupta, T.K. Von Recklinghausen's disease: a clinicopathological study. *Ann. Surg.* 175: 86–104, 1972.
Carey, J.C., Lamb, J.M, and Hall, B.D. Penetrance and variability in neurofibromotosis: a genetic study of 60 families. *Birth Defects 15*(5B): 271–281, 1979.
Riccardi, V. Von Recklinghausen neurofibromatosis. *N. Engl. J. Med.*, 305: 1617–1627, 1981.

M.R. [+ / few]

- multiple cafe-au-lait spots
- axillary / inter-triginous freckling
- multiple neurofibromas
- bony abnormalities

Neurofibromatosis
[von Recklinghausen disease]

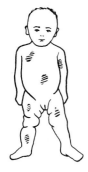
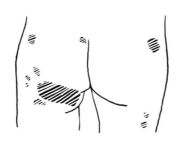
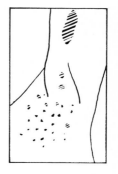

Six or more cafe-au-lait spots at birth and axillary freckling in a child

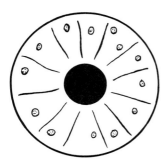

Lisch nodules in iris

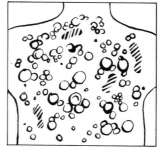

Multiple neuro-fibromas about back

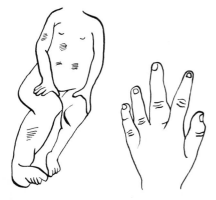

Hypertrophy of leg and fin-gers, pseudoarthrosis of tibia

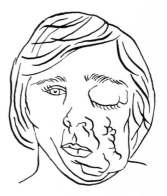

Unilateral neuro-fibromatosis

193. NEVOID BASAL CELL CARCINOMA SYDROME

Clinical Features This syndrome involves not only the skin but also the ocular, skeletal, central nervous, and endocrine systems. Eye findings present at birth include dystopia canthorum, hypertelorism, and congenital blindness due to corneal opacity, cataract, glaucoma, or colobomas of the choroid and optic nerve. Numerous skeletal anomalies present at birth may be observed clinically or by radiographic studies. Such alterations consist of rib anomalies (bifurcation, splaying, synostosis, partial agenesis, and cervical rudimentary ribs), scoliosis, cervical or upper thoracic vertebral fusion, bridging of sella, spina bifida, syndactyly, oligodactyly, polydactyly, arachnodactyly, short fourth metacarpal, Sprengel deformity, defective medial clavicle, pectus excavatum or carinatum, pes planus, and hallux valgus. Calcification of the dura and choroid is frequent. Mental retardation, congenital communicating hydrocephaly, nerve deafness, and agenesis of the corpus callosum have been described. During childhood multiple jaw cysts begin to develop. Later in life patients have a characteristic facial appearance due to mild mandibular prognathism, frontal and temporoparietal bossing, sunken eyes, and a broad nasal root. From childhood to the mid-thirties, multiple basal cell carcinomas appear. The early lesions appear as flesh-colored or brownish dome-shaped papules on the face, neck, upper trunk, and upper limbs. Later these lesions frequently ulcerate. Other cutaneous lesions are milia, comedones, epithelial and sebaceous cysts, lipomas, and palmoplantar pits. The pits are usually shallow holes (1–3 mm), discrete or confluent with red bases. Ovarian fibromas and/or cysts, hypogonadism, cryptorchidism, female pubic escutcheon in males, and gynecomastia have been reported. Other findings include cleft lip and/or palate, fibrosarcoma of the jaw, ameloblastoma, medulloblastoma, lymphomesenteric cysts, cardiac fibroma, kidney malformation, inguinal hernia, and Marfanoid habitus.

Specific Diagnosis Eye and skeletal alterations described above in an infant who has a family history of affected members strongly suggests that he or she may also be affected. In childhood the presence of multiple basal cell carcinomas should prompt the radiographic study of the jaws, chest, and vertebrae. Chromosomal breakage has been observed in fibroblasts from the uninvolved skin of affected patients.

Differential Diagnosis If the jaw cysts are few they may be mistaken for conventional *dentigerous cysts* or isolated *keratocysts*. Multilocular cystic changes of the mandible are found in *cherubism*. Dystopia canthorum and prognathism are part of the *Waardenburg syndrome*.

Prenatal Diagnosis Not yet available in this syndrome.

Basic Defect, Genetics, and Other Considerations The basic defect in this autosomal dominant disorder is not known. The syndrome is probably present in 0.5% of patients with basal cell carcinoma. The gene shows a high degree of penetrance with variable expressivity. There may be possible linkage with the Rh blood group locus.

Prognosis and Treatment The prognosis is generally good but dependent on location and invasiveness of the basal cell carcinomas and other less common tumors. All basal cell carcinomas must be removed early by surgical methods including excision, curettage, and electrocautery.

REFERENCES

Anderson, D.E., Taylor, W.B., Falls, H.F., and Davidson, R.J. The nevoid basal cell carcinoma syndrome. *Am. J. Hum. Genet. 19:* 12–22, 1967.

Donatsky, O., Hjørting-Hansen, E., Philipsen, H. et al. Clinical, radiologic and histopathologic aspects of nevoid basal cell carcinoma syndrome. *Int. J. Oral Surg. 5:* 19–28, 1976.

Gorlin, R.J. and Sedano, H.O. The multiple nevoid basal cell carcinoma syndrome revisited. *Birth Defects 7(8):* 140–148, 1972.

- **dystopia canthorum / eye anomalies**
- **jaw cysts / prognathism**
- **frontal / parietal bossing**
- **basal cell carcinomas / face and upper trunk**

Nevoid Basal Cell Carcinoma Syndrome

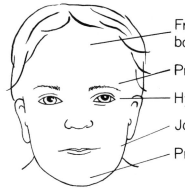

Frontal and temporoparietal bossing

Prominent supraorbital ridges

Hypertelorism

Jaw cysts

Prognathism

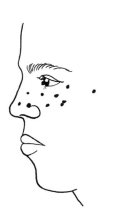

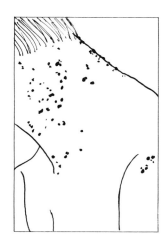

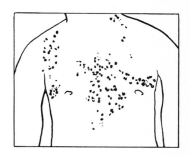

Numerous basal cell carcinomas appearing around puberty

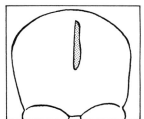

Calcification in falx cerebri

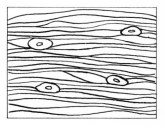

Close up of palmar pits

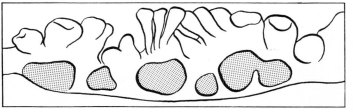

Multiple cysts of mandible

194. PACHYONYCHIA CONGENITA SYNDROMES

Clinical Features There has been considerable discussion in the literature regarding the extent of genetic heterogeneity in this disorder. Two syndromes have been posited as being distinct:

Type I—Jadassohn-Lewandowski Syndrome At birth or early in infancy the nails appear thickened, tubular, and hard, due to the accumulation of a horny, yellowish-brown material. Frequently the nails become hypoplastic or even absent. Paronychia is common. Hyperkeratoses of the palms and soles appear in half the affected patients by the age of three years. This is usually associated with hyperhidrosis involving the same areas while the rest of the dermal surface is dry. Other skin lesions appearing early in life include small follicular papules (keratosis pilaris) over the elbows, knees, and buttocks. A horny plug is present in the center of each papule. There is thickening of the skin due to acanthosis and parakeratosis mainly about the pilosebaceous apparatus. The hair is usually dry. Sparse body hair, eyebrows, eyelashes, and alopecia have been noted. The dorsal surface of the tongue is thickened and has a white or grayish-white appearance. The buccal and oral mucosa may also be involved. Hoarseness due to thickening of the posterior commissure of the larynx has been described.

Type II—Jackson-Lawler Syndrome This form shares with Type I the nail changes, palmoplantar hyperkeratosis, and follicular keratosis but differs in that oral leukokeratosis is never found. Patients with Type II also have natal teeth and multiple cysts which appear around puberty. These cysts are localized mainly on the trunk, axillae, neck, scalp, and face. Most observers consider these cysts to be steatocystoma multiplex. The natal teeth are poorly calcified and are lost by four to six months. Corneal dystrophy has also been reported.

Specific Diagnosis Diagnosis is based solely on the clinical features described above since no specific laboratory findings have been reported.

Differential Diagnosis Natal teeth may be an isolated finding or associated with other conditions such as *cleft lip/palate, Ellis-van Creveld syndrome,* and *Hallermann-Streiff syndrome.* The nail findings are distinctive, whereas similar oral lesions have been noted in *white sponge nevus, dyskeratosis congenita, hereditary benign intraepithelial dyskeratosis,* and other disorders.

Prenatal Diagnosis This is not available presently.

Basic Defect, Genetics, and Other Considerations The basic defect in this hereditary disorder of hyperkeratosis is not known. Both Types I and II are transmitted as autosomal dominant traits. We are currently doubtful regarding their legitimate separation. There is no good evidence that these disorders are more common in Jews, an often repeated statement in the literature. Personal experience and an extensive review of the literature suggest that there are a number of isolated cases of pachyonychia congenita associated with a variety of multiple congenital malformations.

Prognosis and Treatment Complications in this disorder include repeated infections about the nails with loss of the nails, corneal opacities, and partial blindness. The oral lesions are not premalignant. Surgical removal of the nails is often indicated. Special shoes may reduce the degree of plantar keratosis.

REFERENCES

Hodes, M.E. and Norins, A.L. Pachyonychia congenita and steatocystoma multiplex. *Clin. Genet. 11:* 359–364, 1977.

Jackson, A.D.M. and Lawler, S.D. Pachyonychia congenita: a report of six cases in one family. *Ann. Eugen. 16:* 142–146, 1951–52.

Stieglitz, J.B. and Centerwall, W.R. Pachyonychia congenita (Jadassohn-Lewandowsky Syndrome): a seventeen-member, four generation pedigree with unusual repiratory and dental involvement. *Am. J. Med. Genet. 14:* 21–28, 1983.

- thick, horny nails
- palmoplantar hyperkeratosis
- follicular keratosis
- oral leukokeratosis / Type I
- natal teeth / multiple body cysts / Type II

Pachyonychia Congenita Syndromes

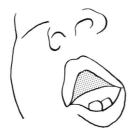

Natal teeth in
Jackson−Lawler type

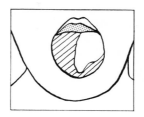

Leukoplakia about the tongue
Jadassohn−Lewandowski type

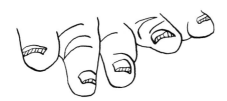
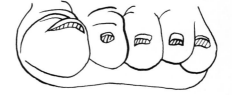

Onychogryposis of finger and toe nails

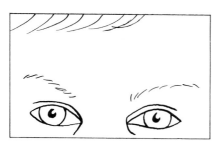

Sparse eyebrows, lashes and
scalp hair in a child−corneal
dystrophy may be present in
the Jackson−Lawler type

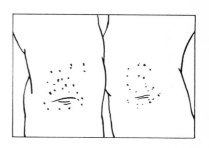

Keratosis pilaris about
the knees of a child

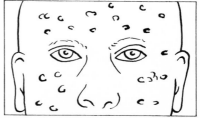

Epidermal cysts about face, sparse
eyebrows, lashes, beard and
alopecia in a young man

413

195. PEUTZ-JEGHERS SYNDROME

Clinical Features During infancy these patients display pigmentary changes consisting of brown to bluish-black macules about the facial orifices, elbows, and extremities. Occasionally such pigmentary findings may also be noted in the umbilicus, axilla, on the shoulder, or even about the nails. As puberty approaches, the pigmentary changes tend to fade. The lower lip is the most frequent site of pigmentary involvement followed by the buccal mucosa. Rarely involved are the palate, gingiva, tongue, and floor of the oral cavity. Pigmentation of other mucosal surfaces such as conjunctival and nasal have been reported. A more important feature of this syndrome is polyposis of the gastrointestinal tract. These polyps are hamartomatous in origin and there are several reports of malignant degeneration. In order of decreasing frequency the polyps are found in the jejunum, ileum, large bowel and rectum, stomach, and duodenum. In actuality they may be found anywhere in the mucus-secreting portion of the gastrointestinal tract. Seventy percent of affected individuals have some gastrointestinal problem by the age of 20 years. Colicky abdominal pain is most common followed by intestinal bleeding. Intussusception, which may spontaneously recede, is a serious complication and iron deficiency anemia may result from chronic blood loss. Polyps have been noted in other parts of the body including the nose, uterus, ureter-bladder, and bronchial mucosa. There does not appear to be any relationship between the amount of oral pigmentation and the degree or distribution of the visceral polyposis. Ten percent of women with this syndrome have ovarian tumors. Granulosa cell tumors may produce precocious puberty. Other tumors include dysgerminoma, cystadenoma, and Brenner tumor.

Specific Diagnosis The clinical findings of pigmentation and polyposis make this a relatively easy syndrome to diagnose. The pigmentary macules vary in size from 1 to 12 mm, while the polyps are from 0.5 to 7.0 cm in diameter. The presence of pigmentary lesions about the face warrants a thorough examination of the gastrointestinal tract.

Differential Diagnosis Polyposis and pigmentation have been described in association with alopecia and nail dystrophy in the *Cronkheit-Canada syndrome*. Other forms of polyposis of the intestinal tract are mainly limited to the large bowel and are not associated with pigmentary changes.

Prenatal Diagnosis Prenatal diagnosis has not been accomplished in this disorder. It is not likely that the pigmentary lesions would be present early in the second trimester of pregnancy to be viewed by fetoscopy.

Basic Defect, Genetics, and Other Considerations The basic defect in this disorder is not known. Genetic transmission is by autosomal dominant inheritance with a high degree of penetrance.

Prognosis and Treatment There is an increased risk of intestinal cancer in these patients, estimated to be about 2–3%. Periodic examination of the gastrointestinal tract of all patients is indicated as well as a yearly examination in affected females for early detection of ovarian tumors. It is important to keep in mind that the pigmentary lesions tend to be absent in adulthood with the exception of those on the labial and buccal mucosa. Surgical treatment is certainly indicated for the ovarian tumor and early recognition of malignant degeneration of a polyp. The presence of intussusception may also warrant such therapy.

REFERENCES

Cochet, B., Carrel, J., Desbaillets, L., and Widgren, S. Peutz-Jeghers syndrome associated with gastrointestinal carcinoma. *Gut 20:* 169–175, 1979.

Dormandy, T.C. Gastrointestinal polyposis with mucocutaneous pigmentation: Peutz-Jeghers syndrome. *N. Eng. J. Med. 256:* 1093–1102, 1141–1146, 1186–1190, 1956.

Steenstrup, E.K. Ovarian tumors and Peutz-Jeghers syndrome. *Acta Obstet. Gynecol. Scand. 51:* 237–240, 1972.

- **pigmentation about lips / elbows / extremities**
- **lower lip most common site**
- **G.I. polyps**

Peutz-Jeghers Syndrome

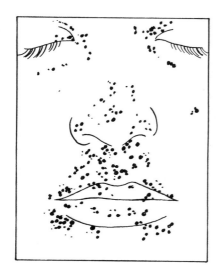

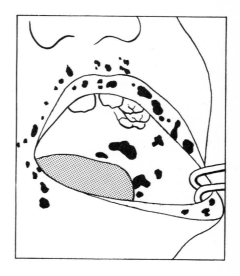

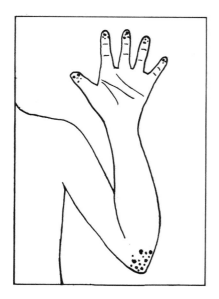

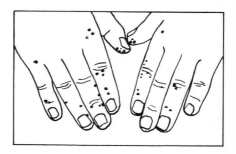

Sites of pigmentary changes about facial orifices, buccal mucosa, elbow and hands

196. POPLITEAL PTERYGIUM SYNDROME

Clinical Features The most striking feature in this syndrome is the pterygium (skin web) which extends from the heel to the ischial tuberosity thus limiting extension, abduction, and rotation of the leg. In most cases the webs are bilateral. Facial features are altered by the presence of cleft lip with or without cleft palate and filiform adhesions between the eyelids. Pits or fistulas of the lower lip and congenital bands extending between the jaws have been described. Several skeletal abnormalities have been described which include hypoplasia or agenesis of the digits, varus or valgus deformation of the foot, soft tissue syndactyly of the second to fifth toes, spina bifida occulta, scoliosis, lordosis, and bipartite or absent patella. The skin over the hallux may have a pyramidal form with one vertex extending to the nail. The toenails, most commonly the second, are hypoplastic. Genital anomálies in the male may include cryptorchidism, absent, cleft, or ectopic scrotum, and inguinal hernia. In the female absence or displacement of the labia majora, enlarged clitoris, and hypoplastic uterus have been reported.

Specific Diagnosis The diagnosis of this disorder is a clinical one and can be made easily in infancy based primarily on the presence of a popliteal web.

Differential Diagnosis Pterygia involving the neck, axilla, antecubital, and popliteal areas occur in the *multiple pterygium syndrome*. Pterygia-like alterations of the lower extremities occur as a finding in the *caudal regression syndrome*.

Prenatal Diagnosis Visualization of the popliteal web during pregnancy with use of a fetoscope could be considered.

Basic Defect, Genetics, and Other Considerations The basic defect in this syndrome is not known. Less than 75 cases have been reported and there is evidence to suggest genetic heterogeneity. Most cases have been isolated but parent-to-child transmission has been noted, thus supporting autosomal dominant inheritance. X-linked inheritance has been ruled out by the presence of male-to-male transmission. Autosomal recessive inheritance has been suggested in severe cases which have occurred in sibs where the parents have been normal.

Prognosis and Treatment Affected individuals are usually of normal intelligence. Cosmetic and orthopedic corrective procedures are indicated. Special caution must be taken in repair of the popliteal web as the sciatic nerve lies free within the pterygium, deep to the fibrous band about halfway between the free edge and the apex. The popliteal vessels are usually located deep in the popliteal space. Frequently muscle groups are absent or muscle insertions are abnormal.

REFERENCES

Bartsocas, C.S. and Papas, C.V. Popliteal pterygium syndrome. *J. Med. Genet. 9:* 222–226, 1972.

Frohlich, G.S., Starzer, K.L., and Tortora, J.M. Popliteal pterygium syndrome: report of a family. *J. Pediatr. 90:* 91–93, 1977.

Gorlin, R.J., Sedano, H.O., and Cervenka, J. Popliteal pterygium syndrome: a syndrome comprising cleft lip-palate, popliteal and intercrural pterygia, digital and genital anomalies. *Pediatrics 41:* 503–509, 1968.

- **popliteal web**
- **cleft lip / lower lip pits**
- **deformed hallucal nails**
- **genital anomalies**

Popliteal Pterygium Syndrome

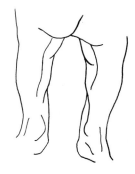 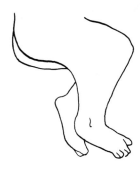 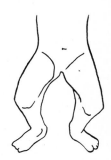

Views of bilateral popliteal pterygia,
on the right note hypoplasia of external
genitalia in a female

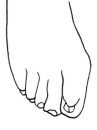 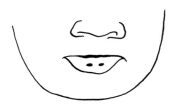 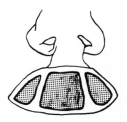

Pyramidal skin
fold extending
to edge of
hallucal nail

Lower lip pits

Bilateral synechiae
between upper
and lower jaws

197. ROTHMUND-THOMSON SYNDROME

Clinical Features The key features are abnormalities of the skin and eyes. The skin findings may be present at birth but usually appear during the first six months of life. They begin on the face and later involve the ears, buttocks, extremities, and finally the entire body. The skin lesion initially appears as erythema of the cheeks and later assumes a marmoreal appearance. Other skin findings include linear telangiectases, brown pigmentation, depigmentation, and punctate atrophy. Sensitivity to sunlight in the form of blister formation is common but usually more severe in early life. Occasionally hyperkeratosis of the palms and soles may be present with verrucous lesions. Approximately half the patients have sparse hair, eyebrows, and eyelashes. Some have total alopecia. The nails are frequently atrophic or rough and ridged. Microdontia along with tooth malformation and failure of eruption are common. Microcephaly and frontal bossing have been noted along with a flat nasal bridge. Zonular cataracts are the most common eye finding. They are present in half the patients and are usually bilateral. They develop rapidly over a period of a few weeks or months and are usually noted by the age of five years. They may appear as early as four months but in some cases they did not make their appearance until the age of 40 years. Degenerative and dystrophic changes of the cornea have also been reported. Other alterations include short stature, scoliosis, and digital anomalies consisting of brachydactyly, syndactyly, and ectrodactyly. Hypoplasia of the ulna and radius and pelvic deformities have also been reported. No specific skeletal alteration is consistently present. Both sexes tend to have poor development of secondary sex characteristics and females are frequently amenorrheic and sterile. Mental retardation has been described in several patients.

Specific Diagnosis No distinct laboratory findings have been reported in this syndrome and thus diagnosis is primarily clinical based on the above features. The histopathology of the skin lesions is not diagnostic, yet the most consistent observations are hyperkeratosis, atrophy of the epidermis, and areas of increased or decreased pigmentation.

Differential Diagnosis In childhood this disorder should be differentiated from the *Cockayne* and the *Bloom syndromes*. The former is characterized by a premature senile appearance with sunken eyes, prognathic mandible, and mental retardation, while in the Bloom syndrome there are various chromosomal findings including breakage. In adults the *Werner* syndrome may be confused with this disorder; however, the presence of severe atrophic changes in skin and muscle along with advanced findings of osteoporosis and arteriosclerosis noted in the Werner syndrome makes the differential diagnosis relatively easy.

Prenatal Diagnosis This is not presently available.

Basic Defect, Genetics, and Other Considerations The basic defect in this rare autosomal recessive disorder is not known. Parental consanguinity has been noted in several cases and the disorder has been reported in identical twins. Possible heterogeneity may exist in this disorder since a mother and son have been reported to be affected. Approximately 70% of patients have been female. Whether this represents true sex predilection or bias of ascertainment is not known.

Prognosis and Treatment The skin lesions tend to be progressive during the early years of life and then become stationary. Carcinomatous changes of the skin may occur in adulthood. Proper skin care with the avoidance of excess exposure to sunlight and other skin irritants is important. Cataract surgery and other surgical procedures may be indicated to correct various congenital malformations.

REFERENCES

Hall, J.G., Pagon, R.A., and Wilson, K.M. Rothmund-Thomson syndrome with severe dwarfism. *Am. J. Dis. Child. 134:* 165–169, 1980.

Hallman, N. and Patiala, R. Congenital poikiloderma atrophicans vasculare in a mother and son. *Acta Derm. Venereol. (Stockh.), 31:* 401–406, 1951.

Kirkham, T.H. and Werner, E.B. The ophthalmic manifestations of Rothmund's syndrome. *Can J. Ophthalmol. 10:* 1–14, 1975.

- **skin lesions on cheeks**
- **sparse eyebrows / lashes**
- **juvenile cataracts**
- **short stature / skeletal anomalies**

Rothmund-Thomson Syndrome

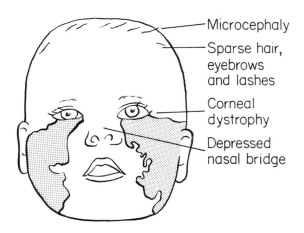

Microcephaly

Sparse hair, eyebrows and lashes

Corneal dystrophy

Depressed nasal bridge

Infant with erythematous skin lesion about cheeks

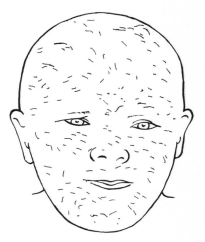

Child with almost total alopecia and reticular pattern to skin lesion

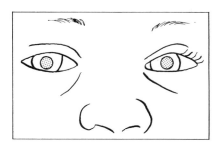

Sparse eyebrows and lashes with zonular cataracts

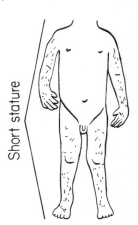

Short stature

Small hands and feet with skin lesion over extremities

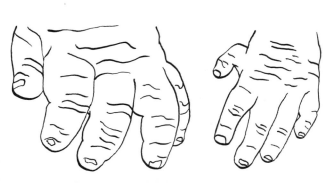

Nail dysplasia, wrinkling of skin and hypoplasia of thumbs

419

198. TUBEROUS SCLEROSIS SYNDROME

Clinical Features Tuberous sclerosis is characterized by the classic triad of epilepsy, "adenoma sebaceum" and mental retardation. During infancy this disorder may present with a tuft of white scalp hair, depigmented macules, or "white spots" plus infantile spasms. "Adenoma sebaceum" appears around the age of five years and occurs in about 65%. They are pink to red nodules with a smooth glistening surface found symmetrically about the nasolabial folds, cheeks, and nose in a butterfly pattern and are really angiofibromas. The chin, ears, forehead, and eyelids may be involved but the upper lip is notably spared. An irregularly shaped plaque of thickened skin, slightly elevated with a *peau d'orange* surface (shagreen patch) may be found in the lumbosacral region in 25%. Periungual fibromas (25%) are common, appearing as smooth buds at the base of the nail or subungually. They are flesh-colored, usually multiple, and may involve both fingers and toes. Depigmented macules are seen in almost 100%. Other skin lesions include multiple skin tags of the neck and axillae, cafe-au-lait spots (15%), poliosis, hemangiomas, and mucosal fibromas. Gingival fibromas and small enamel pits are common oral lesions. The usual symptom is epilepsy. Although the seizures are primarily major motor, focal, psychomotor, and petit mal variants have been noted. Mental retardation of a moderate to severe degree occurs in approximately 65% of patients. It is more prone to occur if seizures are present before two years of age. There is a direct correlation between the severity of skin lesions and neurologic manifestations. About half the patients have unilateral or less common bilateral retinal tumor (phakoma). Congenital blindness, cataract, chorioretinitis, and optic atrophy are other eye manifestations of the disease. Renal hamartomas are found in about 15% of the cases. Rhabdomyomas of the heart may account for death in childhood.

Specific Diagnosis For infants and young children without the typical skin lesions it is suggested that the skin be examined with a Wood's lamp for hypomelanotic macules. Fluorescein angiography of the fundus should be done to rule out retinal phakomas. More recently, CT has been established as a useful noninvasive diagnostic technique. Subependymal nodules occur in some 80% of patients and these provide the most characteristic of all CT findings in this disease. These nodules are multiple, about 1 cm or less in size, often mineralized, and usually adjacent to the lateral and third ventricles. There is no correlation between mental retardation or seizures and positive CT scans or skull radiographic changes. Biopsy of the cutaneous angiofibromas, roentgenogram of the skull showing calcifications in the area of the basal ganglia, and altered electroencephalograms may also be helpful in making a diagnosis. More than half of the patients have cyst-like areas in the phalanges and irregular periosteal new bone formation along the shafts of the metacarpals and metatarsals.

Differential Diagnosis The facial angiofibromas in tuberous sclerosis should be distinguished from those lesions in *multiple trichoepitheliomas, colloid milia* and *atypical xanthomas*. Intracranial calcification may be seen in the *Sturge-Weber anomaly, calcifying subdural hematoma, calcifying neoplasms, cytomegalic inclusion disease, toxoplasmosis,* and *hyalinosis cutis et mucosae*.

Prenatal Diagnosis This is not presently available.

Basic Defect, Genetics, and Other Considerations The basic defect in this autosomal dominant disease is not known. Tuberous sclerosis is found in about 0.1–0.6% of individuals institutionalized for mental retardation and epilepsy and in about 1 in 100,000 to 200,000 in the general population. It has been estimated that the majority of cases result from new mutations with no increase noted in paternal age. However, CT studies have shown findings compatible with tuberous sclerosis in normal parents previously thought not to be affected. Thus the number of cases due to a new mutation may not be as great as thought and asymptomatic parents of an affected child should have a CT scan before genetic counseling is given.

Prognosis and Treatment This disorder tends to be slowly progressive and most patients die by the age of 25 years. Yet it is important to know that the disease in some patients is compatible with normal intelligence and life span. Surgical removal of isolated tumors and use of anticonvulsants and tranquilizers may be helpful.

REFERENCES

Berberich, M.S. and Hall, B.D. Penetrance and variability in tuberous sclerosis. *Birth Defects* 15(5B): 297–304, 1979.

McWilliam, R.C. and Stephenson, J.B.P. Depigmented hair. The earliest sign of tuberous sclerosis. *Arch. Dis. Childh.* 53: 961–963, 1978.

Scotti, L.N., Bartoletti, S.C., Rosenbaum, A. et al. The value of CT in genetic counseling in tuberous sclerosis. *Pediatr. Radiol. 9:* 1–4, 1980.

M.R. [+ / most]

- **angiofibromas about face**
- **white leaf-shaped skin lesions**
- **subungual fibromas**
- **seizures**

Tuberous Sclerosis Syndrome

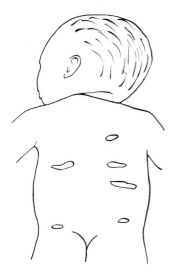

Multiple white macules
on back of infant

Angiofibromas about nasolabial folds

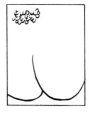

Shagreen patch
lumbosacral area

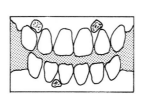

Gingival fibromas

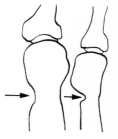

Lytic lesions of
hand bones

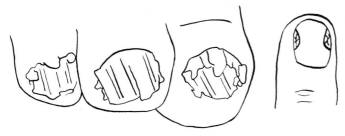

Subungual fibromas about toes and finger

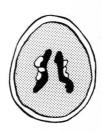

CT scan with
periventricular
calcifications

199. WAARDENBURG SYNDROME

Clinical Features Genetic heterogeneity is known to exist in this syndrome and presently three types are known. Type I, the most common form, can be recognized at birth by the presence of certain facial features which include broad nasal root, loss of frontonasal angle, hypoplastic nasal alae, slightly upturned tip of nose showing the columella, dystopia canthorum, blepharophimosis, lateral displacement of inferior lacrimal points, hyperplasia of medial portion of eyebrows, synophrys, heterochromia irides, and mild mandibular prognathism. Other eye anomalies seen less frequently include microphthalmia, ptosis, and cataracts. A white forelock is observed in 40% of the patients—in some only a few white hairs are present. This finding tends to disappear with age. Premature graying of the hair, eyebrows, and lashes may also occur. Pigmentary anomalies such as vitiligo and hyperpigmentation have been reported as well as hypertrichosis. "Cupid bow" configuration of upper lip, full lower lip, cleft lip/palate, and high-arched palate are other facial features of this syndrome. Congenital sensorineural hearing loss has been observed in 20% of the patients and this may be unilateral or bilateral. Malformations of the external ear have also been described. Several cases have recently been reported to have aganglionic megacolon (Hirschsprung disease).

Type II is characterized by the absence of lateral displacement of the medial canthi (dystopia canthorum) with a much higher occurrence of hearing loss.

In Type III, referred to as the Klein form, the facial and auditory findings observed in Type I are present and, in addition, bilateral involvement of the upper extremities as manifested by hypoplastic changes in the musculoskeletal system, flexion contracture deformities, fusion of carpal bones, and syndactyly are present.

Specific Diagnosis Eye measurements (inner and outer canthal and interpupillary distances) should be made in all suspected individuals. Tables are available for the normal ranges in males and females. The inner canthal distance divided by the interpupillary is greater than 0.6 with dystopia canthorum. Audiologic studies should also be made as some individuals are not always aware of their unilateral hearing loss.

Differential Diagnosis A white forelock (poliosis) can be seen in other disorders such as *Fanconi anemia, piebaldism,* and *rare syndromes* or it may occur as an isolated finding in normal individuals. Heterochromia irides may be acquired, inherited as an autosomal dominant trait, or associated with the *Romberg syndrome. Partial albinism with deafness* is known to occur as an X-linked recessive disorder. Dystopia canthorum can be seen in a variety of conditions.

Prenatal Diagnosis This is not presently available.

Basic Defect, Genetics, and Other Considerations The basic defect in any form of this disorder is not known; however, several investigators favor an alteration in neural crest cell development and/or migration. Types I and II are transmitted as an autosomal dominant with complete penetrance and variable expressivity. Estimate of prevalence of Type I suggests that the syndrome is found in approximately 2% of all congenitally deaf persons in the United States. The incidence of Type II is not known but it is thought to be much rarer than Type I. It is postulated that Type III is also inherited as an autosomal dominant but further documentation is necessary. A syndrome similar to the Waardenburg syndrome (with cutaneous albinism and deafness) is known to exist in cats, dogs, mice, mink, cattle, and horses.

Prognosis and Treatment No form of this syndrome is life threatening. The congenital hearing loss in Type I tends to be static while in Type II it is progressive. Early recognition of a hearing loss is important for proper development of speech and education. All patients with any form of the syndrome should have proper audiometric studies done as early as possible. The upper limb musculoskeletal anomalies in Type III can be disabling and often require orthopedic intervention.

REFERENCES

Goodman, R.M., Lewithal, I., Solomon, A. et al. Upper limb involvement in the Klein-Waardenburg syndrome. *Am. J. Med. Genet. 11:* 425–434, 1982.

Hageman, M.J. and Delleman, J.W. Heterogeneity in Waardenburg syndrome. *Am. J. Hum. Genet. 29:* 468–485, 1977.

Omenn, G.S. and McKusick, V.A. The association of Waardenburg syndrome and Hirschsprung megacolon. *Am. J. Med. Genet. 3:* 217–223, 1979.

- **broad nasal root / hypoplastic alae**
- **dystopia canthorum / synophyrs**
- **pigmentary anomalies / heterochromia iridies**
- **"cupid bow" upper lip / full lower lip**

Waardenburg Syndrome

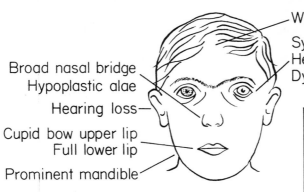

White forelock
Synophrys
Heterochromia iris
Dystopia canthorum

Broad nasal bridge
Hypoplastic alae
Hearing loss
Cupid bow upper lip
Full lower lip
Prominent mandible

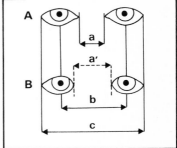

A) normal, B) dystopia canthorum, a) medial canthal distance, a') displacement of medial canthi b) pupillary distance, c) outer canthal distance

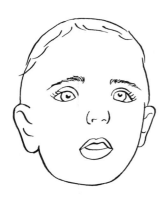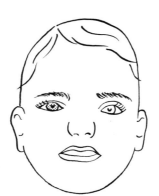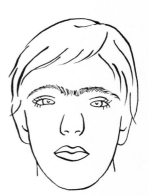

Facial features in other affected children

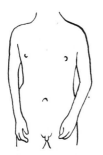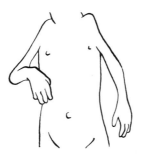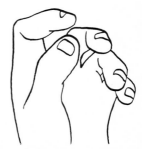

Klein type-hypoplasia of muscles of shoulders, upper limbs and contractures

200. XERODERMA PIGMENTOSUM SYNDROMES

Clinical Features In the most common form of this disorder patients in early infancy display an acute sensitivity of the skin in areas exposed to sunlight. Erythema combined with freckling are commonly noted about the face, ears, neck, hands, and forearms. As the disorder progresses, nonexposed areas of the skin, about the trunk and lower extremities, also become involved. Increased pigmentation interspersed with white parchmentlike areas, atrophy, dryness, scaliness, and telangiectasia are usually seen before the age of two years in the sun-exposed areas. During childhood and adolescence degenerative changes in the skin may occur with the formation of basal cell and squamous cell carcinomas. Melanoma, keratoacanthoma, angiosarcoma, fibrosarcoma, and other benign and malignant lesions have been reported. Early eye findings include photophobia, lacrimation, and conjunctivitis. The bulbar conjunctiva frequently shows pigmentation and telangiectasia; it may undergo malignant degeneration. The cornea may cloud and ulcerate with secondary iritis resulting in synechiae or iris atrophy. As eye involvement progresses, the eyelids lose their cilia, and ectropion, entropion, or symblepharon may occur.

In another form of this disorder termed the *De Sanctis-Cacchione syndrome,* intelligence is severely impaired. Autopsy findings have shown microcephaly with a small brain and diffuse mild cerebral and olivopontocerebellar neuronal loss. Neurological findings may include spastic ataxic gait, athetoid movement of head and arms, areflexia, disturbed speech, sensorineural deafness, and pyramidal and extrapyramidal signs. Such patients are frequently below normal in height and have small external genitalia. Delayed or deficient sexual maturation is common.

Specific Diagnosis In addition to the above clinical findings and distinct histopathologic changes in the skin, the most specific laboratory test shows a failure of DNA excision repair of ultraviolet-induced thymine dimers. Other laboratory studies have shown increased chromosomal breakage in cultured fibroblasts, elevation of IgE, and excessive accumulation of glycogen and subsarcolemmal mitochondrial aggregates in muscle. Cranial CT scan has shown ventricular dilatation, cerebral cortical atrophy, small brainstem, and thickening of the calvarial bones in the De Sanctis-Cacchione syndrome.

Differential Diagnosis Multiple nevi and basal cell carcinomas are seen in patients with the *nevoid basal cell carcinoma syndrome* but this condition is transmitted as an autosomal dominant disorder. Some features of the De Sanctis-Cacchione syndrome may be confused with *Bloom syndrome,* but in the latter there are no extensive skin atrophy and hyperpigmentation changes.

Prenatal Diagnosis Prenatal diagnosis is possible in this syndrome based on the fact that normal cultivated skin fibroblasts have the ability for excision repair, which is absent in this disorder. Assays for excision-repair deficiency or postreplication repair deficiency require relatively few cells; thus, prenatal diagnosis can be accomplished as early as one week after amniocentesis. Heterozygotes tend to have excision repair levels within the range of normal cells and their detection is not always reliable.

Basic Defect, Genetics, and Other Considerations Although the basic defect involves a failure of DNA excision repair of ultraviolet-induced thymine dimers, the exact enzymatic alteration remains unknown. Hybrid cells containing genes from xeroderma pigmentosum (XP) and De Sanctis-Cacchione cells may synthesize the full complement of normal enzymes as evidenced by the enhanced repair levels. Further use of this technique has led to the recognition of five subclasses of XP, each probably caused by a mutation at a different locus. Not all five types are clinically distinct entities and more types may be detected. The De Sanctis-Cacchione type, like all forms of XP, is inherited as an autosomal recessive disorder. It is considered to be quite rare and fewer than 60 cases have been reported.

Prognosis and Treatment Survival to adulthood is unusual and early death is caused by metastatic disease. There is no satisfactory treatment, but patients should avoid sunlight and use solar protective creams. Early surgical removal of malignant growths is indicated.

REFERENCES

Cleaver, J.E. Xeroderma pigmentosum variants with normal DNA repair and normal sensitivity to ultraviolet light. *J. Invest. Dermatol. 58:* 124–128, 1972.

Halley, D.J.J. et al. Prenatal diagnosis of xeroderma pigmentosum (group C) using assay of unscheduled DNA synthesis and postreplication repair. *Clin. Genet. 16:* 137–146, 1979.

Handa, J., Nakano, Y., and Akiguchi, I. Cranial computed tomography findings in xeroderma pigmentosum with neurologic manifestations (De Sanctis-Cacchione syndrome). *J. Comp. Assisted Tomography 2:* 456–459, 1978.

- **skin lesions / exposed areas**
- **hyperpigmentation / atrophy / scarring**
- **skin cancers later**
- **photophobia / conjunctivitis / ectropion**

Xeroderma Pigmentosum Syndromes

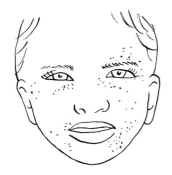 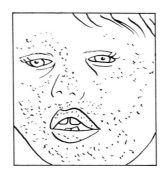 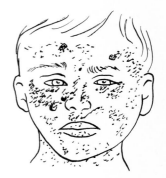

Stages of skin involvement with freckle-like lesions,
hyperpigmentation, keratotic, malignancy and atrophic scarring

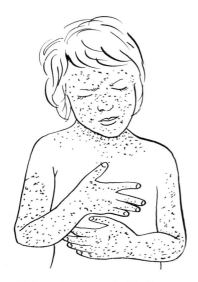 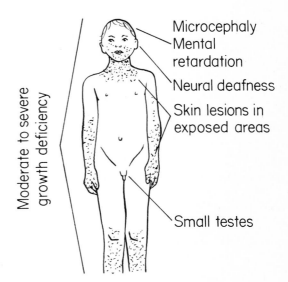

Skin changes initially
limited to sun-exposed
areas of the body

Moderate to severe
growth deficiency

Microcephaly
Mental
retardation
Neural deafness
Skin lesions in
exposed areas
Small testes

De SANCTIS-CACCHIONE SYNDROME
progressive nervous system
deterioration with seizures
spasticity and incoordination

APPENDIX

General Principles for Measuring Body Parts

Guidelines for Head and Facial Measurements

Figures, Tables, and Charts on Body Measurements

Glossary of Medical Terms

Selected Book References

General Principles for Measuring Body Parts
General Guidelines

1. A steel tape or some other type of nonstretching device should be used for measuring. When unilateral, the measurement should be obtained on the right side.
2. When presenting data, if percentiles are used, standard deviations should also be stated.
3. Centimeters should be used instead of inches.
4. For individuals less than 2 years, height measurements should be done while in the supine position. Individuals over 2 should be standing on a rigid, flat surface with the knees held straight and the head facing directly forward.
5. If there is a slant of the palpebral fissure it should be described as being upward or downward in relationship to the lateral aspect of the palpebral fissure (a mongoloid slant is an upward slant while a patient with Treacher Collins syndrome has a downward slant).

HEAD AND FACIAL MEASUREMENTS

Head circumference the measurement of the circumference with the tape just above the eyebrows anteriorly and at the maximum point of the occiput posteriorly.

Head length distance from the glabella (a prominence on the frontal bone above the root of the nose and on the level of the superior orbital ridges) to the prominence of the occiput (measured by spreading calipers).

Head width maximal biparietal distance (spreading calipers).

Skull height distance from nasion (the deepest depression at the top of the nose) to superior head point.

Total facial height distance from the nasion to menton with the teeth in occlusion.

Upper facial height distance from the nasion to the subnasion (the deepest point of concavity at the base of the nose).

Midface height distance from subnasion to cheilion.

Lower face height distance from cheilion to menton.

Facial width the maximal distance between the zygomas as measured by calipers.

Mandible width (maximum) the bigonial width.

Mouth width (at rest) distance from cheilion to cheilion.

Outer canthus the distance between the outer canthi of both eyes.

Inner canthus the distance between the inner canthi of both eyes.

Interpupillary distance (IPD) the distance between the centers of the pupils with the eyes looking straight ahead. In younger children for accurate measurements it may be necessary to use the formula: IPD = .7 + .59 inner canthal distance + .41 outer canthal distance.

Nose length the distance from the nasion to the subnasion (measured with a caliper).

Nasal width the distance between the most lateral aspects of the alae nasi.

Columella length the distance from the tip of the nose to the subnasion.

Philtrum the base of the columella to the midline depression of the vermilion border.

Ear length maximum distance from the superior aspect to the inferior aspect of the ear (pinna).

Ear rotation an angle measured between two lines: one is the Frankfort horizontal plane (the line extending from the external auditory canal to the infraorbital ridge below the pupil), and the other is the line connecting the superior and inferior attachments of the ear.

Ear position the extent to which the superior attachment of the pinna falls above or below the horizontal line drawn between the medial canthi.

OTHER BODY MEASUREMENTS

Chest anteroposterior diameter the distance measured from the sternum at the nipple line to the vertebrae at the same place while at rest.

Chest circumference the measurement of the circumference with the tape placed over the nipples while at rest.

Internipple distance the distance between the centers of the nipples.

Chest width the distance between the midaxillary lines at the level of the nipples (measured with a caliper).

Thoracic index anteroposterior diameter/chest width.

Sternal length the distance from the top of the manubrium to the lowest palpable edge of the sternum.

Upper body segment total body length minus the lower body segment.

Lower body segment distance from the upper pubis to the floor.

Sitting height the distance from the chair seat to the most superior aspect of the head which is held straight (the patient should be sitting on a hard, flat surface with the legs hanging free).

Crown-rump distance distance from the vertex of the head to the lowest part of the trunk which corresponds to either the perineum or the lowest surface of the buttock.

Arm span distance from the tip of the third finger of one hand to the tip of the third finger of the other with arms fully extended.

Arm length distance from the acromion to the tip of the third finger with the arm in full extension and parallel to the body.

Upper segment of the arm the distance from the acromion to the olecranon with the elbow bent at 90 degrees.

Lower arm segment the distance from the olecranon process to the distal end of the styloid process with the elbow bent at 90 degrees.

Upper arm girth circumference measured at the level midway between the acromial and olecranon processes with the arm hanging loosely and with the tape not deforming the skin contour.

Lower arm girth measured at the maximum circumference of the forearm just below the elbow with the arm hanging loosely and the tape not deforming the skin contour.

Angle of the elbow the angle determined by a goniometer using the longitudinal axis of the upper and lower segments of the arm.

Width of the hand the maximum distance from the second to the fifth metacarpal at the metacarpal–phalangeal junction with the fingers together.

Biacromial distance maximum distance between the right and left acromions.

Hand length the distance between the distal wrist crease and the tip of the middle finger.

Total lower limb length the distance from the greater trochanter to the lateral femoral condyle.

Lower segment distance of lower limb distance from the lateral femoral condyle to the lateral malleolus.

Foot length the distance from the posterior prominence of the heel to the tip of the big toe (measured while sitting).

Penile length the distance from the pubic ramus to the tip of the glans of the penis with the penis outstretched.

Guidelines for Head and Facial Measurements

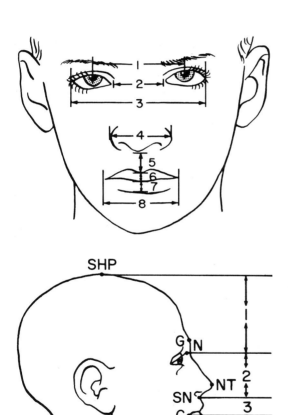

1. interpupillary distance
2. inner canthal distance
3. outer canthal distance
4. interalar distance
5. philtrum length
6. upper lip thickness
7. lower lip thickness
8. intercommissural distance

1. skull height
2. upper face height
3. midface height
4. lower face height
SHP, superior head point
G, glabella
N, nasion
NT, nose tip
SN, subnasion
C, cheilion
M, menton

Figures, Tables, and Charts on Body Measurements

Normal Fontanel and Suture Closure

Fontanel or Suture	Closure Time
Anterior fontanel	1 yr ± 4 mo
Posterior fontanel	Birth ± 2 mo
Anterolateral fontanel	By 3rd mo
Posterolateral fontanel	During 2nd yr
Metopic suture	By 3rd yr (10 % never)
Clinical closure of sutures	6–12 mo
Anatomic closure of sutures	By 30th yr

Head Circumference in Boys and Girls*

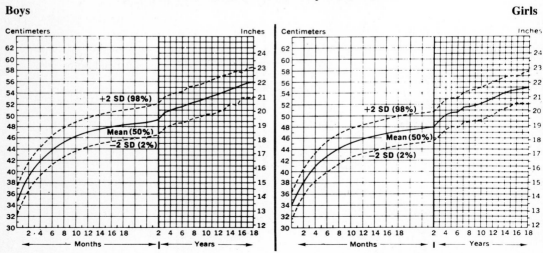

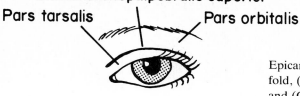

Sulcus orbitopalpebralis superior

Pars tarsalis   Pars orbitalis

A

Epicanthal variations: (A) absence of epicanthal fold, (B) epicanthal fold in Oriental populations, and (C) epicanthal fold in Down syndrome.

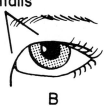

Pars orbitalis

B

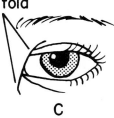

Epicanthal fold

C

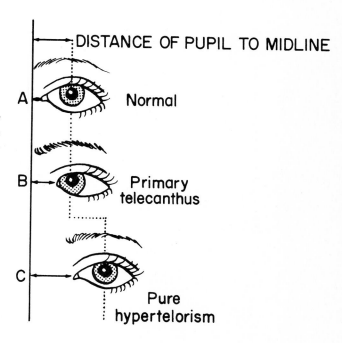

The eye: (A) normal, (B) primary telecanthus, and (C) hypertelorism.

DISTANCE OF PUPIL TO MIDLINE

A — Normal

B — Primary telecanthus

C — Pure hypertelorism

Outer Canthal Distance*

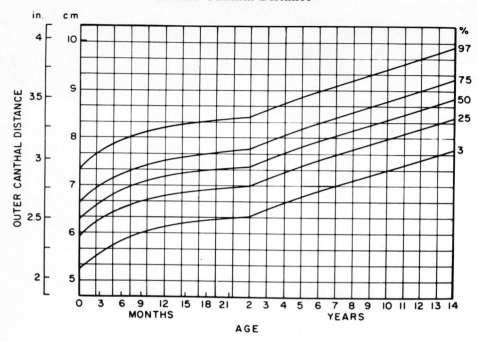

Inner Canthal Distance*

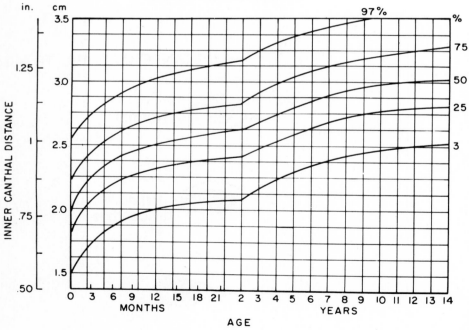

*Figures with asterisks from Feingold, M. and Bossert, W.H. *Normal Values for Selected Physical Parameters: An Aid to Syndrome Delineation*. Bergsma, D. (ed). White Plains: The National Foundation—March of Dimes, Birth Defects X(13), 1974.

Interpupillary Distance*

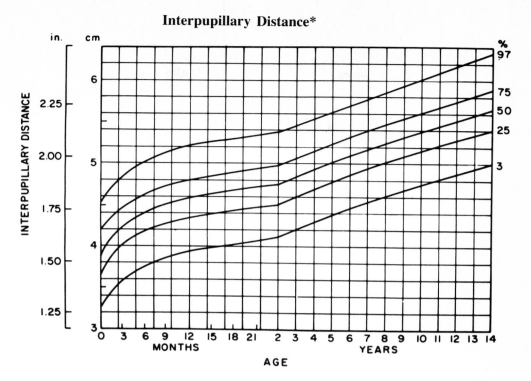

Palpebral Length and Width

Age (yr)	Length (mm) Average	(Range)	Width (mm) Average	(Range)
1	19	(18–21)	8.2	(8–8.5)
1–10	25	(19–29)	8.7	(8.5–9)
11–60	28	(23–33)	9.0	(8–11.2)

435

Anatomical landmarks, external ear.

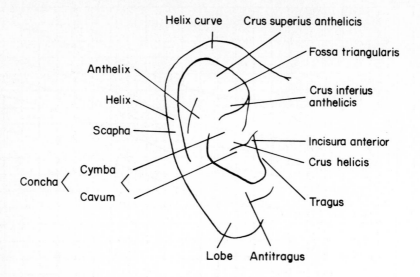

Helix curve — Crus superius anthelicis
Fossa triangularis
Anthelix
Helix
Scapha
Crus inferius anthelicis
Incisura anterior
Crus helicis
Cymba
Concha
Cavum
Tragus
Lobe   Antitragus

Ear measurements.

Height, tip of lobe to most superior part of helical rim
Width, anterior base of tragus to margin of helical rim
Protrusion, greatest distance of the most superior position of the helix from the mastoid area

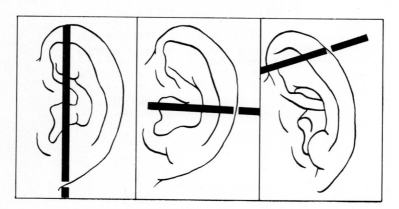

Illusion of low-set ears due to posterior rotat of pinna and reduction in chin size.

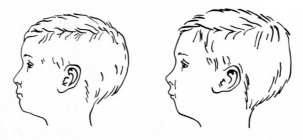

Total Ear Length*

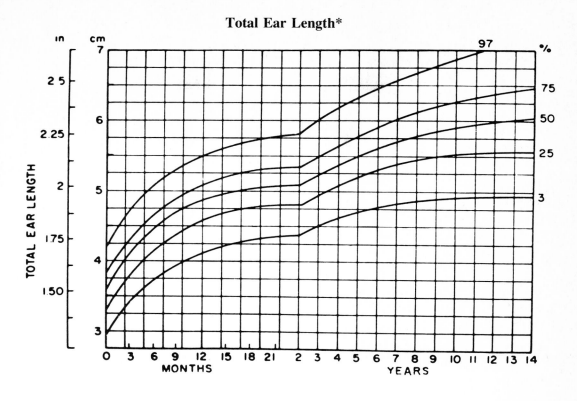

Mean Value of Auricular Size (mm)

Age (yr)	Auricular height		Auricular width	
	Male	**Female**	**Male**	**Female**
0–9	44	41	27	25
1	50	47	31	28
2	50	49	32	31
3	51	50	32	31
4	52	51	32	32
5	54	52	33	32
6	55	53	33	33
7–8	56	56	34	33
9–10	58	57	35	33
11–12	60	58	35	33
13–14	60	58	35	33
15–16	63	58	36	33
17–18	64	59	36	33
18–20	65	59	36	33
20–30	67	59	36	33
30–40	67	61	36	33
40–50	68	63	36	33
50–60	69	64	36	33
60–70	70	68	36	33
70–80	74	68	36	34

Mean and Range of Nasal Dimensions in Whites (mm)

Age (yrs)	Vertical height (n-sn)		Anteroposterior Length (prn-sn)		Alar width (al-al)	
	Male	Female	Male	Female	Male	Female
0–15 wks.	22 (18–25)	23 (20–24)	7 (5–9)	7 (5–9)	21 (18–24)	21 (18–24)
1	32 (29–38)	34 (25–38)	10 (8–14)	10 (4–13)	27 (25–32)	27 (23–30)
3	36 (29–42)	36 (31–41)	12 (9–16)	12 (9–15)	28 (25–33)	28 (23–32)
6	41 (35–47)	40 (32–45)	14 (11–17)	13 (8–16)	30 (25–35)	29 (26–34)
9	43 (37–47)	43 (37–52)	15 (11–19)	14 (11–20)	31 (28–36)	30 (26–35)
12	47 (41–53)	46 (40–50)	16 (12–19)	16 (12–20)	32 (28–36)	32 (28–39)
15	51 (45–58)	48 (40–55)	18 (14–22)	18 (13–22)	35 (30–40)	32 (28–39)
18	52 (45–61)	48 (44–55)	20 (16–24)	18 (15–22)	35 (32–40)	32 (29–39)

Length of Philtrum or Nasal–Labial Distance*

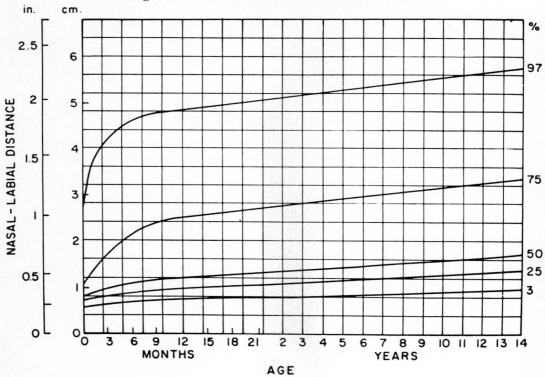

Intercommissural Distance of White Children and Adults

Age (yr)	Males (mm)	Females (mm)
0–1	32	27
2–3	35	30
4–5	39	36
6–7	42	40
8–9	44	42
10–11	46	43
12–13	48	45
14–15	50	47
Adult	52	50

Eruption of Primary Teeth

Teeth	Eruption time (months)	Mean time (months)
Lower central incisor	4½–10	8
Upper central incisor	6–12	9½
Upper lateral incisor	8½–14	11½
Lower lateral incisor	9–16	12
Upper first molar	12–18	15
Lower first molar	12–18½	15½
Lower canine	14½–22	18
Upper canine	14½–22	18
Lower second molar	22–30	26
Upper second molar	22–30	26

Chest Circumference*

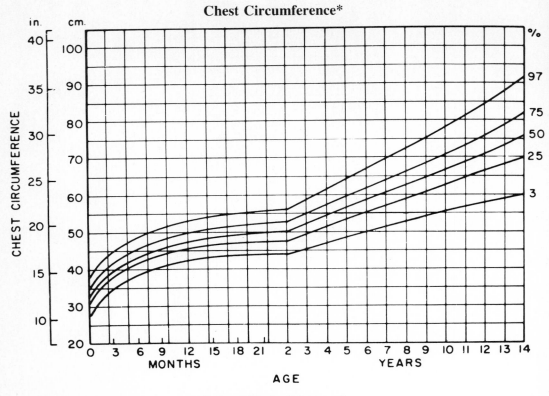

Inter Nipple Distance*

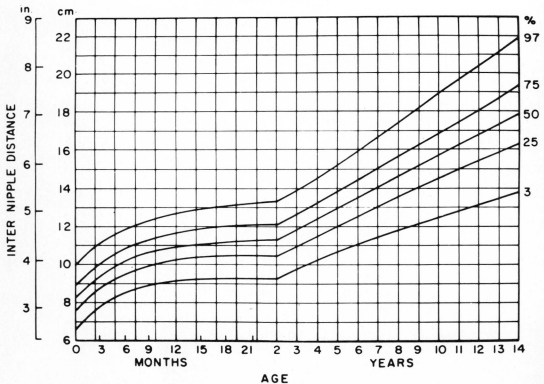

Stretched Penile Length (cm)
in Normal Males

	Mean + SD	Mean − 2½SD
Newborn: 30 weeks	2.5 ± 0.4	1.5
34 weeks	3.0 ± 0.4	2.0
term	3.5 ± 0.4	2.5–2.4
0–5 months	3.9 ± 0.8	1.9
6–12 months	4.3 ± 0.8	2.3
1–2 years	4.7 ± 0.8	2.6
2–3 years	5.1 ± 0.9	2.9
3–4 years	5.5 ± 0.9	3.3
4–5 years	5.7 ± 0.9	3.5
5–6 years	6.0 ± 0.9	3.8
6–7 years	6.1 ± 0.9	3.9
7–8 years	6.2 ± 1.0	3.7
8–9 years	6.3 ± 1.0	3.8
9–10 years	6.3 ± 1.0	3.8
10–11 years	6.4 ± 1.1	3.7
Adult	13.3 ±1.6	9.3

Normal Testicular Volume

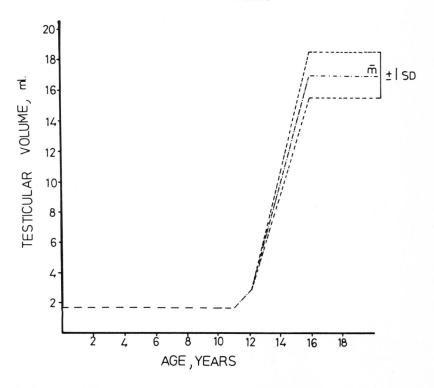

Total Hand Length*

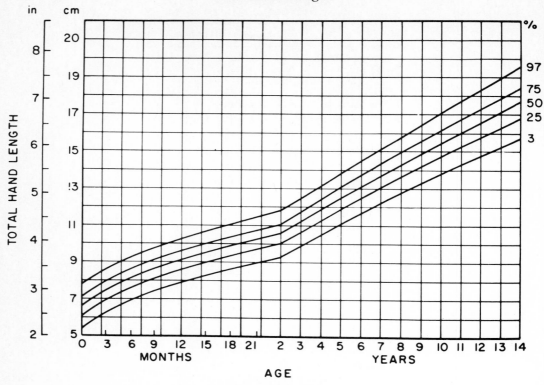

Palm Length*

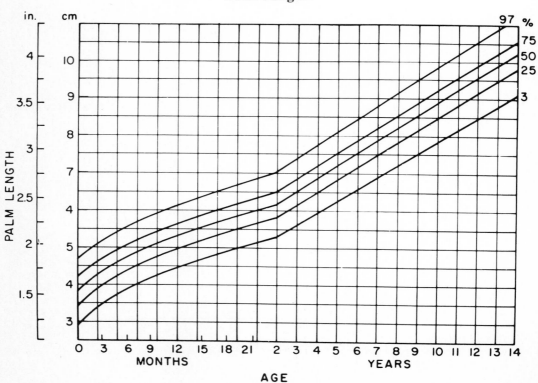

Glossary of Medical Terms

achalasia Failure to relax on the part of a bodily opening, such as a sphincter or the esophagus.

acrocephaly A condition in which the top of the head is pointed, with a vertical index above 77; referred to as acrocephaly, turricephaly, steeple head, and tower head.

acrocyanosis A condition marked by coldness and cyanosis of the hands and feet.

acroosteolysis Dissolution of bone involving the terminal digits of the hands and feet.

acroparesthesia Symptoms of tingling, numbness, and stiffness in the extremities, chiefly the fingers, hands, and forearms; may be associated with pain, pallor of the skin, or slight cyanosis.

adactyly Congenital absence of fingers or toes.

agenesis Defective development or absence of part(s) of the body.

akinesia Absence, loss, or weakness of motor function; the temporary paralysis of a muscle by the injection of procaine.

alopecia Baldness; deficiency of hair, natural or abnormal.

amblyopia Dimness of vision; partial loss of sight.

angioid streak A crack in Bruch's membrane of the retina appearing as a vessel-like structure on fundiscopic examination.

angiomatosis A diseased state of vessels with formations of multiple angiomas.

aniridia Absence of the iris.

ankyloblepharon The adhesion of the ciliary edges of the eyelid to each other.

ankylosis Abnormal immobility and consolidation of a joint.

anodontia Absence of the teeth.

anonychia Congenital absence of a nail or nails.

anophthalmia Congenital absence of one or both eyes.

anosmia Absence of the sense of smell.

antimongoloid slant of eyes Referring to a downward slant of the palpebral fissure of the eye in contrast with the upward slant of the palpebral fissure in patients with Down syndrome.

aphakia Absence of the lens of the eye.

apraxia A disorder of voluntary movement, consisting in a more or less complete incapacity to execute purposeful movements, notwithstanding the preservation of muscular power, sensibility, and coordination in general.

arachnodactyly Unusually long and thin fingers and toes classically observed in the Marfan syndrome.

arhinencephaly Congenital absence of the rhinencephalon.

arhinia Congenital absence of the nose.

arthrogryposis The state of a persistent flexure or contracture of a joint. In arthrogryposis multiplex congenita there is a congenital generalized fibrous ankylosis of the joints of the upper and lower extremities.

atresia Imperforation; absence or closure of a normal opening.

bathrocephaly A condition characterized by a step-like posterior projection of the skull, caused by external bulging of the squamous portion of the occipital bone.

bicornuate or bicornate Having two horns, commonly used to describe a malformation of the uterus.

blepharochalasis Relaxation of the skin of the

443

eyelid, caused by atrophy of the intercellular tissue.

blepharophimosis A narrowing of the slit between the eyelids.

brachycephaly A shortening of the skull; cephalic index is 81.0 to 85.4.

brachymelia A shortening of the limbs.

brachymesophalangy A shortening of the middle digits of the hands and feet.

brachyturricephaly The combination of shortening of the skull along with towering or oxycephaly.

Brushfield spots Spotting of the iris due to increased density of its anterior border layer; this increased density is due to deposition of aggregates of stromal fibrocytes; observed in 85% of patients with Down syndrome. When noted in the normal population (about 25%), they are termed Wöllfflin-Krückmann spots.

buphthalmos Congenital glaucoma; keratoglobus, or enlargement of the eye.

calcaneovalgus A clubfoot that is dorsiflexed, everted, and abducted.

calvaria The upper, dome-like portion of the skull.

camptodactyly Flexion deformity of one or more digits usually involving the middle phalangeal joints but may involve any of the joints of the digits.

cebocephaly A form of holoprosencephaly; the face is characterized by ocular hypotelorism and a centrally placed nose with a single blind-ended nostril.

Chvostek sign A spasm of the facial muscles resulting from tapping the muscles or the branches of the facial nerve.

clinodactyly Incurving of one or more digits of the hand or foot most commonly involving the distal phalanges.

clubfoot A deformity of the foot in which it is twisted out of shape or position, referred to medically as talipes. The various shapes and positions produce such deformities as talipes equinus, talipes calcaneus, talipes cavus, talipes varus, talipes equinovarus, talipes calcaneovarus, talipes valgus, talipes calcaneovalgus, and talipes equinovalgus.

coarctation of the aorta Narrowing or constriction of the aorta, usually near its junction with the ductus arteriosus.

coloboma A fissuring defect especially of the eye, usually congenital, but may be of traumatic origin.

columella nasi The fleshy external termination of the septum of the nose.

concha A structure resembling a shell in shape, as the hollow of the external ear or turbinate bone.

corectopia Abnormal location of the pupil.

corneal nebulae Mild corneal opacity.

coxa valga Deformity of the neck of the femur, the opposite of coxa vara, producing in the limb marked external rotation, increased abduction, and decreased adduction.

coxa vara "Bent hip," bending downward of the neck of the femur.

craniorachischisis Congenital fissure of the skull and spinal column.

cryptophthalmos Congenital complete adhesion of the eyelids.

cryptorchidism A developmental defect in which the testes are found in the abdominal cavity; commonly referred to as undescended testes.

cubitus valgus Deformity of the forearm in which it deviates inwardly when extended.

cyclopia Synophthalmia; a congenital defect in which the two orbits merge to form a single cavity usually containing one eye, which is likely to show more or less evidence of its origin by fusion of the right and left optic primordia.

dacrocystitis Inflammation of the tear sac; especially an acute suppurative inflammation of the submucous tissue, with painful swelling and chronic discharge of pus.

Dandy-Walker anomaly Anomaly in which the primary defect involves atresia of the foramina of Luschka and Magendie; the fourth ventricle becomes dilated into a large cyst in the posterior fossa.

dextrocardia Transposition of the heart to the right side of the thorax.

diastema A space or cleft.

dolichocephaly Elongation in the shape of the skull; cephalic index is 75.9 or less.

dolichostenomelia Long, thin extremities.

dysphagia Difficulty in swallowing.

dystopia canthorum Lateral displacement of the medial canthi of the eyes.

eclabium Eversion of the lips or lip.

ectopia lentis Displacement of the crystalline lens of the eye.

ectrodactyly Total or partial absence of fingers or toes. Synonym: ectromelia.

extropion Eversion or turning out of the edge, as of an eyelid or of the lip.

encephalocele Hernia of the brain, manifested by protrusion through a congenital or traumatic opening of the skull.

enophthalmos Abnormal retraction of the eyes in the orbit producing deeply set eyes.

entropion The inversion of the edge of the eyelid or of any similarly situated structure.

epicanthal folds A congenital deformity consisting of a vertical fold of skin on either side of the nose, sometimes covering the inner canthus.

epiphora An abnormal overflow of tears down the cheek; mainly caused by stricture of the nasolacrimal duct.

epispadias A congenital defect in which the urethra opens on the dorsum of the penis.

equinovarus A blending of pes equinus with pes varus.

esotropia Inward deviation of an eye when both eyes are open and uncovered; convergent strabismus.

ethmocephaly A form of holoprosencephaly in which there are two separate but hypoteloric eyes and a supraorbital proboscis.

euryopia Abnormally wide opening of the eyes.

exophthalmos Abnormal protrusion of the eyeball.

exostosis A bony growth projecting outward from the surface of a bone.

exotropia Outward deviation of an eye when both eyes are opened and uncovered; divergent strabismus.

frenulum A small fold of the integument or of the mucous membrane that limits the movement of an organ or part.

frontal bossing Prominence of the anterior portion of the frontal bone of the skull.

gastroschisis A congenital malformation in which the abdomen remains open.

genu valgum A deformity in which the knees are abnormally close together. Synonym: knock-knee

genu varum A deformity in which the knees are abnormally separated. Synonym: bowleg.

gibbus Extreme kyphosis or hump; a deformity of spine in which there is a sharply angulated segment, the apex of the angle being posterior.

glabella The smooth area on the frontal bone between the superciliary arches.

glossoptosis Downward displacement or retraction of the tongue.

hallux valgus Displacement of the great toe towards the other toes.

hallux varus Displacement of the halluces medially.

hammer toes Contractural deformity of the distal phalanges of the toes.

hemiatrophy Atrophy of one side of the body or of one half of an organ or part.

hemimelia A condition marked by defects in the limbs on one side.

hemiplegia Paralysis of one side of the body.

hexadactyly The occurrence of six fingers (or toes) on a hand (or foot).

hirsutism Abnormal hairiness.

holoacrania A congenital skull defect in which bones of the vault are absent.

holoprosencephaly Impaired midline cleavage of the embryonic forebrain, the most extreme form being cyclopia.

Hutchinson teeth Notched and narrow-edged permanent incisors; regarded as a sign of congenital syphilis, but not always of such origin.

hydramnios Excess of amniotic fluid, same as polyhydramnios.

hydranencephaly Internal hydrocephalus.

hydrocephaly A condition characterized by abnormal increase in the amount of cerebral fluid accompanied by dilation of the cerebral ventricles.

hyperhydrosis or **hyperhidrosis** Excessive sweating.

hyperopia Farsightedness; the lack of refracting power sufficient to focus parallel rays on the retina.

hypertelorism Abnormal distance between two organs or parts; commonly used to describe increased interpupillary distance.

hypertrichosis An abnormal growth of hair; excessive hairiness.

hypoacusis Decreased perception of sound.

hypodontia Absence of a few teeth.

hypogeusia Impairment of the sense of taste.

hypohidrosis Diminished sweating.

hypomentia Decreased mentation.

hypospadias The congenital opening of the urethra on the undersurface of the penis; may also refer to the opening of the urethra into the vagina.

hypotonia Diminished tension or tonicity, or reduction in muscle tone.

hypotrichosis Presence of less than the normal amount of hair.

inanition The physical condition that results from complete lack of food.

iniencephaly A malformation consisting of a cranial defect at the occiput, the brain being exposed.

iridodonesis Tremor of the iris usually due to dislocation of the lens.

keratoconus A conical protrusion of the cornea.

koilonychia A condition in which the nail is concave; spoon nail.

kyphoscoliosis Backward and lateral curvature of the spinal column.

lentigines Brownish pigmented spots on the skin due to increased deposition of melanin and associated with an increased number of melanocytes at the epidermodermal junction.

leukoma A dense, white opacity of the cornea.

leukonychia A whitish discoloration of the nails.

lingua plicata Fissured tongue.

lissencephaly A smooth brain or a brain without convolutions or with only shallow convolutions.

445

livedo reticularis A peripheral vascular condition characterized by a reddish blue net-like mottling of the skin of the extremities.

lordosis Curvature of the spinal column with a forward convexity.

lymphangiectasis Dilation of the lymphatic vessels.

macrocheilia Abnormal or excessive size of the lips.

macroglossia Hypertrophy of the tongue.

macrosomia Enlarged body size.

marasmus Progressive wasting and emaciation, especially such as wasting in infants when there is no obvious or ascertainable cause.

Meckel diverticulum An occasional sacculation or appendage of the ileum, derived from an unobliterated yolk stalk.

megacolon Abnormally large colon, due to dilation and hypertrophy.

meningoencephalocele Hernial protrusion of the brain and meninges.

meroacrania Congenital partial absence of the cranium.

mesomelic Pertaining to the midportion of the arms or leg.

microcephaly Abnormal smallness of the head.

microglossia Abnormal smallness of the tongue.

micrognathia Abnormal smallness of the lower jaw, with recession of the chin.

micromelia A developmental defect characterized by abnormal smallness or shortness of the limbs; short limbs without absence of bone elements. Synonym: brachymelia.

microphthalmia Abnormal smallness of the eyes.

microstomia A congenital defect in which the mouth is unusually small.

milium A small, whitish nodule in the skin, especially on the face. Milia are usually retention cysts of sebaceous glands or hair follicles.

monilethrix A genetic disorder of hair in which the hairs exhibit bead-like enlargements with fracturing at these raised points resulting in sparse to absent hair over the body.

myotonia Increased muscular irritability and contractility with decreased power of relaxation.

nystagmus An involuntary rapid movement of the eyeball, which may be horizontal, vertical, rotatory, or mixed.

N.T.D. Neural tube defect.

oligodactyly Absence of some fingers or toes. Synonym: hypodactylia.

oligodontia Severe deficiency of teeth.

omphalocele Protrusion, at birth, of part of the intestine through a large defect in the abdominal wall at the umbilicus, the protruding bowel being covered only by a thin transparent membrane composed of amnion and peritoneum.

ophthalmoplegia Paralysis of the eye muscles.

opisthotonus A tetanic spasm in which the spine and extremities are bent with convexity forward, the body resting on the head and heels.

osteopathia striata Linear striations seen by X-ray in the metaphyses of long bones and also flat bones.

osteopenia Decreased calcification or density of bone.

osteopoikilosis A condition characterized by the presence of multiple sclerotic foci in the ends of long bones and scattered stippling in round and flat bones.

oxycephaly See acrocephaly.

ozena A condition characterized by intranasal crusting, atrophy, and fetid odor.

pachygyria Unusually thick convolutions of the cerebral cortex, related to defective development.

pachyonychia Thickening of the nails.

paronychia Inflammation of the nail fold with separation of the skin from the proximal portion of the nail; may be due to bacteria or fungi.

pectus carinatum Undue prominence of the sternum, often referred to as pigeon breast.

pectus excavatum Undue depression of the sternum, often referred to as funnel breast.

peromelia Congenitally malformed limb; usually refers to absent hand or foot.

pes cavus Exaggerated height of the longitudinal arch of the foot, present from birth or appearing later because of contractures or disturbed balance of the muscles.

pes equinovarus A clubfoot that is plantar flexed, inverted, and adducted.

pes planus A deformed foot in which the position of the bones relative to each other has been altered, with lowering of the longitudinal arch producing undue flatness of the sole, commonly referred to as flatfoot.

pes valgus The outward angulation of the foot, sometimes referred to as talipes valgus.

phenotype Observed trait in an individual.

philtrum The vertical groove in the median portion of the upper lip, extending from beneath the nose to the outer surface of the upper lip.

phocomelia In its extreme form, direct attachment of hands or feet to the trunk. The term may also be applied to cases of partial absence of any proximal region of the limbs.

plagiocephaly An asymmetric craniostenosis due to premature closure of the lambdoid and coronal sutures on one side; characterized by an oblique deformity of the skull.

platyspondyly Flatness of the bodies of the vertebrae.

poikiloderma A variegated hyperpigmentation

and telangiectasia of the skin, followed by atrophy.

poliosis Premature grayness of the hair.

polydactyly A developmental anomaly characterized by the presence of supernumerary digits on the hands or feet.

polyhydramnios Excess amount of amniotic fluid during pregnancy.

polyphagia Excessive or voracious eating.

polythelia The occurrence of more than one nipple on a breast.

porencephaly The occurrence of cavities in the brain substance, communicating usually with the lateral ventricles.

prognathism Protrusion of the jaw with a gnathic index above 103.

prolabium The prominent central part of the upper lip, in its full thickness, which overlies the premaxilla.

pseudoarthrosis Motion in the shaft of a long bone between the two ends, following an ununited fracture; a false joint.

pterygium A patch of thickened conjunctiva extending over a part of the cornea. The membrane is usually fan-shaped, with the apex toward the pupil and the base toward the inner canthus.

pterygium colli A thick fold of skin on the lateral aspect of the neck, extending from the mastoid region to the acromion, producing congenital webbing of the neck.

ptosis A falling or sinking down of any organ; specifically a drooping of the upper eyelid due to a fault of development or to paralysis of the levator palpebral muscle, a weighting of the lid by a tumor, or recession of the eyeball.

retrognathia Position of the jaws back of the frontal plane of the forehead.

rhizomelic Pertaining to the hip or shoulder joints—the proximal part of the extremities.

Robertsonian translocation Translocation involving two acrocentric chromosomes and leading to their fusion at the centromere or adjacent regions.

saber-shin A tibia with a marked anterior convexity as seen in hereditary syphilis and in yaws.

saddle nose A nose with a sunken bridge.

scaphocephaly A condition in which the skull is abnormally long and narrow, as a result of premature closure of the sagittal suture, with heavy centers of ossification in the line of the suture.

scoliosis An appreciable lateral deviation in the normally straight vertical line of the spine.

sequela Any lesion or affection followed or caused by an attack of disease.

shagreen patches Raised, thickened connective tissue plaques found characteristically in the lumbosacral region, most commonly in tuberous sclerosis.

sirenomelia Union of the legs with partial or complete fusion of the feet.

situs inversus Transposition of the viscera.

Sprengel deformity Congenital upward displacement of the scapula.

staphyloma Protrusion of the cornea or sclera resulting from inflammation.

strabismus Deviation of the eye; the visual axes assume a position relative to each other different from that required by the physiologic conditions. The various forms of strabismus are spoken of as tropias, their direction being indicated by the appropriate prefix, as esotropia, exotropia, etc.

submental Situated below the chin.

symblepharon Adhesion of one or both lids to the eyeball.

symbrachydactyly A condition in which the fingers and toes are short and adherent; webbed fingers or toes.

syndactyly The condition in which two or more fingers or toes are partially or completely adherent due to fusion of the skin or fusion of skin and bone. Cutaneous syndactyly of the second and third toes is a very common genetic finding in the general population and also noted in various syndromes.

synechia Adhesion of parts; especially, adhesion of the iris to the cornea or to the lens.

syneresis The contraction of a gel, e.g. a blood clot, by which part of the dispersion medium is squeezed out.

syngnathia Intraoral bands, possibly remnants of the buccopharyngeal membrane.

synkinesis An associated movement; an unintentional movement accompanying a volitional movement.

synophrys The condition in which the eyebrows grow together.

synostosis A union between adjacent bones or parts of a single bone formed by osseous material, such as ossified connecting cartilage or fibrous tissue.

talipes equinovarus A deformity of the foot in which the heel is turned inward from the midline of the leg and the foot is plantar flexed. This is associated with the raising of the inner border of the foot and displacement of the anterior part of the foot so that it lies medially to the vertical axis of the leg. With this type of foot the arch is higher and the foot is in equinus. This is a typical form of clubfoot.

telangiectasis Dilation of the capillary vessels and minute arteries forming a variety of angiomas.

telecanthus Increased distance between the inner canthi of the eyes.

tetralogy of Fallot The most common form of cyanotic congenital heart disease, the t. consisting of pulmonic stenosis, ventricular septal defect, dextroposition of the aorta, and right ventricular hypertrophy.

tetraphocomelia A defect in which all four extremities are involved and in which the hands and feet are directly attached to the trunk. In milder forms, there may be partial absence of any proximal region of the limbs.

T.O.R.C.H. Toxoplasmosis, other, rubella, cytomegalovirus, herpes.

torticollis A contracted state of the cervical muscles, producing twisting of the neck resulting in an unnatural position of the head. The most common causes for this condition are trauma, inflammation, or congenital malformation involving the cervical vertebrae and/or the sternocleidomastoid muscle on one side.

torus palatinus A bony mass sometimes present on the median hard palate.

trigonocephalus A triangular deformity of the head resulting from premature synostosis of the portions of the frontal bone; the front part of the head is compressed.

Trousseau sign In latent tetany, typical attitude of the hand that is assumed when the upper arm is compressed, as by a tourniquet, or blood pressure armlet.

turricephaly See oxycephaly.

urachus That portion of the reduced allantoic stalk between the apex of the bladder and the umbilicus. Postnatally it is normally merely a fibrous cord, but occasionally the old allantoic lumen may persist as a vesico-umbilical fistula.

varus Bent inward; denoting a deformity in which the angulation of the part is toward the midline of the body, such as talipes varus. The term *varus* is an adjective and should be used only in connection with the noun it describes.

verrucous nevus A mole with a warty surface.

vitiligo A condition characterized by failure of the skin to form melanin, with patches of depigmentation often having a hyperpigmented border and enlarging slowly.

widow's peak A pointed frontal hairline which may be transmitted as an autosomal dominant trait or associated with various syndromes, mainly those involving ocular hypertelorism.

Wormian bones Small, irregular bones in the sutures between the bones of the skull.

xerostomia Dryness of the mouth.

Selected Book References

I GENERAL

Bergsma, D. (ed). *Birth Defects Compendium,* 2nd ed. New York, Alan R. Liss, 1979.

Goodman, R.M. and Gorlin, R.J. *Atlas of the Face in Genetic Disorders.* 2nd ed. St. Louis, C.V. Mosby, 1977.

Gorlin, R.J., Pindborg, J.J., and Cohen, M.M. *Syndromes of the Head and Neck,* 2nd ed. New York, McGraw-Hill, 1976.

McKusick, V.A. *Mendelian Inheritance in Man. Catalogs of Autosomal Dominant, Autosomal Recessive and X-Linked Phenotypes,* 5th ed. Baltimore, Johns Hopkins University Press, 1978.

Smith, D.W. *Recognizable Patterns of Human Malformation. Genetic, Embryologic and Clinical Aspects,* 3rd ed. Philadelphia, W.B. Saunders, 1982.

Vogel, F. and Motulsky, A.G. *Human Genetics: Problems and Approaches.* Berlin, Springer-Verlag, 1979.

Warkany, J. *Congenital Malformations.* Chicago, Year Book Medical Publishers, 1971.

II SPECIFIC AREAS

Chromosome

Borgaonkar, D.S. *Chromosomal Variation in Man. A Catalog of Chromosomal Variants and Anomalies.* New York, Alan R. Liss, 1983.

de Grouchy, J. and Turleau, C. *Clinical Atlas of Human Chromosomes.* New York, Wiley, 1977.

Yunis, J.J. (ed). *New Chromosomal Syndromes.* New York, Academic Press, 1979.

Connective Tissue/Skeletal

Beighton, P. *Inherited Disorders of the Skeleton.* London, Churchill Livingstone, 1978.

Maroteaux, P. *Bone Diseases of Children.* Philadelphia, Lippincott, 1979.

McKusick, V.A. *Heritable Disorders of Connective Tissue,* 4th ed. St. Louis, C.V. Mosby, 1972.

Spranger, J.W., Langer, L.O., Jr., and Wiedemann, J.R. *Bone Dysplasias. An Atlas of Constitutional Disorders of Skeletal Development.* Stuttgart, Gustav Fischer Verlag, 1974.

Wynne-Davies, R. *Heritable Disorders in Orthopaedic Practice.* Oxford, Blackwell, 1973.

Deafness

Konigsmark, B.W. and Gorlin, R.J. *Genetic and Metabolic Deafness.* Philadelphia, W.B. Saunders, 1976.

Eye

Goldberg, M.F. (ed). *Genetic and Metabolic Eye Diseases.* Boston, Little, Brown, 1974.

Sorsby, A. *Ophthalmic Genetics.* London, Butterworth, 1970.

Waardenburg, P.J., Franceschetti, A., and Klein, D. *Genetics and Ophthalmology.* Springfield, Ill., C.C. Thomas, 1961 (Vol. 1) and 1963 (Vol. 2).

Fetus

Galjaard, H. *Genetic Metabolic Disease. Early Diagnosis and Prenatal Analysis.* Amsterdam, Elsevier/North Holland, 1980.

Golbus, M.S. and Hall, B.D. (eds). *Diagnostic Approaches to the Malformed Fetus, Abortus, Stillborn and Deceased Newborn.* New York, Alan R. Liss, 1979.

Milunsky, A. (ed). *Genetic Disorders and the Fetus: Diagnosis, Prevention, and Treatment.* New York, Plenum Press, 1979.

Genetic Counseling

Harper, P.S. *Practical Genetic Counseling.* Bristol, John Wright and Sons, 1981.

Lubs, H.A. and De La Cruz, F. (eds). *Genetic Counseling.* New York, Raven Press, 1977.

Milunsky, A. and Annas, G.J. (eds). *Genetics and The Law.* New York, Plenum, 1976.

Murphy, E.A. and Chase, G. *Principles of Genetic Counseling.* Baltimore, Johns Hopkins University Press, 1975.

Reed, S. *Counseling in Medical Genetics.* New York, Alan R. Liss, 1980.

Hand Malformations

Temtamy, S.A. and McKusick, V.A. *The Genetics of Hand Malformations.* New York, Alan R. Liss, 1978.

Immune System

Feigin, R. and Cherry, J. *Textbook of Pediatric Infectious Diseases.* W.B. Saunders, Philadelphia, 1981.

Fudenberg, H.H., Pink, J.R.L., Wang, A.C., and Douglas, S.D. *Basic Immunogenetics,* 2nd ed. New York, Oxford University Press, 1978.

Rose, N.R., Bigazzi, P.E., and Warner, N.C. (eds). *Genetic Control of Autoimmune Disease.* Amsterdam, Elsevier/North Holland, 1978.

Stehm, R. and Fulginiti, V. *Immunologic Disorders in Infants and Children.* 2nd ed. W.B. Saunders, Philadelphia, 1980.

Mental Retardation

Holmes, L.B., Moser, H.W., Halldorsson, C.S., Mack, C., Paint, S.S., and Matzilevich, B. *Mental Retardation: An Atlas of Diseases with Associated Physical Abnormalities.* New York, Macmillan, 1972.

Tsuang, M.X.T. and Vandermey, R. *Genes and the Mind. Inheritance of Mental Illness.* New York, Oxford University Press, 1980.

Warkany, J., Lemire, R.J., and Cohen, M.M. *Mental Retardation and Congenital Malformations of the Central Nervous System.* Chicago, Year Book Publishers, 1981.

Metabolic/Endocrine

Harris, H. *The Principles of Human Biochemical Genetics,* 3rd ed. Amsterdam, Elsevier/North-Holland Biomedical Press, 1980.

Rimoin, D.L. and Schimke, R.N. *Genetic Disorders of the Endocrine Glands.* St. Louis, C.V. Mosby, 1971.

Scriver, C.R. and Rosenberg, L.E. *Amino Acid Metabolism and Its Disorders.* Philadelphia, W.B. Saunders, 1973.

Stanbury, J.B., Wyngaarden, J.B., Fredrickson, D.S., Goldstein, J.L., and Brown, M.S. *The Metabolic Basis of Inherited Disease,* 5th ed. New York, McGraw-Hill, 1982.

Neoplasia

Lynch, H.T. (ed). *Cancer Genetics.* Springfield, C. C. Thomas, 1976.

Mulvihill, J.J., Miller, R.W., and Fraumeni, J.F. (eds). *Genetics of Human Cancer.* New York, Raven Press, 1977.

Schimke, R.N. *Genetics and Cancer in Man.* Edinburgh, Churchill Livingstone, 1978.

Nervous System

Baraister, M. *The Genetics of Neurological Disorders.* Oxford, Oxford University Press, 1982.

Vinken, P.J. and Bruyn, G.W. (eds). *Handbook of Clinical Neurology.* Amsterdam, Elsevier/North Holland. Vol. 10, 1970: *Leukodystrophies and poliodystrophies;* Vol. 13, 1972: *Neuroretinal degenerations;* Vol. 14, 1972: *The phakomatoses;* Vol. 43, 1982: *Neurogenetic directory.*

Oral

Stewart, R.R. and Prescott, G.H. (eds). *Oral Facial Genetics.* St. Louis, C.V. Mosby, 1976.

Populations/Ethnic Groups

Eriksson, A.W., Forsius, H., Nevanlinna, H.R., Workman, P.L., and Norio, P.K. *Population Structure and Genetic Disorders.* London, Academic Press, 1980.

Goodman, R.M. *Genetic Disorders Among the Jewish People.* Baltimore, Johns Hopkins University Press, 1979.

Sex Differentiation

Federman, D.D. *Abnormal Sexual Development: A Genetic and Endocrine Approach to Differential Diagnosis.* Philadelphia, W.B. Saunders, 1967.

Simpson, J.L. *Disorders of Sexual Differentiation: Etiology and Clinical Delineation.* New York, Academic Press, 1976.

Skin

Der Kaloustian, V.M. and Kurban, A.K. *Genetic Diseases of the Skin.* Berlin, Springer-Verlag, 1979.

Gottron, H.A. and Schnyder, V.W. *Vererbung von Hautkrankheiten.* Berlin, Springer-Verlag, 1955. Vol. 7 of Jadassohn Handbuch.

Teratology

Shepard, T.H. *Catalog of Teratogenic Agents,* 3rd ed. Baltimore, Johns Hopkins University Press, 1980.

Wilson, J.G. and Fraser, F.C. (eds). *Handbook of Teratology,* Vols. 1–4. New York, Plenum, 1977.

Index